# LOSING WEIGHT
# PERMANENTLY
## WITH THE
# BULL'S-EYE FOOD GUIDE

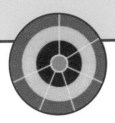

Josephine Connolly Schoonen, M.S., R.D.

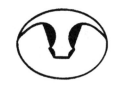

BULL PUBLISHING COMPANY
BOULDER, COLORADO

LOSING WEIGHT PERMANENTLY WITH THE BULL'S-EYE FOOD GUIDE

ISBN: 0-923521-85-2

Bull Publishing Company
P.O. Box 1377
Boulder, CO 80306
www.bullpub.com
800-676-2855

Distributed to the trade by:
PGW
1700 Fourth Street
Berkeley, CA 94710

**Library of Congress Cataloging-in-Publication Data**
Connolly Schoonen, Josephine.
Losing weight permanently with the bull's-eye food guide:
your best mix of carbs, proteins, and fats
by Josephine Connolly Schoonen.
p. cm.
Includes bibliographical references and index.
ISBN 0-923521-85-2
1. Reducing diets. I. Title.
RM222.2.C578 2004
613.2'5—dc22

MANUFACTURED IN THE UNITED STATES OF AMERICA
Publisher: Jim Bull
Editor: Erin Mulligan
Cover Design: Lightbourne
Interior Design and Composition: Shadow Canyon Graphics

# Contents

# Introduction to the Bull's-Eye Food Guides

The Bull's-Eye Food Guide is a powerful, innovative tool developed at Stony Brook University Hospital and Medical Center. Its development has been based on research literature—without industry influence. It organizes foods into groups based on nutrients a food *does* have (such as fiber, vitamins, minerals, phytochemicals, and omega-3 fatty acids) and chemicals it *doesn't* have (such as hydrogenated fats, saturated fats, and added sweeteners). Therefore, you can quickly, easily, and accurately identify foods that are the most healthy and those that are the least healthy.

*Empowered with this information, you can decide how to balance the foods you eat to maximize your health and manage your weight. Using the Bull's-Eye Food Guide is as easy as 1-2-3!*

**1. Take a look at the six different food groups.** There are six triangle-shaped food groups. Foods are placed into one of these groups based on the relative amounts of carbohydrates, proteins, and fats they contain. There are three versions of the Bull's-Eye Food Guide to represent three healthy styles of eating—high-carb, moderate-carb, and lower-carb. Sizes of the six different food groups vary in each of these three guides to represent how foods from these six groups should be balanced in each style of eating. In the high-carb Bull's-Eye Food Guide, the Grain & Starch Group is the largest, and the Fruit Group is also large. These groups get increasingly smaller in the moderate-carb and lower-carb Guides. In the lower-carb Bull's-Eye Food Guide, the Protein Group and the Fat Group are largest, and they get increasingly smaller in the moderate-carb and high-carb Guides. The Vegetable group is large in all versions of the Guide. The Milk & Yogurt Group remains just about the same size in all Guides, because these foods are high in both carbohydrates and proteins. To maximize your nutrient intake and lose weight, it is important to eat foods from all food groups.

**2. Within each food group, note the three sections.** Foods within each food group are divided into 3 sections based on their overall health promoting power. Foods in the green inner circle are the healthiest—"Go Foods." They have the most vitamins, minerals, and phytochemicals that improve health and prevent disease. Most are also high in fiber. They are low in saturated and hydrogenated fats, added sweeteners, and sodium. Most of the foods you eat each day should be from the green inner circle of each of the six food groups. Foods in the yellow middle circle have some nutrients. However, they also have greater amounts of saturated fats, cholesterol, and sodium and less fiber and healthy omega-3 and monounsaturated fats. These foods are "OK Foods." Foods in the red outer circle contain the least amounts of nutrients, fiber, phytochemicals, and healthy fats. They also have the most factors that negatively impact health, such as saturated and hydrogenated fats, added sweeteners, and sodium. These highly processed foods are labeled "Stop & Think Foods." You do not have to completely stop eating them, but you should stop and think carefully before selecting a food in this red section. Consider how many other foods you have had from that section in a day, and try to limit it to one or two selections. In addition, think about serving sizes of these foods carefully, and choose small portions.

**3. Putting it all together.** *Quality*—Use the Bull's-Eye Food Guide to quickly select the healthiest foods. . . most of the time. *Balance*—Use the Guide to balance your food selections and get a wide variety of health promoting nutrients. *Don't forget the water!*—Water is an essential nutrient, but often forgotten. Drink at least 8 cups a day.

# The Lower-Carb Bull's-Eye Food Guide ©®

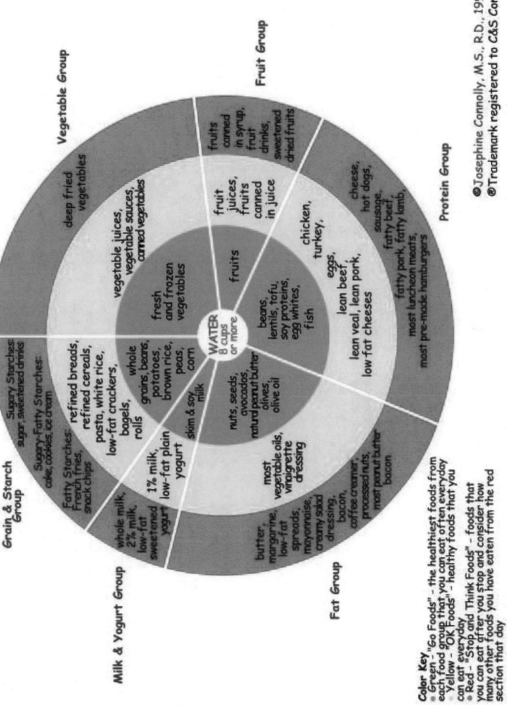

Grain & Starch Group

Vegetable Group

Milk & Yogurt Group

Fruit Group

Fat Group

Protein Group

Sugary Starches: sugar, sweetened drinks

Sugary-Fatty Starches: cake, cookies, ice cream

Fatty Starches: French fries, snack chips

refined breads, refined cereals, pasta, white rice, low-fat crackers, bagels, rolls

whole grains, beans, potatoes, brown rice, peas, corn

deep fried vegetables

vegetable juices, vegetable sauces, canned vegetables

fresh and frozen vegetables

fruits

fruit juices, fruits canned in juice

fruits canned in syrup, fruit drinks, sweetened dried fruits

WATER 8 cups or more

chicken, turkey,

eggs,

lean beef,

lean veal, lean pork, low-fat cheeses

cheese, hot dogs, sausage, fatty beef, fatty pork, fatty lamb, most luncheon meats, most pre-made hamburgers

beans, lentils, tofu, soy proteins, egg whites, fish

nuts, seeds, avocados, natural peanut butter olives, olive oil

most vegetable oils, vinaigrette dressing

butter, margarine, low-fat spreads, mayonnaise, creamy salad dressing, bacon, coffee creamer, processed nuts, most peanut butter bacon

skim & soy milk

1% milk, low-fat plain yogurt

whole milk, 2% milk, low-fat sweetened yogurt

©Josephine Connolly, M.S., R.D., 1996-2004
®Trademark registered to C&S Consultants

**Color Key**: 
- Green – "Go Foods" - the healthiest foods from each food group that you can eat often everyday
- Yellow – "OK Foods" - healthy foods that you can eat everyday
- Red – "Stop and Think Foods" - foods that you can eat after you stop and consider how many other foods you have eaten from the red section that day

# The Moderate-Carb Bull's-Eye Food Guide®

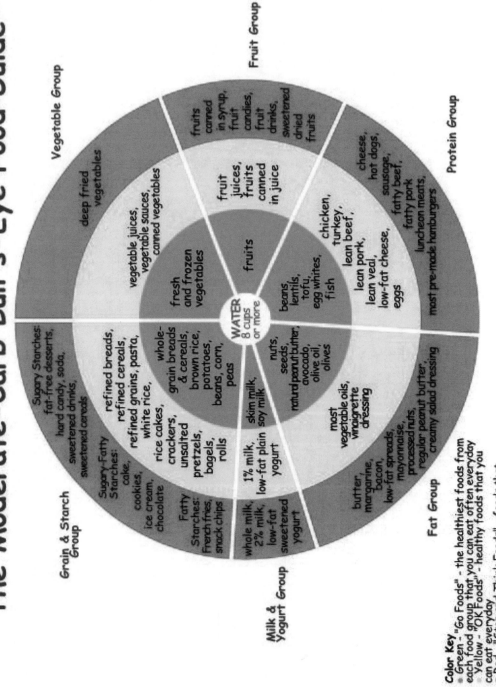

Vegetable Group

Fruit Group

Protein Group

Fat Group

Milk & Yogurt Group

Grain & Starch Group

**Vegetable Group**
- fresh and frozen vegetables
- vegetable juices, vegetable sauces, canned vegetables
- deep fried vegetables

**Fruit Group**
- fruits
- fruit juices, fruits canned in juice
- fruits canned in syrup, fruit candies, fruit drinks, sweetened dried fruits

**Protein Group**
- beans, lentils, tofu, egg whites, fish
- chicken, turkey, lean beef, lean pork, lean veal, low-fat cheese, eggs
- cheese, hot dogs, sausage, fatty beef, fatty pork, luncheon meats, most pre-made hamburgers

**Grain & Starch Group**
- whole-grain breads & cereals, brown rice, potatoes, beans, corn, peas
- refined breads, refined cereals, refined grains, pasta, white rice, crackers, unsalted pretzels, bagels, rolls
- Sugary Starches: fat-free desserts, hard candy, soda, sweetened cereals
- Sugary-Fatty Starches: cake, cookies, ice cream, chocolate
- Fatty Starches: French fries, snack chips

**Milk & Yogurt Group**
- skim milk, soy milk
- 1% milk, low-fat plain yogurt
- whole milk, 2% milk, low-fat sweetened yogurt

**Fat Group**
- nuts, seeds, natural peanut butter, avocado, olive oil, olives
- most vegetable oils, vinaigrette dressing
- butter, margarine, bacon, low-fat spreads, mayonnaise, processed nuts, regular peanut butter, creamy salad dressing

**WATER 8 cups or more**

©Josephine Connolly, M.S., R.D., 1996-2004
®Trademark registered to C&S Consultants

**Color Key**
- Green - "Go Foods" - the healthiest foods from each food group that you can eat often everyday
- Yellow - "OK Foods" - healthy foods that you can eat everyday
- Red - "Stop and Think Foods" - foods that you can eat after you stop and consider how many other foods you have eaten from the red section that day

# The High-Carb Bull's-Eye Food Guide®©

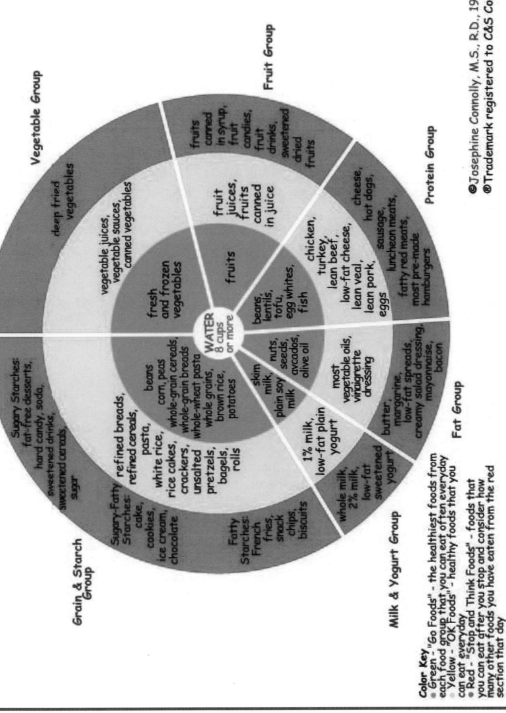

©Josephine Connolly, M.S., R.D., 1996–2004
®Trademark registered to C&S Consultants

**Color Key**
- Green – "Go Foods" – the healthiest foods from each food group that you can eat often everyday
- Yellow – "OK Foods" – healthy foods that you can eat everyday
- Red – "Stop and Think Foods" – foods that you can eat after you stop and consider how many other foods you have eaten from the red section that day

# Preface

This book is the result of my 14 years of work helping patients manage their weight. I use the term manage, because the long-term maintenance of weight loss is a management process that I liken to a journey. This book does not promise fast weight loss but holds the clues to successful permanent weight loss. In my many years of clinical practice, the individuals who lose weight and keep it off do the following:

- Take the time to learn about nutrition and stay engaged in this process for a minimum of 6 months

- Improve the quality of their diet while decreasing their calorie intake

- Work to tease apart long-term habits associating eating with other things

- Learn to include some favorite junk foods on a regular basis without guilt

- Increase their regular physical activity

Throughout this book I empower you with tools to lose weight in a step-wise fashion, taking breaks along the way to change key underlying habits. Learning to use the tools to manage this process will enable you to craft a realistic, healthy eating style you can live with and enjoy. This process is like taking a journey in which you have mapped out a route with lots of exciting places to stop and enjoy on the way to your final destination. As you progress along your journey, your eating style will evolve and you will become free of habits associated with excessive calorie intake. Thousands of people have used this approach to lose 10 to 100 pounds over the last 14 years. You can be the next person to do the same. Simply open your mind to new ideas, and get ready to start your journey.

The Bull's-Eye Food Guide approach is an innovative weight management process in that it *empowers you* to do the following:

⦿ Improve the quality of the food you eat to include a large variety of delicious whole foods. Rather than using one quality of a food, such as carbohydrate content or glycemic index, a holistic approach is used to guide your food choices. The Bull's-Eye Food Guide helps you identify the healthfulness of a food quickly and easily. Eating a high-quality base diet, while including some favorite less healthy foods, is the first step in crafting a diet that will lead to permanent weight loss.

⦿ Determine the best mix of carbohydrates, proteins, and fats for *you*. Whether you need a lower-carbohydrate, moderate-carbohydrate, or high-carbohydrate style of eating is dependent on the genes you were born with, your health status, your current lifestyle, and your food preferences. Your needs may change as you lose weight and improve your health, therefore you are guided through a process of evaluating your results and modifying your plan as needed. This is an individualized approach—not a one-size-fits-all approach.

⦿ Determine the right amount of calories you need each day to lose weight. Your calorie needs depend largely on your height and weight. Whether you are eating a lower-carbohydrate or high-carbohydrate diet, calories do matter—a lot! Selecting the right eating style can help you control your calorie intake, while correcting metabolic problems. You are provided a structured eating plan and menus based on your calorie needs, and the best mix of carbohydrates, proteins, and fats. After following the structured plan and learning the best mix and amount of foods for you, try to wean yourself off the structured plan and use a variety of other tools that you can realistically make a part of your lifestyle forever. These tools help you to permanently structure new eating habits and develop a healthy relationship with food.

⦿ Determine the best pattern of weight loss for you. If you have a small amount of weight to lose (10 to 20 pounds), you may be able to lose all the weight in 8 to 16 weeks. If you have more weight to lose, you will be guided through a process of managing your weight loss over a longer period of time. In either case, this process will help you make the weight loss permanent, because you foster the necessary changes in your metabolism needed to make the weight loss last. In addition, this process allows you to emotionally and psychologically process the resulting changes in habits, routines, and relationships with other people. This process is typically ignored, yet critical for long-term success.

There are plenty of daily menus and recipes for you to follow to get your weight loss started. The book guides you through an easy process to change the given menus and create a lifetime supply of daily menus. You are strongly encouraged to read the background material so you understand your plan. Having an in-depth understanding is necessary for you to negotiate the food market place and to resist falling prey to the latest diet craze or food manufacturers' offerings. This information distinguishes the Bull's-Eye approach from all others and empowers you to manage your weight while maximizing your health. You may find that reading the background chapters a few times during your journey is helpful, because they are packed with useful information.

In working with the Bull's-Eye Food Guide program, you do not need to read the book cover to cover to get started. The following approach, as shown in Figure P-1, is recommended. Read Chapters 1 and 2 to get a general understanding of the rationale and philosophy of this program, as well as to understand the primary tool—the Bull's-Eye Food Guide. Next, if you want to get the weight loss started right away, go to Chapter 5 to select your calorie level and eating style. You can then refer to the Menus and Recipes section and start following the appropriate menus. As you start following the menus, read Chapters 3 and 4. Chapter 3 provides important background nutrition information. Chapter 4 presents detailed information on the Bull's-Eye Food Guide that you will need in order to follow and modify your plan. As you continue to follow your selected menus and modify them to suit your taste preferences, your weight loss will continue. Next read the chapter on your selected eating style: Chapter 6 for the lower-carb style, Chapter 7 for the moderate-carb style, and Chapter 8 for the high-carb style. These chapters will further guide you in following your structured eating plan to ensure the best mix of carbohydrates, proteins, and fats for you, within your best calorie range. Although some diet gurus imply that calories do not matter, this is simply not true and not backed up by the research in this area. Calorie balance is essential for weight loss. Getting the right mix of carbohydrates, proteins, and fats helps with weight loss, but equally as important helps correct your metabolism in a way to support weight loss, maintenance of weight loss, and optimal health. Follow the structured plan until you learn to serve yourself the appropriate amounts and mix of foods—at least 4 weeks. In the meantime, read Chapters 9 and 10 to learn and practice tools that will empower you to balance your calories in a more flexible manner and without measuring foods and drinks. Most importantly, these tools help you to focus on internal signals of hunger and fullness, and to tease apart habits that tie eating to other activities (such as television viewing) or emotions (stress, boredom, frustration, sadness, or loneliness). Practicing and mastering these tools is a key to long-term success. You are encouraged to work through these processes over an extended period of time. In other words, this should be a book whose pages get worn over months or years as you practice these skills and keep the weight off. Individuals who have followed this plan have lost 5 to upwards of 20 pounds in 12 weeks. More importantly, however, is that individuals have had long-term success by staying engaged in the processes presented in these chapters for 6 months to 2 years—long enough for these processes to positively influence metabolism and foster truly new habits and ways of thinking about food!

Chapter 11 presents a very new concept in weight loss: a step-wise approach to weight loss. This means that you lose about 15 to 20 pounds and then take a break from the weight loss. This is like taking an interesting side trip on your journey to a healthy weight. During this break, your body's metabolism recovers from the negative impact of dieting. At the same time, you practice the new habits you have started to get to this point of weight loss. You also take the time to consider and process other changes that may have occurred, such as flattering comments or strains in relationships. It is important to process both these changes in your body's chemistry and your way of thinking about yourself and relating to people. Taking time for these adaptive processes is critical for long-term success.

Lastly, Chapter 12 provides examples of other people's weight management journeys using this approach. These scenarios can provide examples for you, as well as help you appreciate the benefits of the long-term approach.

Now it is time to get ready for your journey. It will be a learning process that will have many long-term positive effects on your weight and health. Take your time, stay engaged in the process, and you too will lose weight permanently!

## Special Thanks

We embark on many journeys during our lifetime and enjoy the company of many travelers along the way. I have learned much from those with whom I have traveled. Many people have influenced the preparation of this book, and to them I am forever grateful—especially my husband Martin, my parents Anna and Tom, my children Jan, Anna, and Martien, and my mentor in the Department of Family Medicine at Stony Brook University Hospital and Medical Center, Dr. Raja Jaber.

In Health,

Josephine Connolly Schoonen, M.S., R.D.
A Fellow Traveler

# Figure P-1

## Your Journey to Optimal Weight and Health

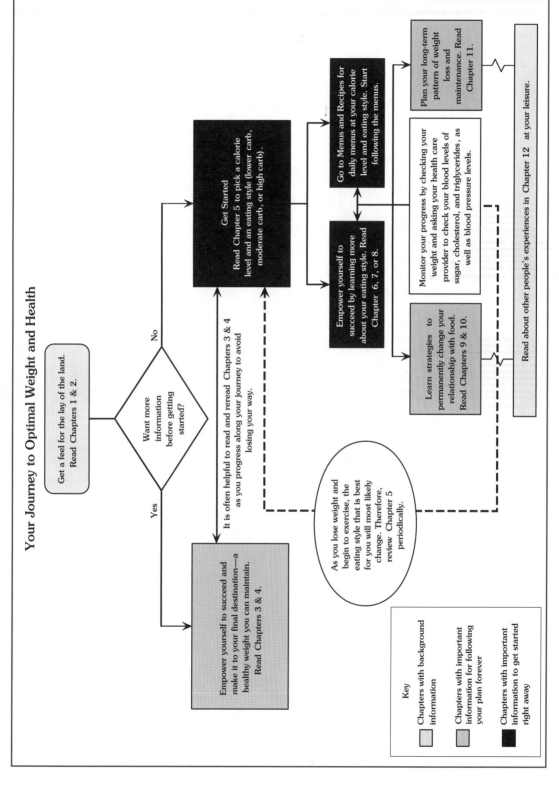

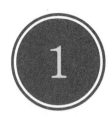

# YOUR WEIGHT MANAGEMENT JOURNEY

## What You Will Discover in Chapter 1

◉ It is essential to balance weight and health goals, and to develop a strategy to manage your weight and optimize your health at the same time.

◉ You need to individualize your eating style in regard to relative amounts of carbohydrates, fats, and protein.

◉ Losing weight in stages, with weight maintenance breaks in between stages, makes the weight loss permanent.

◉ The Bull's-Eye Food Guide is an innovative method of organizing foods to empower you to make informed decisions about food choices, despite a confusing food marketplace.

◉ *Losing Weight Permanently with the Bull's-Eye Food Guide: Your Best Mix of Carbs, Proteins, and Fats* is organized into 12 chapters, swap lists, menus and recipes, and one appendix (body mass index).

## Getting Started

This book will be your guide as you develop a personalized healthy long-term weight management plan based on your medical history and lifestyle. Personalization is the key to success. Information emerging from the Human Genome Project and based on the new field of nutritional genomics tells us that no single diet plan is right for everybody because of differences in our genetic blueprints. Fortunately, you do not need to understand genetics to craft an eating style that will help you lose weight. You simply need to follow the guidelines in this book and match up your personal health characteristics to one of three eating styles.

The following chapters provide a balance between practical information and the background information you need to maximize your health while losing weight. If you want the background information first, read on. If you want to get started right away, go to Chapter 5 to pick a daily calorie level and select an eating style then go to Menus and Recipes for menus. If you take that route, make sure you understand the concept of maintenance breaks (refer to Chapter 11 for detailed information on weight maintenance breaks) before you lose 15 to 20 pounds, because at that point you will need to modify your plan.

Whether you want to get started right away or read the background information first, it will be important for you to read the background information at some point so you understand your eating plan. The background information empowers you to create the plan that will work best for you and to modify this plan as necessary. The information, especially in this chapter and Chapters 2, 3, and 4, is very thorough. You may find that you will need to read it a few times and refer back to it as you are following your plan and losing weight—especially if you want to really understand how to make the weight loss permanent and maximize your health.

Consider your efforts to manage your weight as a journey. Along the way you will be learning more about your health, food, and nutrition. Your success may not always be straightforward, as journeys are often along windy paths and roads. However, you will get to your destination if you stay focused, determined, objective, and optimistic. For some, the journey will be longer than others, and this may be due to differences in genetic blue-prints. One of the keys to long-term success is the development of a positive self-concept and self-confidence as you change your relationship with food. As you learn more, you will be able to make more and more changes in your diet and exercise habits that will make you feel great. Do not be concerned if you choose not to follow the plans described in Chapters 6, 7, and 8 or menus in Menus and Recipes 100% to the letter. You can make a lot of progress with weight loss by just moving in the right direction and getting close. In fact, *changes in current eating habits that move you gradually toward the suggested eating plan often result in more permanent changes in eating habits.* There is always time for improvements as your journey progresses. Whether you give up your old eating habits cold-turkey or gradually change your eating habits is up to you. You may start off one way, and then decide to change course. Allow yourself to be flexible, and adopt the style that works best for you at any given time.

## A Research-Based Weight "Management" Plan That Works

Most "diets" promote eating styles that simply do not lead to optimal health and promote short-term weight loss followed by weight gain in the long run. Rather than focusing on weight loss, decide to "manage" your weight over time. Taking on this goal and the associated necessary self-education will empower you to make dramatic improvements in your health and weight.

Most of us can follow a popular diet long enough to lose weight. The tricky part is finding a style of eating that is flexible and works in the long run to promote a healthy weight and optimal overall health for a lifetime. Recent research demonstrates that there is no one-size-fits-all approach to eating healthy, and that there are at least three different healthy styles of eating—moderately-low-carbohydrate/moderately-high-fat (lower-carb), moderate-carbohydrate/moderate-fat (moderate-carb), and high-carbohydrate/low-fat (high-carb). *In addition to the amount you eat, the quality of carbohydrates, fats, and proteins are essential factors in all three eating styles.* Which style will work best for you depends on your current lifestyle, age, weight, family medical history, your medical history and health status, as well as your level of physical activity. This book will guide you as you develop and follow a style that promotes maximal health and an optimal weight for you.

Recent research also demonstrates that your pattern of weight loss, that is how much weight you lose over a given period of time, is also critically important. Most diets promote relatively fast, continuous weight loss over just weeks or months. Considering that it usually takes years to gain excess weight this does not make much sense. Such a pattern of weight loss does not allow your body to adjust to new food and calorie intake levels along the way. Instead it leads your body into a starvation or energy-conservation state. In this state your body becomes a more efficient machine, conserving as much of the calories you eat as it can and making weight loss more difficult. Once you have a slip or go off your plan, weight creeps back on, frustration settles in, and you throw in the towel and go back to your old style of eating. Before you know it you are back to your old weight or at an even higher weight. Continuous fast weight loss also does not give you enough time to get used to the new behaviors needed to support your new eating style. You lose weight fast by quickly and dramatically changing many of these behaviors at once. You may be doing any or all of these—buying only low-calorie foods, preparing food differently, giving up many favorite foods, eating out less, and exercising more. These are new behaviors, and you need time to adjust to them. In addition, you may not have time to process changes in relationships that may occur or the attention you may receive. Making behavioral and emotional adjustments to weight loss is a crucial component of success—and something that many diet plans do not take into account at all.

The unique approach to managing your health and weight that follows in this book includes losing weight in stages. In the material that follows, you will be instructed to lose about 15 to 20 pounds, and then gradually increase your food intake enough to stop the weight loss and maintain your new weight for at least 2 to 4 weeks. This time off from actively losing weight is called a *maintenance break*. After the first break, you will be instructed to lose the next 15 to 20 pounds and then take a second maintenance break. You continue this process until you reach a weight at which you are comfortable and healthy. With this approach it is much easier to keep off the weight you lose.

In Figure 1-1, time in months is represented along the bottom of the graph. Vertically along the side, weight is represented. The lines represent changes in weight over time. The black dotted line reflects what happens when most people follow a diet. They lose weight fairly quickly, but because most diets do not promote a realistic and healthy long-term eating style, most people gravitate back to their old high-calorie style of eating shortly after reaching their goal weight. Also remember that after quick weight loss the body goes into a starvation mode and needs fewer calories, so gaining weight is easier than ever. The increased calorie intake associated with the old eating style, combined with a reduced calorie need after quick

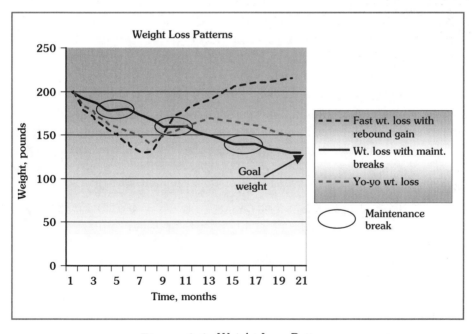

**Figure 1-1.** Weight Loss Patterns

continuous weight loss, leads to weight regain. People resume their old eating habits easily, because sticking to drastic changes in buying, preparing, and eating food is simply too difficult. The experience of weight gain makes the dieter feel like a failure when it comes to weight management, and the resulting bad feelings can further erode attempts to control calorie intake. Often the weight gain continues. Before you know it, you weigh more than when the diet started.

Some people, represented by the gray dotted line in Figure 1-1, lose weight in a yo-yo pattern. They lose weight at a moderate pace and then after reaching a goal weight, they experience some rebound weight gain. Luckily, they are usually able to stop the weight gain before returning back to their prediet weight. Some are even able to resume the old diet or start a new one, and begin to lose weight again. Many people go through this process a number of times. Eventually, some stumble upon a balance between calories consumed and calories used. They get to a healthy weight and stay there, but this can be a very stressful and emotionally draining experience—when weight is down you feel good, and when weight is up you feel lousy. If you fall into this category, you might be thinking, "Is there a healthier, less emotionally stressful way to lose weight?" The answer is yes.

The healthiest, least stressful, and most successful pattern of weight loss, represented by the thick black line in Figure 1-1, is the recommended way to manage your weight. In this scenario, you lose about 15 to 20 pounds in the first 3 to 4 months. At this first short-term weight goal, you stop the weight loss by gradually increasing calories consumed until weight stabilizes. Then you take a break from losing weight—in other words, on your journey you stop off at a scenic place. During this maintenance break, your body adjusts physiologically and you adjust psychologically and emotionally to the lifestyle changes you had to make to get to that point. You practice the new habits you established to get to this point. People around you, adults and children, can also use this time to adjust to changes in your routine and habits. They may need to learn how to support your efforts, and adjust their habits accordingly. For example, your spouse may have to learn to enjoy different types of meal preparation or make time for you to exercise. Children may need to learn that for a half-hour in the morning they need to play independently while you are on your exercise machine. A minimum time for maintenance breaks is 2 to 4 weeks, although they can be as long as a few months or even a year or so. Planning the length of a maintenance break requires consideration of your health status, lifestyle, anticipated time constraints or pressures on your schedule, and your level of patience. With this process there are no psychological set-backs, no blows to the self-esteem—just gradual and permanent improvements in your health and weight. By the time you get to your ultimate goal weight, you have practiced most of your new habits, and those around you have adjusted as well, so maintenance is pretty easy. In this way you are set up for success. Now, let's move to an introduction to the tools used in this book to facilitate changes in eating and exercise behaviors.

## An Overview of the Tools

There are a variety of tools in this book to help you change your eating and exercise habits. The most important tool is the Bull's-Eye Food guide, which you can use to make healthy food choices in a market place that is often very confusing. Other tools will help you modify your behaviors, such as the hunger-fullness scale, journaling, food-mood dominos, goal ladders, and experiential eating exercises. These other tools can be found in Chapters 9 and 10.

The Bull's-Eye Food Guide is a unique tool that will empower you to create an individualized, comprehensive, life-long eating pattern that will maximize your health while you manage your weight. It is based on the latest research in the fields of nutrition, food science, and medicine. Perhaps most importantly, it is free of corporate bias—it is not influenced by the food and beverage industry or by associations of growers or producers. The Bull's-Eye Food Guide was developed at a leading university hospital and medical center over a 12-year period and has benefited from input from researchers, health care practitioners, students, and patients during this time. It is a time-tested tool that has been used by thousands of people to create personal eating plans, improve their health, and manage their weight. As research in the area of genetics evolves, it has become clear that no one diet is best for everyone. Your genes determine your body's basic capacity to metabolize your food and the amount of calories your body uses at rest. The food and physical activity choices you make modify this basic capacity. The Bull's-Eye Food Guide system enables you to develop a personalized eating style, monitor your body's response, and make appropriate changes until your eating style supports optimal health and a healthy weight. Refer to the Bull's-Eye Guides for pictures of the three versions of the Bull's-Eye Food Guide. The Bull's-Eye Food Guide encourages intake of a variety of foods from the six food groups, with the vast majority of healthy food selections from the green inner circle, some selections from the yellow circle and only a few if any from the red outer circle. The details of the guide and how to use it to craft a new eating style will be discussed at length in Chapters 2 and 4.

The Bull's-Eye Food Guide is an innovative way of organizing foods that gives a clear indication of how healthy a food is compared to other foods in the same food group. The grouping system does not consider just one factor, such as glycemic index, fat content, or carbohydrate content. Rather the grouping system is based on many concepts, such as nutrient density, level of processing, and relative amounts of carbohydrates, fats, and proteins, as well as quality of carbohydrates, fats, and proteins. Nutrient density simply refers to how many nutrients, such as vitamins and minerals, are in a food relative to the amount of calories that food provides. Therefore, foods with a high nutrient density are considered healthy and provide a lot of vitamins, minerals, and other nutrients for the calories they provide (such as broccoli, salmon, kidney beans, and walnuts). Foods with a lower nutrient density are considered unhealthy and provide few nutrients relative to the amount of calories they provide (such as soda, cake, and candy). Most people like to eat at least some foods with a low nutrient density, and with this approach you can learn how to work in some of these foods.

The approach to long-term healthy eating is twofold: (1) learn how to quickly identify healthy and unhealthy foods, and (2) learn how to create a base diet made up of mostly foods that have high nutrient densities with some other favorite foods added for pure satisfaction. As you eat healthier foods and feel healthier and lose weight, you will learn to prefer them.

Thus, over time, your food preferences will change and evolve. Think of this process as training your taste buds, just as you train your bicep muscles. If you change the stimulus your taste buds are exposed to (healthy food), you can modify their response (appreciation of healthy food). Some of the highly processed unhealthy foods you like now will become less appealing, and some healthy foods will become more appealing. These changes take time, a lot of time, and require consistent exposure to healthy, less processed foods. So be patient, and be sure to keep trying new healthy foods along your weight management journey.

The organization of the Bull's-Eye Food Guide empowers you to gradually craft long-term eating styles that are personalized to be just right for you. All of us need a diet high in vitamins, minerals, and fiber. However, the amount of calories, as well as the source of those calories (i.e., carbohydrates, fats, and proteins), each of us needs varies based on medical history, family history, current health status, current food intake, and activity level. The Bull's-Eye Food Guide groups foods with relatively similar amounts of carbohydrates, fats, and proteins together, so you can develop eating styles that best fits your needs—a lower-carb style, a moderate-carb style, or a high-carb style. How precisely you want to plan and monitor your eating style on a day-to-day basis depends on your needs, preferences, and lifestyle. Chapters 5, 6, 7, and 8 provide detailed structured eating plans. Chapters 9 and 10 provide more casual approaches focused on internal perceptions and feelings of hunger and fullness.

The goal of this book is to provide the tools you need to develop an eating plan that works for you now, and a strategy to modify the plan if necessary for long-term success. Such a system provides a path to health, prevention or management of chronic illnesses, and lifelong weight management.

## Why a New Food Guide Is Necessary

There is no doubt about it—now is the time for a completely new way of organizing our thoughts about food and how we plan our meals and snacks. Confusion reigns when it comes to the definition of healthy eating.

At the same time, the burden of weight-related chronic illnesses threatens the health care system. Many chronic illnesses that are on the rise, such as diabetes, hypertension, and some cancers, are related to poor dietary habits. More than half of American adults, approximately 64%, are overweight or obese, and about one in four children are overweight or at risk for overweight. The personal suffering as well as the economic burden of such trends is staggering.

Obviously, there are many interrelated reasons for these trends, such as aggressive marketing by fast food and soft drink companies, increased restaurant portion sizes (super-sizing), increased use of sweeteners in manufacturing foods and beverages, increased dependence on convenience foods, and increased sedentary activities such as television viewing and computer activities. Although there are certainly genetic predispositions that increase the risk for obesity and other illnesses among some people, genetic causes are not at the heart of the current obesity epidemic. The genetic pool of the population can simply not change that fast. Changes in the amount, frequency, and quality of foods available in our day-to-day living environments are often overlooked. Take a look around your community. Are there vending machines in your worksite or where you take your children to participate in various clubs and sports? Does your school district have a contract with a soda company to sell only their beverages in exchange for donations? Do children in your school district or the children of co-workers sell candy to fund club activities? Are there more fast food restaurants or restaurants with children's menus without whole fruits and vegetables? When you start taking a closer look around, you will probably notice that there are more junk foods available now than you remember 10 or 20 years ago.

An additional factor contributing to the increase in obesity that I think is of equal importance is the lack of clear advice about nutrition and recommendations that reflect the current research literature. Most recommendations made by government agencies and health care organizations are too vague. This is not an accident. Rather, the confusion is largely planned and created by the food and beverage industry—one might think of it as *engineered confusion*. It is to the food industry's advantage to keep nutrition recommendations as vague and loose as possible, that is, "There are no good foods or bad foods—just eat everything in moderation." What does that mean? Should I eat my fruits and vegetables in moderation just as I moderate my intake of soft drinks, sweetened cereals, purple catsup, and colored yogurt with candy toppings? What is a moderate amount of soda, 12 ounces or 22 ounces? If the vending machine in my office only sells the new 22 ounces bottles, am I supposed to drink half today and drink the rest warm tomorrow?

At first these questions may sound a bit funny, but in reality you face these types of decisions every day. In order to eat healthily you need some firm advice from someone. Try this. Remove the judgmental terms *good* and *bad* in the phrase "there are no good foods or bad foods." Replace *good* with *healthy* (having a high nutrient density), and *bad* with *unhealthy* (having a low nutrient density). With this in mind, it is reasonable to recognize that there are healthy (nutrient dense) and unhealthy (not nutrient dense) foods. In addition, a healthy diet would include mostly healthy foods and only some unhealthy foods. Foods can be grouped in a meaningful way that gives an indication of their relative healthfulness, as in the Bull's-Eye Food Guide. This empowers you to quickly decide if a food is healthy or unhealthy, and then you can decide whether you should select it or not based on how many other unhealthy foods you have already had that day. It is unrealistic to think that you will never eat unhealthy foods, but to get to a healthy weight and stay there you need to first recognize them and then limit them.

All foods provide calories, an adequate amount of which are necessary for health. Most foods have some vitamins or minerals, and even overall unhealthy foods may be high in one to two vitamins or minerals because manufacturers purposefully add these nutrients. One reason for doing so is for marketing purposes, to confuse potential buyers and to infuse their foods with an air of healthfulness. For example, food manufacturers add a lot of vitamins and minerals to cookie-type or cartoon character cereals that have high-fructose corn syrup and hydrogenated fats but no fiber. This makes the cereals appear healthy. However, overall healthfulness is related to the types of carbohydrates, amount of fiber, types of fats, types and amounts of colorings, additives and preservatives—not just the amount of vitamins and minerals. In other words, cookie-type cereals are really not part of a healthy breakfast as advertised.

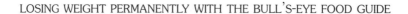

Current national nutrition recommendations do not help consumers clearly identify healthy foods. Some consumers make food choices based on convenience, cost, and taste with little thought about nutritional value. However, many consumers trying to make healthy choices mistakenly purchase foods that have been represented by national food guides and recommendations as healthy but aren't, such as fruited yogurts, sweetened cereals, hot dogs, kids frozen entrees, highly sweetened flavored milks, bagels, and French fries. A food guide that clearly indicates the relative healthfulness of foods enables consumers to make better food choices— to balance more frequent selections of healthy foods with less frequent selections of favorite unhealthy foods. The least healthful foods need not be avoided altogether, but should be clearly identifiable. The food industry spends billions of dollars to make unhealthy foods appear healthy, such as vitamin fortified cookie-type breakfast cereals. Recommendations made by experts need to counterbalance such deception in a clear, concise, objective way. Due to food manufacturer's development and aggressive marketing of more and more foods of poor nutritional quality, consumers are increasingly confused and consuming lots of unhealthy foods. Food manufacturers drive perceived needs and food choices in their efforts to increase profits. They do so through advertising, and also by influencing government recommendations. Advertising is a legitimate business practice. However, the level of influence food and beverage manufacturers have over national nutrition recommendations and policies is of grave concern.[1,2] Some health care professionals at the national level have responded by lowering the standards of what is considered healthy. For example, a panel of experts drafted new United States Department of Agriculture (USDA) guidelines for sugar and sweeteners intake in 2003. The panel increased the recommended limit on added sugar intake from 10% of total calories to 25% of total calories. In other words, the USDA now states that it is okay for a full quarter of your total calories to come from added sugar—that is, sugar above and beyond the sugar naturally provided by fruit and milk. For somebody eating 1800 calories per day, this means that 450 calories could come from sugar or sweeteners: 112.5 grams of sugar per day. Eating this many highly sweetened foods a day would certainly make it difficult to get the optimal amounts of vitamins, minerals, fiber, and phytochemicals in your diet each day while maintaining a healthy weight. Such standards open the door for manufacturers to promote highly sweetened foods and beverages as healthy.

Rather than further weaken nutrition recommendations in the midst of a national obesity epidemic, nutrition professionals need to raise the bar of nutrition standards with empowering tools that consumers can use to craft a healthy diet. Once armed with these tools, it is then up to consumers to make their own food choices—some of which will be healthy and others of which will not. With such tools, at least consumers stand a chance in managing their weight and maximizing their health.

The field of nutrition is an active and complicated area of research that is continuously evolving. It is not advisable for consumers to change their diets in response to every new study or claim. However, it is important for consumers to develop a conceptual framework based on research that has accumulated over years, and to carefully adjust this framework as scientific evidence accumulates. Such is the nature of the Bull's-Eye Food Guide. The initial framework was developed 12 years ago. Over the years, it has been revised to incorporate advances in nutrition research. Most recently, the author has developed tools for people to create individualized eating plans based on personal medical information and preferences. These tools have been used in university hospital weight management groups, individual counseling sessions and research studies. Individuals participating in these activities are guided to consider genetic predispositions, accumulated effects of past eating and exercise patterns, and current lifestyle factors when crafting their individualized plan. Next, people are guided to monitor their response to this initial plan, and modify it until optimal effects are realized. Now readers of this book have the same opportunities to craft lifetime healthy eating styles.

The Bull's-Eye Food Guide is a new paradigm for organizing foods and creating healthy patterns of eating that reflect the current research in nutrition independent of food industry influence. This new model conveys the nutrition information necessary to maximize health, prevent chronic illnesses and maximize the treatment of existing chronic illnesses. It also has the built-in flexibility to empower individuals to create an individualized program that works for them.

# What's to Come

The remainder of this book is based on the Bull's-Eye Food Guide and my 12 years of practice in clinical nutrition. Chapter 2, "The Bull's-Eye Food Guide: Your Compass," introduces the guide in detail. Chapter 3, "Supplies You Will Need on Your Journey," explains nutrient categories, including macronutrients (carbohydrates, proteins, and fats) and micronutrients (vitamins and minerals), water, and phytochemicals. The information in this chapter is quite detailed. You do not have to read it before getting started. However, the concepts are important to guide your decision making for long-term success. You may find that you get the most out of this chapter when you read it a few times as you progress. In Chapter 4, "Learning to Use the Compass," each of the major food groups (Vegetable Group, Fruit Group, Grain & Starch Group, Protein Group, Fat Group, and Milk & Yogurt Group) and their corresponding subgroups (green inner circle, yellow middle circle, and red outer circle) are thoroughly explained. Chapter 5, "Mapping Out Your Journey," presents a system to guide you in the development of your personal eating style. Information in this chapter will help you to select a daily calorie level and one of three eating styles. Each of these three eating styles—lower-carb, moderate-carb, and high-carb—are described in detail in Chapters 6, 7, and 8, respectively. The advantages and disadvantages of each approach are also presented. In Chapter 9, "Getting a Better Sense of Direction," the concept of hunger and fullness scaling is discussed in detail. This technique offers an alternative to weighing and measuring food intake to control the amount of food consumed. Controlling consumption is a strategy that is important for long-term success and optimal well-being. Rules of thumb for estimating appropriate portion sizes are also presented in Chapter 9. Supportive techniques critical to restructuring eating habits permanently are discussed in detail in Chapter 10, "Tools, Tools, and More Tools." This includes tools to decrease the frequency of lapses and to decrease the length of lapses that do occur. These tools include guided imagery, journaling, food-mood dominoes, experiential eating, and goal setting. Chapter 11, "Your Internal Engine and Fuel Efficiency Ratings," explains issues regarding metabolic rate, calorie needs, and patterns of weight loss. This chapter guides you through the process of maintenance breaks to favorably manipulate your metabolic rate to facilitate long-term maintenance of weight lost. Exercise is discussed in this chapter, because it has an important impact on metabolisms and calorie balance. Chapter 12, "Travelers' Diaries," provides examples of diet makeovers for you to consider when improving your own eating and exercise habits. Three different versions of the Bull's-Eye Food Guide, one that is consistent with each of the eating styles (lower-carb, moderate-carb, and high-carb) are presented in the front of the book. The Swap Lists of all the foods in each of the food groups and subgroups are presented just before the Menus and Recipes. The Menus and Recipes section includes menus for each of the three eating styles at five different calorie levels, along with recipes. Appendix 1 includes body mass index charts that are helpful in determining health risks associated with weight and short-term weight loss goals.

## *Important Points To Remember from Chapter 1*

- ◉ A successful weight management strategy includes selection of the most appropriate eating style, as well as the appropriate weight loss pattern that includes maintenance breaks between intervals of weight loss.

- ◉ The Bull's-Eye Food Guide is a unique nutrition education tool that represents the most recent nutrition research without influence from the food industry or growers. This decreases confusion and empowers you to create a healthy eating style.

- ◉ The Bull's-Eye Food Guide is flexible to allow consumers to individualize their eating plan based on medical history, family history, current eating plan, and level of physical activity.

- ◉ This book addresses the following main issues: (1) food quality using the Bull's-Eye Food Guide, (2) distribution of calories among carbohydrates, proteins, and fats, (3) techniques to determine and monitor appropriate quantity of food intake, (4) patterns of weight loss to maximize long term success, and (5) swap lists and sample menus to help you stay on course.

# BULL'S-EYE FOOD GUIDE: YOUR COMPASS

## What You Will Discover in Chapter 2

- The Bull's-Eye Food Guide places foods in six major food groups, based on their relative amounts of carbohydrates, proteins, and fats.

- Each of the six major food groups of the Bull's-Eye Food Guide is divided into three subgroups (green inner circle, yellow middle circle, and red outer circle) based on overall nutrition quality.

- A new graphic food guide is needed to empower you to create a healthy eating style based on foods that have high nutrient densities, while enabling you to include smaller portions of less nutrient-dense favorite foods.

## The Major Themes of the Bull's-Eye Food Guide

The Bull's-Eye Food Guide is a system of organizing foods to maximize health based on the most up-to-date nutrition research. It will be your compass on your weight management journey, pointing you to the healthiest foods. Within the guide, foods are placed into six major food groups: the Vegetable Group, the Fruit Group, the Grain & Starch Group, the Protein Group, the Fat Group, and the Milk & Yogurt Group. Each major food group comprises a triangular-shaped piece of a target. The size of the area covered by each group depends on the style of eating plan selected. (See Chapter 5 for an introduction to the three eating styles.) Each of these major food groups has three subgroups, which divide foods in the six major groups by nutritional quality. Refer to the front of the book for pictures of the three versions of the Bull's-Eye Food Guide consistent with the three eating styles.

The colors of a stoplight are used to emphasize the concept of quality. The inner green circle, closest to the bull's-eye of the target, includes foods of the highest nutritional quality for that major food group. These are the *Go Foods* and should make up the foundation of your diet. The middle yellow circle includes foods of moderate nutritional quality, called OK *Foods*. OK Foods provide a fair amount of nutrients for the calories they provide. However, they also have significant undesirable qualities, such as low fiber contents or more than a moderate amount of saturated fat or sodium. Over time it is recommended that you train your taste buds to like foods in the green group that you can use as substitutes for foods in the yellow group (such as brown rice for white rice, whole-wheat pasta for white pasta, olive oil for corn oil). The outer red circle includes foods of the lowest nutritional quality for that major food group, referred to as *Stop and Think Foods*. These foods are typically highly processed, and offer few nutrients for the calories they provide. Often they are high in components known to increase the risk for chronic illnesses, such as saturated fat, trans/hydrogenated fats, sugar or other sweeteners, or sodium. You may have difficulty avoiding these foods completely, and it is reasonable for you to work in one or two of these foods a day. However, you are encouraged to stop and think before eating a food or beverage located in the outer circle. Specifically, you need to consider how many other foods you have eaten from the outer circle on that particular day. Try to work down to one to two choices a day. In addition, you should consider the serving size of foods from the outer circle very carefully because small amounts of these foods provide a lot of calories or undesirable components.

Water is at the center of the Bull's-Eye Food Guide for many reasons. First, water is an essential nutrient, and individuals should strive to drink at least 8 cups of water each day. This requirement may be met with water or seltzer. However, other unsweetened beverages can count towards meeting the required amount. Naturally fruit-flavored, unsweetened waters and herbal teas are also good choices to contribute to the water requirement. Adequate water consumption prevents mild dehydration, a common problem that can lead to fatigue. Another important reason for increasing water intake is to displace other beverages typically consumed, which are usually high in calories, sugar, fat, alcohol, and artificial sweeteners. In addition, for some people thirst may be perceived as hunger. For these people, drinking enough water may decrease feelings of hunger or delay unnecessary eating.

The two graphic themes—the target and the stoplight color scheme— are used to help orient you to the food guide. Foods from all six major groups of the food guide are important, and the closer you get to the bull's-eye the higher the nutritional quality. Nutritionally, the guide is organized to do the following:

◉ Encourage a high intake of vitamins and minerals, especially highlighting trace minerals not added to enriched or fortified grain products;

◉ Encourage a high fiber intake;

◉ Encourage the intake of least-processed foods;

◉ Encourage a plant-based diet high in phytochemicals;

◉ Discourage the intake of foods high in added sugar, sweeteners, and sodium; and

◉ Discourage the intake of trans/hydrogenated and saturated fats.

## Placement of Foods

Foods are grouped based on their nutrient content. For a detailed discussion of nutrients provided in each food group and foods placed in each group and subgroup refer to Chapter 4. A full list of the foods in each group and subgroup are in the Swap Lists beginning on page 263. A brief description follows here.

Carbohydrates, proteins, and fats are the components of foods that provide calories. Foods are placed in one of the six main food groups depending on the relative amounts of these components in a particular food. Within each of the six main food groups, there are three subgroups. The criteria for placement within subgroups are based on amounts of vitamins, minerals, fiber, and phytochemicals, as well as quality of carbohydrates and fats. The criteria are specific for each food group. Full lists of foods in each of the main six food groups and subgroups are found in the Swap Lists.

Foods in the Vegetable Group have a small amount of carbohydrate and protein and no significant amount of fat. Fresh and plain frozen vegetables have the most vitamins, minerals, and fiber and are placed in the inner circle. Canned vegetables as well as vegetable juices and sauces are in the middle group. These types of foods lose fiber and usually have added sodium, sugar, and fats. Deep-fried vegetables are in the outer circle because of their high fat content and the loss of nutrients and phytochemicals associated with this type of frying.

The Fruit Group includes foods that get all of their calories from simple carbohydrates. Fresh, plain, frozen, or plain dried fruits are in the green inner circle, because they contain high amounts of vitamins, minerals, and fiber. Canned fruits and fruit juices are in the middle circle because some of their vitamins and fiber is lost in processing and sugar derived from fruit juice is usually added. Fruit-type products with added sugars or sweeteners belong in the red outer circle. Foods that are technically fruits but have a lot of fat, such as avocados, are considered part of the Fat Group. Foods that are technically a fruit but low in carbohydrate, such as tomatoes, are likely placed in the Vegetable Group.

A diverse group of foods are in the Grain & Starch Group. They derive the majority of their calories from carbohydrates, but they also have some protein and a little bit of fat. Whole grain breads and cereals (whole-wheat pasta and brown rice), starchy vegetables (potatoes, peas, and corn), and other whole grains (millet and amaranth) are in this group. This group also includes some whole-wheat, low-fat products, such as low-fat whole-grain waffles. Processed grains (white bread, regular pasta, white rice, and bagels) typically have low fiber and trace mineral contents, and they are placed in the middle of this group. They may have added sodium and fats, especially small amounts of unhealthy trans/hydrogenated fats. Foods in the outer circle are further subdivided. Sugary starches get almost all of their calories from sugar. Fat-free cake, cookies, and ice cream belong in this subgroup, as well as jelly, jams, syrup, and soda. Sugary-fatty starches derive calories from sugars and fats, and therefore are associated with additional fat servings as noted in the swap list for this group (see Swap Lists). Examples of these foods include cake, cookies, and chocolate. Starchy-fatty foods have complex carbohydrates, rather than sugars, and fats. They also are associated with additional fat servings as noted on the Swap Lists. Potato chips, French fries, biscuits, and fatty crackers are examples from this group.

Foods in the Protein Group provide a lot of protein, variable amounts of fat, and typically no carbohydrates. Placement in the green inner circle emphasizes vegetarian sources of protein that provide fiber and health-promoting phytochemicals. Healthy omega-3 polyunsaturated fats are also encouraged by the organization of this group with the placement of fish in the green inner circle. The middle yellow circle includes the leanest sources of animal protein that provide a lot of vitamins and minerals, including lean meats, white-meat skinless poultry, eggs, and low-fat cheeses. The outer circle includes high-fat meats and poultry, regular cheese, and processed peanut butter.

Foods in the Fat Group provide virtually no carbohydrates and protein, and a lot of fat. Fats in the inner circle are highest in healthy fats, such as monounsaturated and omega-3 polyunsaturated fats, which do not pro-mote heart disease. Specific oils, such as olive oil, cold-pressed canola oil and peanut oil, avocados, nuts, and seeds belong to this inner subgroup. The middle circle includes fats that are high in other types of polyunsatu-rated fats, such as vegetable oils not listed in the green inner circle and salad dressings made from them. The outer circle includes foods that are high in trans/hydrogenated fats and saturated fats. These fats have been

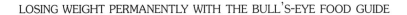

shown to increase the risk of heart disease in genetically susceptible people. Foods that are high in such fats include margarine, butter, bacon fat, and heavy cream.

The Milk & Yogurt Group includes foods that are high in carbohydrates, protein, and calcium. The lowest-fat types of cow's milk and low-fat soymilk are placed in the inner circle, as well as fat-free yogurt. The middle circle includes 1% fat milk, soymilk, and low-fat yogurt. The outer circle includes high-fat and highly sweetened cow's milk, yogurt, and soymilk.

## *Important Points To Remember from Chapter 2*

◉ The Bull's-Eye Food Guide divides foods into one of six major food groups based on each food's relative amounts of carbohydrates, proteins, and fats.

◉ Each of the six major food groups is divided into three subgroups based predominately on nutrient density, fiber content, and quality of carbohydrates, proteins, and fats.

◉ Water is at the center of the Bull's-Eye Food Guide to promote optimal hydration and decrease the intake of beverages with added sugar, alcohol, and artificial sweeteners.

◉ The stoplight color theme and target concept reinforce the location of nutrient-dense foods in the center of the graphic.

# SUPPLIES YOU WILL NEED
# ON YOUR JOURNEY

### *What You Will Discover in Chapter 3*

◉ There are three well-established nutrient categories: macronutrients (carbohydrates, proteins, and fats), micronutrients (vitamins and minerals), and water. In addition, phytochemicals are compounds in plant foods that are increasingly recognized as important for optimal health. Each of these categories of nutrients and phytochemicals has different effects on your health.

◉ The nutritional quality of a food is based on its cumulative nutrient densities, fiber content, phytochemical content, types of carbohydrates and fats, and level of processing.

◉ Foods have varied types of carbohydrates and fats that affect your health differently.

◉ You will benefit most by getting your vitamins and minerals from whole foods.

(continued on next page)

---

### *What You Will Discover in Chapter 3 (continued)*

- Water is often overlooked as an essential nutrient, and you need to make a conscious effort to consume an optimal amount.

- In the beginning of your weight management journey, you may eat many processed, calorie-modified foods to help you decrease your calorie intake, such as diet soda and low-fat desserts. As you progress, however, the goal is to use less of these foods and more nutrient-dense whole foods.

---

When most people are trying to lose weight or prevent weight gain, they usually focus on calories and calories only. Many diet programs and food manufacturers drive this focus. Most foods created for and marketed to dieters are highly processed and often contain fat and sugar substitutes. In many cases, these foods lack the nutrients and phytochemicals naturally found in whole foods. Your body needs many of the natural nutrients and phytochemicals lost in processing to create energy, maintain health, and support the many biochemical systems that regulate energy storage and balance. Calcium, for example, has recently been found to influence fat storage. Keep in mind that health should not be defined as simply the absence of disease, but rather as optimal functioning and well-being. The best way to achieve this optimal level of health, as well as to slow aging, is by consuming foods with a large array of nutrients and phytochemicals, in addition to getting daily physical activity. The Bull's-Eye Food Guide arranges foods in a way that makes it easy to plan a diet high in nutrients and phytochemicals.

In the beginning of your weight management journey you may find processed, calorie-modified foods helpful. This is likely because they can help you reduce calorie intake without necessarily decreasing the total amount or volume of food you eat. However, as you explore and change your relationship with food over an extended period of time, you will be able to decrease your calorie intake by decreasing the volume of food you eat. This can be done by decreasing both your portion sizes and the number of times you eat in a day. As this point your eating will appropriately be guided by your level of hunger as opposed to emotions, habits, and external cues. As this occurs you can enjoy the flavor of nutrient-dense whole foods in smaller portions that allow you to manage your weight— even if some of these foods are occasionally high in calories. So throughout this program you will be working to decrease your calorie intake while increasing your nutrient intake.

The rest of this chapter provides background information, which is important in the long run to guide your decision-making processes regarding food and beverage choices. In other words, when planning your weight management journey you need to know what supplies, or nutrients, you need to pack. The type of information provided here will help you to understand your body's nutrient needs and to develop a long-term weight management strategy that will optimize your overall health and weight. However, it is not necessary to read this chapter before you get started. If you want to start on your journey right away, go to Chapter 5 to pick a calorie level and eating style. Then go to Menus and Recipes for menus, and you can be on your way. As you are following your eating style and selected menus, read and reread this chapter to understand as much as you can about the importance of your food choices on your health and weight. Armed with all of this knowledge, you can make the best personal choices in the very confusing market places along your way. In other words, you will be less likely to fall prey to food and beverage manufacturers' persuasive marketing tricks.

## Why Do We Need to Eat?

You eat for many reasons, such as for taste, pleasure, and comfort. However, you *need* to eat to get the nutrients your body requires. Nutrients are components of food that your body must have to work properly. There are three categories of nutrients: macronutrients (which provide calories), micronutrients, and water. A calorie is a measure of the energy content of food. Your body needs energy to perform mechanical acts, such as pumping your heart and expanding your lungs. It also needs energy to perform the millions of chemical reactions that occur inside your cells every day to make new body tissues and repair damaged tissue. The chemical energy in food is the source of all energy for your body and allows it to keep going day after day. This is different from plants, which derive energy from light. The chemical energy in food is stored in the macronutrients called carbohydrates, fats, and proteins. In order to get the energy, food must first be digested into its smallest building blocks by your stomach and intestines. These products of digestion then pass into your blood. Sugars are the building blocks of carbohydrates, amino acids of proteins, and fatty acids of fats.

Alcohol also provides energy. It provides calories but no nutrients, and is therefore considered an empty calorie. Alcohol in excess of one drink a day for women and two drinks a day for men increases your risk for many chronic illnesses, such as certain types of cancer and liver disease. In addition, alcohol intake above these amounts provides excessive amounts of calories that would make weight loss difficult.

Micronutrients include vitamins and minerals. Vitamins and minerals are necessary to support all of the essential functions described above, but they do not provide calories or energy. Foods and beverages are also the source of all micronutrients. They are released as food is digested and absorbed into your blood stream. Vitamins and minerals enter each one of your body's cells where they perform their essential work in supporting all cellular activities. Without the appropriate kinds and amounts of vitamins and minerals, the cell's activities are interrupted.

We often overlook water as a nutrient, even though it is a component of every body tissue. All of your cells' chemical reactions occur in water. A watery-based fluid also surrounds your body's cells. A relatively small amount of water is actually produced by your cells as a byproduct of their many chemical reactions. The majority of your water needs are, however, met by consuming foods and beverages. Water is at the center of the Bull's-Eye Food Guide to remind you to drink water often.

Phytochemicals are compounds in food that are not considered nutrients, because they have not been shown to be absolutely essential for life. This means that your body can function without them, and you will not develop known deficiency diseases such as anemia or rickets if your diet is low in phytochemicals. However your body is likely not functioning optimally without adequate phytochemicals. Scientists are actively researching the role of phytochemicals in preventing chronic illnesses, such as heart disease, cancer, and diabetes. The majority of foods in the green inner circle of the Bull's-Eye Food Guide are high in phytochemicals.

Eating fewer calories than you use on average is the key to weight management. However, you also need to know how to maximize your nutrient intake while creating this negative calorie balance to ensure that your permanent weight loss also leads to optimal health. The Bull's-Eye Food Guide helps you do this. This tool categorizes foods in a way that empowers you to maximize your micronutrient and phytochemical intake, while creating the balance of macronutrients that is right for you to manage your weight. The chapters that follow reveal the practical information and skills you need to apply the Bull's-Eye Food Guide and create delicious meals and snacks. Increasing the calories you use for physical activity each day is also of critical importance (further discussed in Chapter 11). First though, you need to understand more about caloric density, nutrient density, and nutrients.

## Caloric Density

Caloric density of a food refers to the number of calories in a given amount of weight of that food—usually 1 gram. As a frame of reference, a paper clip weighs approximately 1 gram. There are about 30 grams in an ounce. In efforts to eat fewer calories than you use a day, it is helpful to eat foods with a low calorie density, because you can eat more of these foods for a given number of calories. For example, for 50 calories you can eat 2 cups of red pepper slices with a sandwich for lunch. The red pepper slices would take a while to eat, and provide a satisfying crunchy texture. If instead, you spend the 50 calories on mayonnaise, you would be able to spread 1 teaspoon of mayonnaise on the sandwich, which would barely be noticeable. Unlike the mayonnaise, the red peppers provide a wealth of micronutrients and phytochemicals, as well as color and texture to the meal. Vegetables have a low caloric density, because of their high fiber and water content. Carbohydrates and proteins, such as those found in vegetables, have a similar caloric density of 4 calories per gram. Fats, such as those found in mayonnaise, are much more calorically dense with 9 calories per gram. Alcohol falls in the middle with 7 calories per gram.

Foods with a high water content have a lower caloric density, because the water adds weight but no calories. Fiber also adds weight with no calories and, therefore, lowers caloric density further. Because vegetables have a high water and fiber content and a low fat content, they have a very low caloric density. Foods high in fat and low in fiber, such as butter, oils, and fatty meats have a high caloric density.

Although the concept of caloric density is useful, it should not be used as the sole criterion for selecting healthy foods to eat. In fact, the concept of caloric density has been inappropriately used to support some low-fat unhealthy diets—diets that are made up of highly processed, fat- and calorie-modified foods that are low in fiber and overall nutritional quality. Examples of such foods include diet meal-replacement bars, low-fat artificially sweetened desserts, low-fat peanut butter and many reduced-calorie frozen foods. If you follow this type of a diet with little concern for portion sizes, it will be difficult to have long-term healthy weight loss, despite the relatively low caloric density.

## Nutrient Density

Nutrient density is an important concept in evaluating the nutritional quality of a food. It refers to the amount of a nutrient provided by a food relative to the amount of calories the food provides. A food would have a specific nutrient density for each nutrient it contains. There is no accepted way of totaling nutrient densities. Rather, different foods' nutrient densities for an array of nutrients are generally compared graphically. Foods with high nutrient densities provide a lot of nutrients in few calories. Healthy foods have high nutrient densities. Foods with low nutrient densities provide few nutrients relative to their high calorie content. Unhealthy foods have low nutrient densities. When evaluating whether a food is healthy, nutrient density is one factor to consider, but other factors should be considered as well. For example, sugar content, fiber content, and quality of fats are also important factors.

Sometimes food manufacturers try to make less healthy foods (such as those high in sugar or hydrogenated fats) look healthier by adding a lot of vitamins and minerals to increase their nutrient densities. These types of foods would only have high nutrient densities for the nutrients that have been added. However because of the poor quality of carbohydrates and fats they contain, they would be considered unhealthy choices. Fat and sugar substitutes can also be used to decrease calorie content, which would also make nutrient densities appear higher. A diet primarily made up of such foods would not promote long-term optimal health.

Figures 3-1, 3-2, and 3-3 show nutrient densities for five sample foods in regard to protein, five minerals and four vitamins. In the figures, higher bars indicate higher nutrient densities. In all three categories, spinach has the highest nutrient density, because it is naturally low in calories and high in nutrients. Plain low-fat milk has a high water content and is a good source of many nutrients. It also has a high nutrient density for many vitamins and minerals. The highly sweetened flavored milks that are becoming increasingly popular would have much lower nutrient densities because of the large amount of extra calories from sugar. Almonds are high in fiber and many vitamins and minerals. They also are relatively high in healthy polyunsaturated and monounsaturated fats. Although their nutrient densities for many vitamins and minerals are high, the high-calorie fats do reduce them somewhat. Keep in mind that you do need healthy fats in your diet, so selecting nutrient-dense foods to provide this fat is a smart choice—just watch the portion sizes. Foods, such as soda and cake, provide a lot of calories and very few nutrients. Therefore, these types of foods have low nutrient densities, except for nutrients that have been added, as in the case with folate in cake. In summary, eating foods with high nutrient densities that also have high-quality carbohydrates and fats is the key to

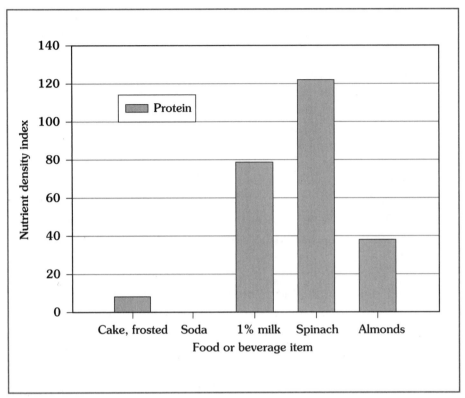

**Figure 3-1.** Nutrient Density in Regards to Protein

losing weight while optimizing health. Foods in the inner green circle of the Bull's-Eye Food Guide have high nutrient densities, those in the yellow have moderate nutrient densities, and those in the red outer circle have low nutrient densities.[1]

## Carbohydrates

All carbohydrates are made up of chains of sugar units. Starch, in particular, consists of very long chains of sugar units. The chains that are in a simple straight line are called amylase and the branched chains are called

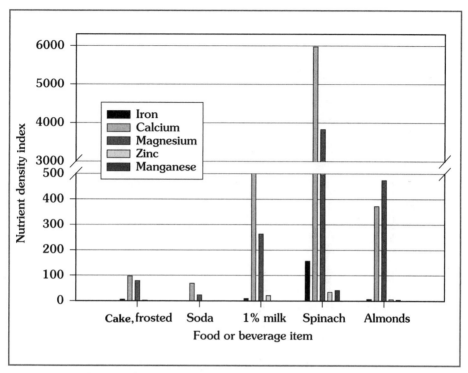

**Figure 3-2.** Nutrient Density in Regards to Minerals

amylopectin. Because dietary sugars are the building blocks of starch, sugars are considered part of the Grain & Starch Group. Fiber, another type of carbohydrate, is made up of long chains of sugar units with cross-links between the chains. Our bodies are not able to break these cross-links, and therefore we cannot digest fiber. They are two types of fiber—soluble and insoluble. Because you cannot digest either type, fiber travels through your gastrointestinal tract and is passed when you have a bowel movement. Fiber never enters your blood stream, thus it provides no calories. However, while it is traveling through your gastrointestinal tract it is involved in many processes that promote health. Resistant starches and oligosaccharides, although not technically fiber, are starch products that are not degraded in the small intestine. They are similar to fiber in that they are passed along to the

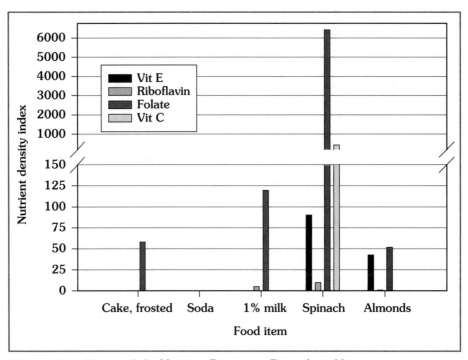

**Figure 3-3.** Nutrient Density in Regards to Vitamins

intestines, and eventually fermented by the bacteria that live there. Although it may be hard to believe, many of these bacteria promote good health. They produce vitamins and short-chain fatty acids that help the cells lining the intestines and the colon. They also help the immune system to work optimally. Fiber and resistant starch are actually the food source for those bacteria, and diets high in fiber and resistant starch promote colonies of these healthy bacteria. The more healthy bacteria you have, the less disease-causing bacteria colonies will form.

Sugar alcohols are another type of carbohydrate that is found in foods. They do not contain the type of alcohol that you drink, called ethanol. They are sugars that have been chemically modified. Due to this modification, they provide fewer calories per gram than regular sugars (about 2 calories per gram instead of 4 calories per gram), but they still offer a sweet taste.

They are digested more slowly than regular sugar, and cause a smaller increase in blood sugar levels. However, when eaten in excess they can cause bloating and diarrhea, have a laxative effect, and cause an increase in blood sugar. Some common sugar alcohols include mannitol, sorbitol, xylitol, lactitol, isomalt, maltitol, and hydrogenated starch hydrolysates. They are found naturally in many fruits and vegetables, and are also man-made from starches. They are used in many diet foods and foods labeled as sugar-free because they are not technically a simple sugar. Recently, they are being used in many foods touted as low-carbohydrate foods. Some manufacturers even subtract them (and fiber) from the total carbohydrate in a serving of a food product and call the resulting number *net carbs* or *impact carbs*. This is misleading, because sugar alcohols do provide calories and can increase blood sugars.

Sugars and sweeteners in Americans' diets have increased dramatically since the early 1980s—with a 28% increase in added sugar consumption between 1983 and 1998. The United States Department of Agriculture estimates that in 2003 the average person ate 142 pounds per person per year (61 pounds refined sugar, 79 pounds of corn sweeteners, and about 1 pound of honey and other sweeteners).[2] There has been a shift in the source of added sugar and sweeteners from table-top use to manufacturer use. Until recently, the USDA recommended that adults limit their added sugars to a maximum of 12 teaspoons a day, yet the USDA estimates that the food supply provided 31 teaspoons of added sugars per person per day in 2000. The largest contributor of added sugars is soft drinks, which provide 33% of all added sugars consumed.[2,3,4]

Sugars and starches can be found in foods that have a lot of fiber or foods that are low in fiber. For example, sugars are found in low-fiber foods like fruit juice, cakes, cookies, soda, and other sweetened beverages. Sugars are also found in fruits, which are high in fiber. White bread, highly processed starches, bagels, and white pasta are sources of starch that are low in fiber. Whole-wheat bread, brown rice, kidney beans, and sweet potatoes are examples of starchy foods that are high fiber. When you eat starches that are low in fiber, you break the starch down very quickly into sugar, and this sugar passes from your intestines into your blood—leading to higher levels of sugar in your blood than before you ate. How high the sugar goes and how long it stays high is largely dependent on your body's ability to make and use a hormone called insulin. Insulin is necessary to facilitate the passage of sugar from the blood into the cells, which need it to produce energy and make various compounds. When you eat starches that are high in fiber, the fiber cross-links make it more difficult for the stomach and intestines to break the starch down—they simply get in the way. So the starches are digested into sugar slowly and absorbed into the blood stream slowly. In summary, low-fiber starches and simple sugars in foods have a similar negative effect on blood sugar levels. However, high-fiber starches lead to a diminished blood sugar response.

Remember, fiber does not provide any calories, but does provide bulk. It, therefore, promotes a feeling of fullness, which helps decrease total calorie intake. Fiber also provides exercise for muscles lining your intestines and in so doing prevents diverticulosis. Diverticulosis is the development of out-pockets along the intestinal tract because of a weak intestinal wall. Fiber also prevents constipation and hemorrhoids, and helps to lower blood cholesterol levels. It is associated with a lower risk for obesity, constipation, heart disease, diabetes, hypertension, and some types of cancers.

High-fiber starchy foods made from whole grains are high in vitamins and minerals, such as thiamin, riboflavin, niacin, chromium, manganese, magnesium, selenium, and zinc. Low-fiber processed and refined starches are much lower in micronutrients relative to their original unprocessed versions. When food manufacturers process and refine grains, they remove the outer bran and germ coatings that contain 17 key nutrients and 25% of the protein originally in the whole grain.[5] Manufacturers are required by law to add only five nutrients back after processing—thiamine, riboflavin, niacin, iron, and folic acid. Many nutrients lost are simply lost for good. Some starches are fortified with nutrients. This means that nutrients not originally present are added to the final product. Food manufacturers often use this tactic to make their highly processed products seem healthier than they truly are. For example, highly processed cereals with lots of sugar, lots of hydrogenated fats, and no fiber are fortified with many vitamins and minerals. This makes them appear healthy, even though they are high in sugar and missing many nutrients originally in the grain.

The intake of carbohydrates affects your blood sugar. Despite individual variability in how various foods affect blood sugar, some general trends for different types of foods can be expected. The glycemic index was developed to describe the effect different foods typically have on blood sugar. It refers to the rise in blood sugar that results after eating a specified amount of food on an empty stomach when compared to eating the same amount of sugar (glucose) on an empty stomach. The glycemic index of glucose is arbitrarily assigned a glycemic index of 100. Foods with a high glycemic index can be expected to lead to a high blood sugar if eaten alone on an empty stomach. This is generally not favorable. Alternatively, foods with a low glycemic index can be expected to result in small increase in blood sugar. Both fat and fiber decrease the glycemic index of a food. Although glycemic index is an interesting and important concept, it should not be used as the sole indicator of the healthfulness of a food for a few reasons. First of all, the glycemic index of a food is not fixed or stable. For example, the glycemic index of pasta varies based on how long it is cooked, and the glycemic index of fruits vary widely based on growing conditions and ripeness. Scientists debate about how to measure glycemic index, and methodological differences may account for differences in reported indices for foods. Refer to the glycemic indices noted in Table 3-1. The foods in the table are organized in columns by category of nutrient density, with foods of high nutrient density in the first column and those with the lowest nutrient density in the last column. The glycemic indices of foods in each column range from low to high values. Therefore, there are some nutrient-dense foods that have a high glycemic index, although most have a low glycemic index. High-carbohydrate foods with moderate and low nutrient densities tend to have high glycemic indicies.

The glycemic index of any one food is changed when that food is eaten in combination with other foods, beverages, or condiments. For example, putting olive oil on pasta changes the glycemic index of the pasta. Most of the foods we eat are part of a meal or snack that has its own composite glycemic index. Lastly, the glycemic response to a food can vary day to day

**Table 3-1.**

Glycemic Index of Foods Grouped by Nutrient Density

| Food | Glycemic Index | Food | Glycemic Index | Food | Glycemic Index |
|------|------|------|------|------|------|
| **High Nutrient Density** | | **Moderate Nutrient Density** | | **Low Nutrient Density** | |
| Potato, baked | 85 | Waffles | 76 | Jellybeans | 78 |
| Bread, whole-wheat | 53 | White bread | 73 | Doughnuts | 76 |
| Banana | 52 | Bagel, white | 72 | Pop Tarts | 70 |
| Corn, cob | 48 | Croissant | 67 | Corn chips | 63 |
| Carrots | 47 | Rice, white | 56 | Ice cream | 37 |
| Kidney beans | 28 | Spaghetti | 44 | M&Ms | 33 |

in the same individual, based on such factors as the previous meal eaten. Therefore, glycemic index is only one characteristic of a food that should be considered when determining its healthfulness. Baked potatoes have a relatively high glycemic index, and have been banned in many diets. Baked potatoes provide fiber, vitamin C, potassium, and vitamin $B_6$, and they are low in sugar and unhealthy fats. They are rarely eaten alone. A medium-sized baked potato eaten in combination with fish and vegetables sautéed in olive oil and garlic would be a very healthy meal, and the glycemic index of the meal would be favorable. Low nutrient-dense, processed foods with a high glycemic index would be considered unhealthy. Therefore, when evaluating the nutritional quality and healthfulness of foods, nutrient density and glycemic index need to be considered, as well as other factors, such as types of fats. The Bull's-Eye Food Guide takes all of these factors into consideration, making it easy for you to identify foods that are most healthy (green section), moderately healthy (yellow section), and least healthy (red section).[6]

In summary, the healthiest food sources of carbohydrates are those that are least processed, high in fiber, and low in unhealthy fats, such as starchy vegetables (whole corn, potatoes, and sweet peas), legumes (dried peas, beans, and lentils), whole grains (whole wheat, whole amaranth, whole or Scotch barley, whole kamut), and whole fruits. Nonstarchy vegetables, such as string beans, broccoli, sweet peppers, and zucchini provide smaller amounts of starch per serving. Milk and yogurt provide significant amounts of carbohydrate. All of these foods have high nutrient densities, and generally have moderate to low glycemic indices.

## Fats

Fatty acids are the building blocks of fats in your body. They are calorically dense, providing 9 calories per gram. This is more than twice the amount of calories provided by carbohydrates. A fat is made up of three fatty acids attached to a sugar-type molecule. Fats in foods have to be digested into their components before they can be absorbed into your body. They can be made up of any combination of four different types of fatty acids: saturated, polyunsaturated, monounsaturated, and hydrogenated fats. No one food has just one type of fatty acid. All foods with fat have a mix of fatty acids. However, foods are usually primary dietary sources of one type of fatty acid, and are often referred to as sources of just that fat. For example, olive oil is referred to as a healthy monounsaturated fat. It is a good source of monounsaturated fat, but it does have polyunsaturated and saturated fats as well.

The types of fats in your diet have a profound effect on your health, because dietary fats determine the makeup of each of your cell membranes, which are primarily made of fat. The fatty acid composition of your cell membranes affects the cells' shape, flexibility, and permeability, as well as the types of chemicals called *eicosanoids* that are produced inside your cells. Eicosanoids are hormone-like substances that regulate many organ systems and processes in your body, such as the level of inflammation, constriction of blood vessels, and the stickiness of your blood. These processes influence the development and progression of many chronic diseases, such as heart disease.

Saturated fatty acids are hard at room temperature, and they are the predominant fat in animal products, such as the fatty marbling in meats, whole milk, cheese, butter, and eggs. Coconut oil, palm oil, and palm kernel oil are plant-based fats that are high in saturated fatty acids. Diets high in saturated animal fats have been linked to the development of heart disease and some types of cancers.

Polyunsaturated fatty acids are liquid at room temperature. There are different types of polyunsaturated fats, such as omega-3 and omega-6 polyunsaturated fats. Two fatty acids are considered essential nutrients, meaning that they are essential for normal growth and development but cannot be made by the body. Linoleic acid is an omega-6 polyunsaturated fat found in high concentrations in seeds, vegetable oils, mayonnaise, and salad dressing. Linolenic acid is an omega-3 polyunsaturated fat found in high concentrations in green leafy vegetables, soybeans, flaxseed, phytoplankton, seaweed, and fish. Some eggs produced by hens fed high omega-3 diets are also high in omega-3s.

The ratio of omega-3 and omega-6 polyunsaturated fats in the American food supply has changed markedly since the 1800s so that there is much more omega-6 polyunsaturated fatty acids relative to omega-3 polyunsaturated fatty acids. This is primarily due to two factors. The first factor is how animals raised for food are being fed. Rather than grazing freely on various greens, some of which are high in omega-3 fatty acids, animals now eat commercially prepared feeds that are high in omega-6 polyunsaturated fats and have virtually no omega-3 fatty acids. Therefore, the fatty acid content of all animal products (meat, milk, cheese, butter) is lower in omega-3 fatty acids. This is also true of farm-raised fish, as opposed to wild fish. The second change in the food supply involves the increased commercial use of vegetable oils from safflower, sunflower, and corn sources, all of which are high in omega-6 polyunsaturated fats. The introduction of margarine exemplifies the increased role of these oils, as does the increased production and promotion of infant formulas. Infant formulas contain these vegetable oils as a source of essential fatty acids and historically have contained no omega-3 polyunsaturated fats. Therefore, when formula replaces breast milk, which does contain omega-3 fatty acids at levels dependent on the mother's diet, the ratio of these fats in infants' diets is negatively affected. Some infant formula manufactures are creating products that have omega-3 fatty acids added, but they are usually significantly more expensive. Foods naturally high in omega-3 polyunsaturated fatty acids, such as seaweed or algae, leafy green vegetables, fatty fish, walnuts, and soybeans, are not common in the American diet. Therefore, there is a negative trend towards the increased intake of omega-6s relative to omega-3s. You do need both omega-6s and omega-3s in your diet, but you need to make a conscious effort to include omega-3s, because they are much more rare in foods.

Monounsaturated fatty acids are also liquid at room temperature. Olive oil is by far the best source of monounsaturated fatty acids. It is also very low in saturated fatty acids. Peanut oil, natural peanut butter, olives, many nuts, soybeans, and soybean oil are also high in monounsaturated fatty acids and relatively low in saturated fatty acids. Meats and chicken have a fair amount of monounsaturated fatty acids as well, but meat is also a good source of saturated fatty acids. In some cultures, olive oil is a dietary staple. Many Mediterranean countries, such as Greece and Italy, have culinary traditions that favor olive oil as well as fruits and vegetables and low intakes of animal fats. Such dietary styles have been associated with decreased chronic illnesses, such as heart disease and cancer.

Hydrogenated, or trans-fatty acids are not naturally found in significant amounts in the food supply. However, food manufacturers commonly add hydrogenated fats to foods in the form of partially hydrogenated vegetable oils. Food manufacturers take liquid polyunsaturated fats and create solid hydrogenated or partially hydrogenated fats, which are more solid and have a longer shelf life. They are often added to cakes, cookies, crackers, breads, chips, and even some breakfast cereals. Food manufacturers are only required by law to list total and saturated fats until 2006, when they will also be required to list trans fats. You do not have a physiological requirement for trans fatty acids, and they should be avoided completely— or as much as possible.

The kinds of fats you consume affect your health in many ways, such as affecting your risk of heart disease. Cholesterol is a fat-like substance that needs to be transported around your body in watery blood. Because fat and water do not mix well, your intestines and liver make structures, similar to suitcases, to carry fat and cholesterol around your body in your watery blood. These suitcases are called lipoproteins. There are many different types of lipoproteins, but two that are important relative to your risk of heart disease are LDL and HDL lipoproteins. A high level of LDLs increases your risk of heart disease, whereas a high level of HDLs decreases your risk of heart disease. The types of fatty acids in your diet affect the levels of these lipoproteins. Saturated fats increase both LDLs and HDLs, but their negative impact is greater than their positive impact. When polyunsaturated fats replace saturated fats in your diet, LDLs are lowered but HDLs are lowered as well. When monounsaturated fats replace saturated fats in the diet, LDLs are lowered but HDLs are protected and stay about the same. When trans fats replace saturated fats, LDLs are increased and HDLs are lowered—the worst possible outcome. Therefore, monounsaturated fats have the most advantageous affect on your risk for heart disease, saturated fats have a negative affect, and trans fats have the most adverse affect.

Another example of the affect of fats on your health is the effect they have on the outer coating of all of your cells, called cell membranes. Cell membranes are made up largely of fatty acids. The fats you eat affect the types of fatty acids on all of your cell membranes. Because the machinery in your cells, called enzymes, uses the fatty acids on your cell membranes as ingredients, the fats in your diet affect the chemicals produced by this machinery. These chemicals are very powerful, and especially influence processes such as inflammation, platelet adhesion (or blood stickiness), and vasoconstriction or dilation (or closing and opening of blood vessels). When omega-3 polyunsaturated fatty acids are more predominant on cell membranes, they are more often pulled off the membrane to be used by the cell's enzymes. This leads to less inflammation and platelet adhesion, as well as vasodilation. When omega-6 polyunsaturated fatty acids are more prevalent in your diet, the result is higher levels of inflammation and platelet adhesion, as well as more vasoconstriction—these processes can increase your risk for conditions such as heart disease, asthma, rheumatoid arthritis, and inflammatory gastrointestinal disorders.[7,8,9,10,11]

# Proteins

Proteins have the same caloric density as carbohydrates, 4 calories per gram. They are made up of amino acid building blocks. There are 22 amino acids that are used by the body. Nine are considered essential, meaning that they must be supplied by the diet because they can't be made by your body. Complete proteins provide all nine essential amino acids in the appropriate ratios. Protein in the food you eat is digested into amino acids, which are then absorbed into your blood stream. Your genetic code then rearranges amino acids in new sequences. After chains of amino acids are assembled, they collapse into three-dimensional shapes unique to each specific protein. Each protein's unique three-dimensional structure enables it to carry out very specific functions.

Unlike carbohydrates and fats, amino acids are chemically unique in that they include nitrogen in addition to carbon, hydrogen, and oxygen atoms. Excessive amounts of nitrogen must be eliminated by the kidney, and this process requires adequate water intake. High-protein animal foods, such as meat, fish, chicken, and milk, provide all essential amino acids. High-protein foods derived from plants do not provide all of the essential amino acids, except for soybeans, which are complete proteins. Therefore, vegetarians need to eat a wide variety of plant-based foods (legumes, grains, nuts, and seeds) or some animal proteins (such as eggs, milk, or cheese) throughout the day to obtain all of their essential amino acids.

A daily supply of protein in the diet is required for growth and repair of body tissues. When decreasing total calorie intake and losing weight, protein needs are increased to minimize the breakdown of muscles for energy. With this higher protein intake, more weight loss is from body fat and less from lean body tissues (such as muscles). This is important, because the more muscle mass you have the more calories your body uses every minute of every day.[12,13] This helps to create a negative calorie balance and weight loss. Most Americans get plenty of protein and meet these increased needs quite easily. However, many popular high-protein foods are also highly processed and high in saturated fats. See Menus and Recipes for sample menus with adequate amounts of high-quality protein foods that will give you the beneficial effects of dietary protein.

## Vitamins and Minerals and Phytochemicals

Vitamins and minerals are needed for every chemical reaction and process in the body. They are needed in relatively small amounts (milligrams or micrograms per day), compared to carbohydrates, proteins, and fats (grams per day). Vitamins help special kinds of proteins called enzymes, which function as the cells' metabolic machinery, function properly. Minerals are also necessary for enzymes to do their jobs. In addition, minerals can become part of body tissues, such as calcium in bones. There are 14 vitamins and 17 minerals known to be essential for life. Vitamins and minerals work together with enzymes and other chemical regulators in your body to keep all bodily functions working. Since the early 1900s, researchers have been uncovering the role of vitamins and minerals in preventing deficiency diseases and, until recently, dietary recommendations have been based on adequate amounts to prevent these types of diseases. Recent revisions to vitamin and mineral recommendations, called Dietary Reference Intakes (DRIs), consider adequate amounts to prevent chronic diseases, such as cancer and heart disease. DRIs include recommendations for adequate intakes, as well as recommended limits on dietary intakes to prevent toxicities. This information is especially helpful for people taking multiple supplements from which the amounts of specific vitamins or minerals may exceed healthy amounts. For information on specific vitamins and minerals, including recommended dietary intakes, upper tolerable limits, functions, and food sources go to the United States Department of Agriculture's Food and Nutrition Information Web page (http://www.nal.usda.gov/fnic/etext/000105.html).

Vitamins are complex compounds that are made by a plant or animal or microbe. There are two categories of vitamins: water-soluble vitamins and fat-soluble vitamins. Water-soluble vitamins travel easily in your watery blood, and extra amounts are excreted in urine. Fat-soluble vitamins need dietary fats to be absorbed well. They also need special transporters to travel through your blood. An excess of fat-soluble vitamins can be stored along with fat in your body, and excessive amounts for long periods of time can more easily cause toxicities. Some vitamins (vitamin C, vitamin E, and beta carotene or pre-vitamin A) function as antioxidants, and prevent potential harmful reactions in your body. Potentially harmful oxidative reactions occur every day during the process of normal metabolism, although some environmental factors such as pollution and exposure to cigarette smoke increase the occurrence of these reactions. Oxidative reactions cause the production of free radicals, which are highly reactive chemical species that can damage your body's cells and tissues. Your body has natural defenses against these free radicals; however, dietary antioxidants boost these defense mechanisms and help prevent potential damage. In addition to the vitamins listed above, some minerals—copper, manganese, selenium, and zinc—are necessary to support your body's own defense systems. Excessive oxidative damage is associated with increased risk for cancer, heart disease, cataracts, and general aging. An example of an oxidative reaction is the browning of apple slices exposed to the air. Dipping the apple slices in lemon juice or orange juice can prevent the browning, because the juices have vitamin C that prevents the oxidation processes.

The minerals that help prevent oxidation are in the category of trace minerals, those minerals needed in the smallest amounts. Major minerals include those that become part of the structure of your body (calcium, phosphorus, and magnesium), as well as electrolytes that regulate water balance and nerve signals (sodium, chloride, and potassium). Plants extract inorganic minerals from the soil and bind them to other molecules produced by the plants. Animals and people consume the plants, and the minerals are incorporated into their tissues. Minerals that are added to foods by manufacturers may be bound to various compounds to facilitate their absorption, for example, calcium can be bound

**Table 3-2.**
Recommended Food Sources of Selected Vitamins and Minerals

| Minerals | Food Source | Vitamins | Food Source |
|---|---|---|---|
| Calcium | Low-fat milk, cheese, and yogurt; calcium-set tofu; broccoli, kale, and Chinese cabbage | Folate (folic acid) | Whole- and enriched-grain products; dark leafy vegetables |
| Chromium | Lean meat; eggs; whole-grain products | Niacin | Lean meat, fish, and poultry; natural peanut butter; legumes; whole- and enriched-grain products |
| Iron | Lean meat; fortified grain products | Vitamin A | Fortified low-fat milk, yogurt and cheese; darkly colored fruits and leafy vegetables; eggs; fatty fish |
| Magnesium | Legumes; nuts; green leafy vegetables; whole-grain products | Vitamin $B_{12}$ (cobalamin) | Lean meat, fish, and chicken; eggs; low-fat milk, yogurt and cheese; fortified-grain products |
| Manganese | Nuts; legumes; whole-grain products | Vitamin C (ascorbic acid) | Citrus fruits; tomatoes; potatoes; Brussels sprouts; sweet peppers; cauliflower; broccoli; strawberries; cabbage; spinach |
| Selenium | Seafood; whole-grain products; vegetables | Vitamin D (calciferol) | Fatty fish; fortified milk products; fortified cereals; eggs (Note: Vitamin D is also produced by body with sun exposure on the skin) |
| Zinc | Lean red meats and some seafood; whole- and fortified-grain products | Vitamin E | Vegetable oils; nuts and seeds; whole grains; leafy green vegetables |

to a carbonate or citrate compound. The mineral content of fruits, vegetables, and grains varies based on the mineral content of the soil in which they were grown. Food sources of selected vitamins and minerals are indicated in Table 3-2. In general, eating a variety of foods from the inner circle of the Bull's-Eye Food Guide is the best strategy to get the vitamins and minerals your body needs to work optimally.

# Water

Water accounts for 55% to 75% of adult body weight, depending largely on age and relative amounts of muscle and body fat. Water is necessary to provide an environment for your cells' chemical reactions, maintain blood volume and the cardiovascular system, regulate body temperature, and remove waste products of metabolism as urine and bowel movements. The human body loses water through sweat, urine, bowel movements, and expired air.

Beverages and solid foods provide the majority of water your body needs, but your body also produces water as a byproduct of many chemical reactions. Men need about 4½ quarts of water per day and women need about 3-3/4 quarts per day. Your water needs are increased with physical activity, exposure to extreme temperatures, and exposure to recirculated air. In addition, as you increase your fiber intake you should also increase your water intake because fiber absorbs water in the gut and increases water losses in bowel movements. Beverages are an obvious source of water, but solid foods provide more than you may think. For example, fruits and vegetables are 80% to 95% water. Fish, meat, and poultry are 65% to 70% water, and grain products are about 40% to 60% water. On the other hand fats, such as butter and oils, are only 16% and 0% water, respectively.

Most adults meet their water needs by responding to their thirst. However, by the time you perceive thirst, you are already mildly dehydrated or low on your water supply. A generally accepted rule of thumb is to drink enough water to make your urine almost clear. Making an effort to drink 8 to 12 cups of fluid a day is consistent with current recommendations, and may facilitate weigh loss if drinking water helps you delay non–hunger-related desires to eat. This is only true if the fluids you select are calorie-free.

Plain water is by far the preferred fluid to meet the majority of your water needs. Fluid low-fat milk may also be consumed to meet 2 or 3 cups of fluid needs, as long as your body can tolerate milk. Drinking greater than 4 ounces of juice a day can be problematic if weight loss is a goal, because of the excessive calories and sugars it can provide. Whole fruits are nutritionally superior to fruit juice, and more filling relative to the calories provided. Artificially sweetened beverages can play a role in meeting your fluid needs, however artificial sweeteners may perpetuate the desire for sweet foods and increase hunger due to an insulin response. Using artificially sweetened beverages early in your weight-loss journey may help you cut back on calories if they are replacing caloric beverages. Over time, it would be helpful to reduce your intake of artificially sweetened beverages and to replace them with water, naturally flavored water and seltzer (without added sweeteners or artificial sweeteners), and iced or hot herbal teas. Sports drinks are a preferred fuel source during and after exercise for competitive athletes who have an increased need for calories and some micronutrients. However, for noncompetitive athletes who are exercising to promote optimal health and weight loss, sports drinks are not recommended because of their sugar and calorie content. For example, if you are walking for a half-hour you may burn 100 to 350 calories (depending on your size and pace). Yet 16 ounces of a sports drink will provide about 100 calories and 28 grams of sugar, thereby working against your goal of creating a negative calorie balance. The caffeine content of beverages may be an issue, especially if you are sensitive to caffeine or if your health care provider has recommended that you decrease your caffeine intake (National Academy of Sciences 2004).[14]

## Phytochemicals

Phytochemicals are found in plants that promote health. Although research in this area consistently finds that the intake of phytochemicals decreases the risk of many chronic illnesses (cancer, stroke, heart disease, and macular degeneration), they have not been found to be essential for life. The most common classes of phytochemicals include carotenoids, flavonoids (including isoflavones and phytoestrogens), inositol phosphates (phytates), lignans (phytoestrogens), isothiocyanates and indoles, phenols, saponins, sulfides and thiols, and terpenes. Phytochemicals occur naturally in fruits, vegetables, whole grains, legumes, nuts, and teas. They co-exist in plant foods and are likely to work in concert to exert their positive effects. Studies in which individuals receive isolated supplemental forms of phytochemicals alone or in combination with one or two other phytochemicals have not consistently had positive outcomes. Some scientists suspect that this is because researchers are not able to replicate the necessary combinations and ratios of phytochemicals necessary to confer their health-promoting effects. This is very likely given that there exist hundreds of phytochemical compounds, with innumerable potential effective combinations. The mechanisms by which they exert their positive effects are not yet fully understood, but it has been proposed that they do the following: serve as antioxidants, enhance immune response, enhance cell-to-cell communication, cause cancer cells to die, and support the liver's detoxification enzyme systems.

Phytochemicals are very stable, and for the most part not destroyed with cooking. However, the refining process does cause a marked decrease in the phytochemical content of whole grains. In order to ensure a phytonutrient-dense diet, eat a wide variety of foods from the inner circle of the Bull's-Eye Food Guide—at least 6 servings of whole vegetables and 2 to 3 servings of whole fruits each day. In addition, select whole grains over refined grains, and use onions, garlic, and herbs liberally in cooking because they also contain phytochemicals.[15]

## Nutrient Supplements

The need for nutrient supplements is somewhat controversial. It is certainly possible and desirable to meet all of your nutrient needs through whole foods and beverages. Unfortunately, Americans eat far too few whole foods. For example, according to the United States Department of Agriculture, Americans consume only 3.3 servings of vegetables a day. This estimate includes French fries, which are not nutrient/phytochemical-dense foods. When only dark green and deep yellow vegetables are considered, the daily serving of vegetables drops to 0.2 servings a day. This is in comparison to the minimum recommended intake of 3 to 6 servings per day. Approximately 48% of Americans consume less than one serving of fruit a day. This is compared to the recommended 2 servings for those who require 2200 calories per day and 3 servings a day for those who require 2800 calories per day.

Taking a nutrient supplement in addition to a high-quality base diet can provide insurance of adequate nutrients on a daily basis. However, taking a nutrient supplement on top of a base diet that is low in fruits, vegetables, and whole grains will not make up for the poor base diet and may provide a false sense of security. In such a scenario, a nutrient supplement may help meet the needs of essential vitamins and minerals, but it will not promote optimal health because it will be lacking in many, many phytochemicals. For example, there are hundreds of carotinoids in fruits and vegetables yet only a few are typically isolated and put in supplements. Therefore, the benefits of taking a full array of phytochemicals from whole foods cannot be replicated with nutrient supplements. Supplements may, however, help meet your needs on off days when your diet is not quite up to par.

## Important Points To Remember from Chapter 3

◉ Many factors need to be considered when determining the healthfulness of a food—caloric density, nutrient density, fiber content, phytochemical content, types of carbohydrates, types of fats, and level of processing.

◉ The Bull's-Eye Food Guide takes all of the above factors into consideration in the placement of foods within groups or subgroups. This helps you to make quick and well-informed food and beverage decisions.

◉ Water is an overlooked essential nutrient that you should make a conscious effort to consume.

◉ It is most beneficial to get your vitamins and minerals from whole foods.

# LEARNING TO USE
# YOUR COMPASS

## What You Will Discover in Chapter 4

◉ Foods are carefully placed in the six food groups of the Bull's-Eye Food Guide in a way that accounts for many aspects of nutritional quality: vitamin and mineral content, quality of carbohydrates and fats, phytochemical content, fiber content, and level of processing. Healthiest foods are in the green inner circle. Moderately healthy foods are in the yellow middle circle, and the unhealthy foods are in the red outer circle. Therefore by selecting foods mostly from the green inner circle, you can craft a healthy diet without having to consider all of these issues separately.

◉ One of the basic ideas of the Bull's-Eye Food Guide system is that a basic eating plan can be developed that has a specified amount of calories, carbohydrates, proteins and fats, as well as built-in flexibility for you to pick the foods you like to create menus based on the plan without counting calories and grams. In order to do this, each food group is assigned an amount of calories, carbohydrates, proteins, and fats. Then, a portion of food in each

(continued on next page)

## What You Will Discover in Chapter 4
### (continued)

group that provides roughly these amounts is defined. These portions are called swaps, because swaps of foods within a group are interchangeable—you can swap one for another. Swaps are not serving sizes, because you may have more than one swap of a food group in a meal. Therefore the serving size (the amount you actually serve yourself and eat) could be one swap or many swaps.

◉ Foods within a particular food group and subgroup provide a similar set of nutrients (vitamins, minerals, and phytochemicals).

◉ When you develop your plan in later chapters, you will know how many swaps you have from each food group for each meal.

◉ You can use the nutrition information on food packages to determine the swap equivalents of a specific food.

## Overview

This chapter provides detailed information about the Bull's-Eye Food Guide—your compass. The Bull's-Eye Food Guide will point you in the right direction to quickly select healthy foods. This information is necessary to start changing your food choices and crafting new eating styles. Similar to Chapter 3, this chapter provides a lot of detailed information regarding foods and nutrients. The chapter is organized by food groups of the Bull's-Eye Food Guide as presented in the front of the book. It would be helpful to go through this chapter—even if it is just quickly—as you begin your weight management program. To begin your weight management journey go to Chapter 5 to select your calorie level and eating style, and then go to Menus and Recipes for specific menus to follow. The information provided in the pages that follow will help you make the best food choices as you follow your menus and program. As you progress, it would be helpful to go back and review this chapter a few times. Throughout this chapter you are also referred back to Chapter 3 for more detailed information on nutrients.

As discussed in Chapter 2, the Bull's-Eye Food Guide is made up of six major foods groups. Each major food group has three subgroups. A food is placed in one of the major food groups based on its relative amounts of carbohydrates, proteins and fats, as well as caloric density (the number of calories per gram). There is a predetermined number of calories associated with each food group as shown in Table 4-1. For example, 60 calories are the assigned number of calories for the Fruit Group. An amount of each food in each food group that provides the predetermined amount of calories is called a swap. The following portions of fruits have about 60 calories and are equal to one swap from the Fruit Group: 10 grapes, 1 apple, ½ banana, or 12 cherries. The amount of calories, carbohydrates, proteins, and fats in a swap of food from each of the six major food groups is also predetermined, and shown in Table 4-1. These portions that provide the predetermined number of calories, carbohydrates, proteins and fats are called swaps, because swaps of foods within a group are interchangeable—you can swap one for another. Swaps are not considered serving sizes because you may have more than one swap of a food group in a meal. Therefore the serving size (the amount you actually serve yourself and eat) could be equal to one swap or many swaps. Refer to the Swap Lists for lists of all foods in each group and subgroup, and the portions of food assigned as a swap.

- Foods in the Vegetable Group also get most of their calories from carbohydrates with a small amount of protein and no fat. Their caloric density is much lower than the foods in the Grain & Starch Group.

- Foods in the Fruit Group get all of their calories from carbohydrates.

- Foods in the Grain & Starch Group get most of their calories from carbohydrates with a small amount of protein and almost no fat.

**Table 4-1**

Selected Nutrient Content of Swaps from Each Food Group and Sample Swaps

| Food Group | Calories (per swap) | Carbohydrates (grams per swap) | Proteins (grams per swap) | Fat (grams per swap) |
|---|---|---|---|---|
| **Vegetable Group** | 25 | 5 | 2 | 0 |
| **Swaps:** ½ cup broccoli, 1 cup sweet pepper slices, ½ cup cooked spinach, 1 large tomato | | | | |
| **Fruit Group** | 60 | 15 | 0 | 0 |
| **Swaps:** 1 apple, ¾ cup blueberries, ½ banana, 1 cup cubed honeydew melon, ½ grapefruit, 10 grapes | | | | |
| **Grain & Starch Group** | 80 | 15 | 3 | 1 |
| **Swaps:** 1 slice whole-wheat bread, ½ cup whole-wheat pasta, ⅓ cup brown rice | | | | |
| **Protein Group** | 55 | 0 | 7 | 3 |
| **Swaps:** 1 ounce salmon, 3 ounces tofu, 1 ounce chicken, 1 ounce eye round steak | | | | |
| **Milk & Yogurt Group (nonfat)** | 90 | 12 | 8 | 0 |
| **Swaps:** 1 cup skim milk, 1 cup plain nonfat yogurt, 1 cup low-fat soymilk, 1 cup 1% milk | | | | |
| **Fat Group** | 45 | 0 | 0 | 5 |
| **Swaps:** 1 teaspoon olive oil, ⅛ avocado, 6 almonds, 2 teaspoons natural peanut butter | | | | |

- Foods in the Protein Group get most of their calories from proteins with some fat as well.

- Foods in the Fat Group get all of their calories from fat.

- Foods in the Milk & Yogurt Group get a lot of calories from carbohydrates and a lot from proteins.

After being placed in one of the six major food groups, foods are then placed in one of the three subgroups of that food group. This placement is based on the amounts of nutrients they provide relative to the calories they offer. Foods in the green inner circle have a lot of nutrients relative to their calorie content. They typically contain high amounts of fiber and low amounts of added sweeteners and sodium. If they have fat, it is the healthiest of the kinds of fats. The foods in this subgroup are the healthiest in each food group. Foods in the yellow middle circle still provide many nutrients, but they contain less fiber and may have some added sweeteners, sodium, and fats. These foods are moderately nutrient dense and moderately healthy. In general, however, they are considered healthier than their nutrient content justifies. Frequent selections from the yellow subgroup instead of the green subgroup (regular pasta over whole-wheat pasta, refined cereals over whole-grain cereals, and white rice over brown rice) lead to a diet markedly low in fiber, micronutrients, and phytochemicals. Don't get lulled into thinking these foods can be the base of a healthy diet. Foods in the red outer circle provide the least nutrients for the amount of calories they provide. They typically are high in added sweeteners, trans or saturated fats, or sodium. These foods are generally recognized as less healthy. See Figure 4-1 for a summary of the relationships among nutrients in foods and the placement of foods into groups and subgroups.

Remember, a swap of any one food in a food group can be traded in for a swap of another food from that same food group, yet about the same amount of calories, carbohydrates, proteins, and fats would be provided. For example, suppose if after reading Chapter 5, you decide you will have two swaps from the Grain & Starch Group for dinner. Either of the following choices would count as two swaps:

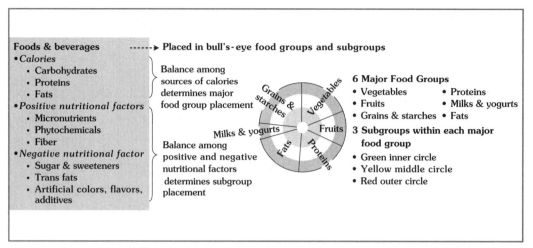

**Foods & beverages** ----→ **Placed in bull's-eye food groups and subgroups**
- *Calories*
  - Carbohydrates
  - Proteins
  - Fats
- *Positive nutritional factors*
  - Micronutrients
  - Phytochemicals
  - Fiber
- *Negative nutritional factor*
  - Sugar & sweeteners
  - Trans fats
  - Artificial colors, flavors, additives

Balance among sources of calories determines major food group placement

Balance among positive and negative nutritional factors determines subgroup placement

**6 Major Food Groups**
- Vegetables
- Fruits
- Grains & starches
- Proteins
- Milks & yogurts
- Fats

**3 Subgroups within each major food group**
- Green inner circle
- Yellow middle circle
- Red outer circle

**Figure 4-1.**
Nutrients in Foods and Placement of Foods into Groups and Subgroups

- ⅔ cup of brown rice (one swap is ⅓ cup, so two swaps would be ⅔ cup);

- ⅔ cup of kidney beans (one swap of kidney beans is also ⅓ cup, so two swaps is ⅔ cup); or

- A combination of ⅓ cup of brown rice and ⅓ cup of kidney beans

Any of these three combinations would provide about 160 calories, 30 grams of carbohydrate, 6 grams of protein, and 2 grams of fat.

The concept of swaps is extremely valuable because it allows you to monitor your calorie intake, as well as balance your intake of carbohydrates, proteins, and fats, *without ever having to count calories or grams.* You simply have to keep track of your swaps during the day. See Table 4-2 for identification of food groups, subgroups, foods, and swaps as shown on the Swap Lists. In addition, Chapters 6, 7, and 8 explain swaps and trading swaps in greater detail. Lastly, the menus in the Menus and Recipes section indicate the food groups and number of swaps in each of the sample meals. Reviewing this information will help review the concept of swaps and trading swaps from within a food group.

## Table 4-2. Sample Bull's-Eye Food Guide Swap List

*See pages 263–276 for complete swap lists for each food group.*

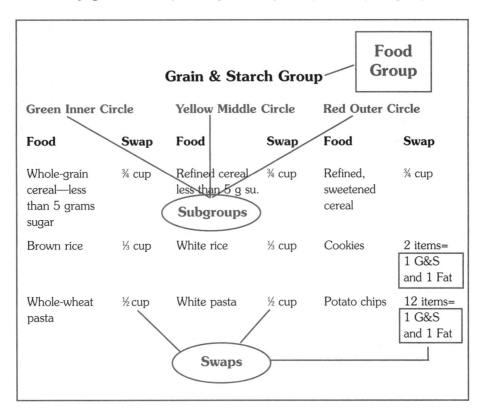

In general you should try to select most foods from the green inner circle. However, if some of your favorite foods are in the red outer circle, you can plan to trade-in these less-healthy alternatives for healthier options occasionally. You should limit selections from the red outer circle to about one time a day if following a lower-calorie plan after reading Chapter 5. If you determine in Chapter 5 that based on your current height and weight you can follow a higher-calorie plan, then you can select two swaps a day from the red outer circle. Just keep in mind that a single food selection from the red outer circle may be counted as two swaps from a food group or a combination of swaps from two different food groups because of the high calorie content. Therefore, make sure you save up enough swaps for such foods. For example a standard-size piece of coffee cake with crumb topping counts as two swaps from the Grain & Starch Group and two swaps from the Fat Group.

In the next six sections of this chapter each food group and its three subgroups are described in detail, and the placement of foods is explained. For each food group there is a three-column swap list of foods in the Swap Lists. The swap lists indicate the foods in each group and subgroup as well as the amount of that food considered a swap. The first column corresponds with the green inner circle, the middle column with the yellow middle circle, and the last outer column with the red outer circle. You should refer to the Swap Lists beginning on page 263 as you read about the food groups. After each food group is described, a summary chart is provided that provides selected nutrient information, swaps, and ranges of recommended swaps per day.

## Introduction—Vegetable Group

The **Vegetable Group** includes plant foods that are very low in calories. The vegetable could come from the stems (such as asparagus), roots (such as carrots and turnips), bulbs (such as onions), leaves (such as lettuce and cabbage), or flowers (such as broccoli and cauliflower). The calories they have come from carbohydrates and proteins. Many vegetables that are biologically fruits, such as tomatoes, cucumbers, zucchini, and sweet peppers, are included in this group rather than the Fruit Group. They are included in the Vegetable Group because these particular fruits are much lower in carbohydrates and calories than other fruits, and in this way more similar in calorie content to vegetables.

Vegetables provide lots of fiber, vitamins (vitamin A, vitamin C, vitamin E, vitamin K, and many B vitamins), minerals (potassium, iron, calcium, and magnesium), and phytochemicals, as well as some carbohydrates and proteins. Phytochemicals are compounds in plant foods that are not as well-defined as vitamins and minerals, yet they are strongly suspected to offer many health benefits. Examples of phytochemicals in vegetables include carotinoids, flavones, phenols, and indols. Cruciferous vegetables, such as broccoli, bok choy, cabbage, kale, Brussels sprouts, and turnips, are good sources of indols. Indols help enzymes in the liver to detoxify and excrete cancer-causing chemicals, and thereby prevent these chemicals from damaging cells. Anthocyanins are phenols that give some vegetables their red or bluish colors. Very powerful antioxidants called anthocyanins can decrease your risk for heart disease and cancer, as well as slow some processes of aging. There are hundreds of phytochemicals found in vegetables, and they are thought to work best in combinations. Almost all studies exploring the role of whole vegetables in health find that people with diets plentiful in whole vegetables have decreased risks for many illnesses, including heart disease, cancer, diabetes, and hypertension. Studies exploring the effects of supplemental forms of some phytochemicals do not consistently find the same health benefits. This is likely because many phytochemicals are necessary to be present in particular ratios to have their beneficial effects. Therefore, supplemental phytochemicals may not be providing the optimal kinds and mixes of phytochemicals—especially if your baseline diet is not high in phytochemicals. It is best to get these health-promoting compounds from eating a variety of vegetables and other plant-based foods.[1,2,3,4,5] For more information on phytochemicals, refer to Chapter 3.

Vegetables contain mostly insoluble fiber. This type of fiber helps increase the speed with which food travels through your gastrointestinal tract. Everybody has potential carcinogens in their digestive tracts that originate from the environment or digestion of food components (especially highly processed foods). Therefore, as fiber moves along your gastrointestinal tract, it drags potential carcinogens from the body more quickly than they would have been excreted without the fiber. As a result, the potential carcinogens have less time to cause damage. This type of fiber also prevents constipation and weakening of the lining of the gastrointestinal tract, which can lead to out-pockets known as diverticuli. This is important because diverticuli can become infected and cause abdominal pain and serious illness.

## The Green Inner Circle

The green inner subgroup of the Vegetable Group includes fresh, unprocessed, nonstarchy vegetables, as well as frozen nonstarchy vegetables without added sauces or flavorings. These foods are high in fiber , vitamins A and C, and folate, and they provide significant amounts of potassium and vitamin E. In addition, they supply major amounts of phytochemicals. Because vegetables are high in fiber and low in calories, they help you feel full. Add them to lunch as a salad, sliced on a sandwich, or as crunchy side dishes. Start your dinner meal with a salad or broth-based vegetable soup (watch the sodium if necessary), and then have 1 or 2 cups of a hot vegetable with your meal. Filling up on low-calorie vegetables makes it easier to cut back on portion sizes of higher-calorie starchy side dishes and protein foods. In addition, vegetables add color, flavor, and texture, making your meals more interesting. Take the opportunity and the challenge to move away from conditioned preferences for salt, sugar, and trans fats and move toward the interesting and diverse flavors that vegetables provide. Try flavoring your vegetables with different herbs and spices. See the sample menus in the Menus and Recipes section.

Frozen and fresh vegetables are both in the green inner circle, because they are generally comparable in nutritional quality. The nutrient content of vegetables is greatest at the time of harvest. Therefore, freshly picked vegetables have the highest vitamin content. Frozen vegetables are typically blanched and frozen shortly after harvest. The blanching and freezing process is associated with the loss of only a small amount of some vitamins, such as vitamin C, folate, and thiamin. Once frozen, the nutrient content is maintained if the vegetables are stored properly at 0 degrees Fahrenheit for 6 months or less. Similarly, the vitamin content of fresh vegetables decreases during transport and storage, and with home cooking. To retain the most vitamins, steam vegetables or microwave with just a little water. Minerals are much more stable, and only small amounts are lost with processing and cooking. For many people, frozen vegetables can be conveniently kept on hand, and may lead to less waste since just the amount needed can be removed and cooked.

Starchy vegetables are not unhealthy or especially fattening, they just provide many more calories and carbohydrates per swap. Therefore, they are more similar to foods in the Grain & Starch Group, and in their unprocessed form are placed in the green inner circle of that group.

## The Yellow Middle Circle

The yellow middle subgroup includes vegetable juices and sauces, as well as canned vegetables. The canning process leads to much greater vitamin losses than the freezing process. In addition, canned vegetables are typically high in sodium and may have added fats and sweeteners. Despite these issues, canned vegetable products are still good sources of many vitamins, minerals, and phytochemicals.

Vegetable juices and sauces are low in fiber and often have added sodium and sweeteners. Fats may be added to vegetable sauces, such as tomato sauce. When selecting such an item, compare different brands. Select the brands with no added trans fats and corn sweeteners, as well as those with the least amount of sugar and sodium.

## The Outer Red Circle

Deep-fried vegetables and vegetables in cream sauces are in the red subgroup, because of the excessive amount of total fat. These vegetables are often high in saturated or trans fats.

## Summary Recommendations for the Vegetable Group

Because vegetables have very few calories per swap but a lot of fiber, vitamins, minerals, and phytochemicals, you should include at least six swaps of a wide variety of whole, unprocessed vegetables in your diet each day. Vegetables also provide a feeling of fullness because of their fiber content. It is virtually impossible to eat too many whole vegetables, unless of course they are deep-fried. Depending on how many vegetables you are currently eating, it may take some time to learn how to include this many vegetables in your diet, but it is certainly a worthy goal. See Table 4-3 for a summary of important information regarding the Vegetable Group.

# Introduction—The Fruit Group

Biologically, fruits are defined as the fleshy reproductive part of a plant that holds the seeds. Technically, many foods generally considered to be vegetables are really fruits, such as tomatoes, cucumbers, zucchini, and

**Table 4-3.** Summary Information for the Vegetable Group

| Summary Nutrient Information for the Vegetable Group | |
|---|---|
| ◉ Calories per serving: 25 | ◉ Protein, grams per serving: 2 |
| ◉ Carbohydrate, grams per serving: 5 | ◉ Fat, grams per serving: 0 |
| **Serving Sizes for Selected Foods from the Vegetable Group** *(For more examples, refer to the Swap Lists beginning on page 263.)* | |
| ◉ ½ cup of most cooked or fresh vegetables | ◉ ⅓ cup of tomato sauce |
| ◉ 1 cup of raw fresh leafy greens | ◉ ½ cup cooked leafy greens |
| **Recommended Number of Swaps per Day** *(See Chapters 6, 7, and 8 for specific recommendations.)* | |
| ◉ 6 servings a day is highly recommended | ◉ 4 servings per day is the recommended minimum |

sweet peppers. Nutritionally, fruits and vegetables are differentiated by the relative amounts of carbohydrate, sugar, and calories per unit of weight. Vegetables are relatively low in carbohydrate, sugar, and calories compared to fruits. Therefore, tomatoes, cucumbers, zucchini, and sweet peppers, which are low in calories, are nutritionally classified as vegetables. The Fruit Group includes fruits that are high in carbohydrate with no significant fat or protein content. Although biologically considered fruits, olives and avocados are high in fat—albeit healthy monounsaturated fat. Therefore, these fruits are in the green inner circle of the Fat Group.

Similar to foods in the Vegetable Group, foods from the Fruit Group offer significant amounts of vitamins (such as vitamin A, vitamin C, and many B vitamins), minerals (potassium) and fiber, as well as phytochemicals. For example, oranges contain more than 170 phytochemicals, including flavinoids, limonoids, carotinoids, and polyphenols. These phytochemicals inhibit inflammation, tumor growth, and harmful oxidation processes. In addition, some of them stimulate enzymes in the liver responsible for detoxifying potential harmful compounds.

## The Green Inner Circle

All whole and dried fruits are in the green inner subgroup because they retain their natural nutrients and phytochemicals, as well as their fiber content. Their high water and fiber contents give whole fruits a high nutrient content with moderate calories. Therefore, they have a moderately high nutrient density—refer to Chapter 3 for more information on nutrient density. Plain dried fruits retain their nutrients and fiber, but the calories are more concentrated because most of the water has been removed. Therefore, the amount of food in a swap of dried fruits is smaller than whole fruits. Only plain dried fruits with no added sugars, sweeteners, or fats are in the green inner circle. Check ingredient lists on dried fruit packages carefully.

Most fruits are high in a type of fiber called water-soluble fiber, which helps lower serum cholesterol levels. The fiber in whole and dried fruits decreases the rate at which the sugars are digested and absorbed into your blood. This is important, because virtually all of the calories and carbohydrates in fruits are in the form of sugars. Without the fiber these sugars would have a greater impact on blood sugar levels. Some individuals are resistant to the action of insulin, a chemical regulator in your body that moves sugar from the blood into cells where it is needed. For these individuals, the decreased rate of absorption associated with fiber helps to maintain normal blood sugar levels. See Chapter 3 for more information on blood sugar responses to foods and insulin.

Although frozen fruits are less common than canned fruits, they are becoming increasingly available. Fruits frozen without any added sweeteners or fruit juice blends retain the majority of their nutrients, phytochemicals, and fiber, without additional unnecessary sugars and calories. Berry combinations and melon combinations are the most common.

## The Yellow Inner Circle

Fruit juices are in the yellow middle section because of their lower fiber content and concentrated sugar. Without the fiber imparting a feeling of fullness, it is far too easy to consume excessive calories from fruit juice. In addition, inadequate fiber intake is a common problem that negatively impacts on intestinal health and indirectly overall health and well-being. Therefore, it is much better to consume whole fruits as opposed to fruit juices.

Many fruit juice blends have added stripped juice. *Stripped juice* is simply the sugar and water originally in the juice, devoid of its nutrients and phytochemicals. In other words, it is really sugar-water. By blending stripped juice with real fruit juice, the sugar and calories are more concentrated and the nutrients diluted. One of the reasons manufacturers use this source of sugar is because the final product can be labeled "100% fruit juice"—even though the stripped juice retains none of the vitamins, minerals, or phytochemicals originally in the fruit. In addition, the stripped juices do not change the color or flavor of the product being sweetened. It is hard to be sure if a fruit juice named on an ingredient list has been stripped of its nutrients or not. However, the following fruit juice ingredients are often stripped: pear, apple, grape, white grape, or pineapple juices. Fruit juice blends with stripped juices are especially high in calories and sugar, and lower in nutritional quality. So don't be fooled into thinking that fruit juice is healthy. Read the nutrition information on food labels of juices carefully, and notice how much sugar is in the fruit juice.

Canned fruits are also often packed with stripped juices. In addition, canned fruits lose some of their vitamins because of the high heat necessary during the canning process. Despite this, canned fruits packed in water or juice can be a source of nutrients, and due to their convenience can help achieve an adequate intake of fruit.

## The Red Outer Circle

Fruit drinks and other fruit-based products with added sugars are in the red outer subgroup. Examples include fruits packed in heavy syrup, sweetened or colored apple sauces, sweetened dried fruits, and fruit drinks. These products typically provide fewer nutrients per calorie. They may, however, be high in a few nutrients, such as vitamin C, due to fortification. Fruit products with significant added sweeteners do not promote good health, despite high levels of a few specific nutrients due to fortification.

## Summary Recommendations for the Fruit Group

Two to four fruit swaps per day are generally recommended. Very tall people or very active people with high calorie needs may be able to include six or more fruits and still maintain a healthy weight. Ideally, all of these fruits would be whole or plain dried fruits, because these products are highest in nutrients without added sugars. Whole and dried fruits also contribute significant amounts of fiber, unlike fruit juices. Fruit juice intake may easily become problematic, because it provides a lot of calories without creating a sense of fullness. In addition, its sweet taste and generally perceived healthfulness makes overconsumption all too easy. Competitive athletes with very high calorie needs may find that fruit juice can help them meet their calorie needs and prevent unwanted weight loss. See Table 4-4 for a summary of important information regarding the Fruit Group.

**Table 4-4.** Summary Information for the Fruit Group

| Summary Nutrient Information for the Fruit Group | |
|---|---|
| ◉ Calorie content per serving: 60* | ◉ Protein, grams per serving: 0 |
| ◉ Carbohydrate, grams per serving: 15 | ◉ Fat, grams per serving: 0 |
| **Serving Sizes for Selected Foods from the Fruit Group** <br> *(For more examples, refer to the Swap Lists beginning on page 263.)* | |
| ◉ 1 small to medium piece of fruit | ◉ ½ banana |
| ◉ ½ cup cut up fruit salad | ◉ 2 tablespoons dried fruit |
| ◉ ½ cup of real fruit juice | ◉ 10 grapes |
| **Recommended Number of Swaps per Day** <br> *(See Chapters 6, 7, and 8 for specific recommendations.)* | |
| ◉ 2 to 4 servings for most individuals (preferably whole fruits) | ◉ 6 or more servings for very active adults or adolescents, such as competitive athletes |
| * Fruits vary considerably in their caloric density. Therefore each fruit has a specific serving size that contains about 60 Calories. | |

## Introduction—The Grain & Starch Group

Grains, starches, and sugars are part of the same group because they are made up of the same building blocks—a single, one-sugar unit building block. Sugars are made of only one or two of these building blocks. Starches are long chains of these building blocks. Grains are a common source of starch, as are legumes (dried peas and beans), winter squashes (acorn, butternut, and spaghetti squash), and starchy vegetables (pota-toes, corn, and peas). Foods in the Grain & Starch Group derive most of their calories from carbohydrates, with just a small amount of protein and an even smaller amount of fat. Depending on the subgroup, the carbohy-drates may be mostly starch, sugar, or fiber. The types of fats added to most breads, crackers, and bakery products are typically unhealthy trans fats. However, there are increasingly more brands of these products available that use liquid oils that have not been hydrogenated. Refer to Chapter 3 for detailed discussions of the quality of carbohydrates and fats.

Unprocessed sources of starch, such as whole grains, starchy vegeta-bles, winter squashes, and beans, are good sources of many vitamins and minerals, as well as fiber. They also do not have the added trans fats. However, processed versions of these products lose many of their nutrients and only some are added back during manufacturing. Therefore, some micronutrients are difficult to get in adequate amounts if you are eating mostly processed or refined sources of starch, such as white bread, white rice, and regular pasta. In addition, processed starches are usually low in fiber, and the resulting carbohydrates are quickly and easily digested. Therefore, these low-fiber starches have a high glycemic index and result in greater blood sugar and insulin responses than higher fiber starches. Again, refer to Chapter 3 for a detailed explanation of blood sugar respons-es to food and the significance of such responses.

## The Green Inner Circle

Foods in the green inner subgroup are the least processed, most nutrient dense, and highest in fiber. They tend to have low glycemic indices. This subgroup includes whole-grain breads and cereals. These types of breads will have a "whole" grain, such as "whole wheat" listed as the first ingredi-ent, and will have at least 3 grams of fiber per serving size as defined on the food label. Do not be fooled by breads and grain products listed as multigrain, which are actually made of mostly refined flours that get their brown color from molasses. Some may also have gums or other ingredi-ents added for fiber, but do not have whole grains and the micronutrients that come with them. You may need to read the labels of breads and cereals available in your supermarket carefully at first to identify those that are whole grain. Once you spend the time to identify them, you will be able to quickly select them on your subsequent shopping trips. Whole-grain breads typically have about 80 to 100 calories per slice, and one slice is considered a swap. Light or low-calorie whole-grain breads have only 40 calories per slice, and therefore two slices are considered one swap.

There are a rich variety of whole grains that you can buy and cook at home, or buy in the form of breads and cereals. Wheat-based whole grains include bulgur and whole couscous. Gluten is the protein found in these grains. Other whole grains that contain the protein gluten include kamut, whole or Scotch barley, spelt, whole rye, and triticale (a hybrid of wheat and rye grain). Some people have an intolerance to gluten and need to avoid grains that contain gluten. Oats may be problematic for some people with gluten intolerance. Grains that do not have gluten include amaranth and teff. Brown rice can also be used to make cereals and flours that are used to make gluten-free breads, crackers, and pastas. Other types of products that are used as grains but are not technically grains and do not contain gluten include buckwheat and quinoa. See the menus in Menus and Recipes for interesting ways to include these grains in your diet.

People who have a gluten intolerance or celiac disease need to eat grains or grain-like products that do not include the protein gluten. For these people, gluten damages their intestines and can cause intestinal disorders. There is also a growing body of controversial scientific literature that links gluten intolerance to systemic disorders such as eczema, psoriasis, infertility, thyroid diseases, and rheumatoid arthritis. Therefore, it is important to avoid wheat- and gluten-containing products (wheat, rye, oats, kamut, barley, spelt, triticale) if you have such an intolerance.

In addition to grain and grain-like products, starchy vegetables (such as potatoes, sweet potatoes, peas, corn, jicama, yucca, and cassava), winter squashes (such as acorn squash, butternut squash, spaghetti squash, and pumpkin), and legumes (kidney beans, navy beans, garbanzo beans, white beans, pinto beans, dried peas, and lentils) are found in this subgroup of the Grain & Starch group. They provide a moderate amount of carbohydrates, some protein, and almost no fat.

In addition to being high in B vitamins, the foods in this subgroup are a significant source of vitamin E, fiber, a wide variety of minerals (such as chromium, selenium, magnesium, and zinc), and phytochemicals (flavinoids, lignins, phenols, phytoestrogens, and saponins). See Chapter 3 for detailed information on these nutrients.

## The Yellow Middle Circle

Foods in the yellow middle subgroup are more processed and refined versions of those foods found in the green inner circle of the Grain & Starch Group, such as refined-flour breads, rolls, cereals, white pasta, white rice, pearl barley, bagels, and most crackers. These foods provide similar amounts of calories, carbohydrates, and proteins per swap as those in the inner circle. These foods do provide many nutrients, especially B vitamins and iron, that are required to be added during processing. However, they are lower in fiber, many trace minerals, and phytochemicals in comparison to foods in the green inner circle. In addition, they tend to have some added sodium, and, although generally low in fat, the fat they do have tends to be trans fats. They also tend to cause a higher blood sugar response than foods in the green inner circle.

## The Red Outer Circle

Foods in the red outer subgroup are low in nutrients relative to the high amount of calories they provide. In addition, they are low in fiber and have added sodium, sugar, and/or saturated or hydrogenated fats. This subgroup is divided into three sections: sugary starches, sugary-fatty starches, and fatty starches.

The sugary starches include foods that get most of their calories from simple carbohydrates and sugars and have very little fat. Examples include heavily sweetened cereals, soda, jelly, jam, syrup, hard candy, frozen yogurt, sherbet, fat-free cake and muffins, and fat-free cookies. These foods tend to have a high glycemic index. A typical portion of these foods may be equal to one or two swaps from the Grain & Starch Group.

The foods in the sugary-fatty starches section of this subgroup include regular cakes, cookies, chocolate, and candies. These foods are high in sugar and hydrogenated or saturated fats. In addition to counting as one or two swaps from the Grain & Starch Group, these foods may also count as one or two swaps from the Fat Group.

Lastly, the fatty-starches section includes foods that have starch rather than sugar and contain saturated or hydrogenated fats, such as biscuits, French fries, and snack chips. See Chapter 3 for a full description of the types of fats and the effects they have on your health. These foods also count as a combination of swaps from the Grain & Starch Group, as well as from the Fat Group.

Highly processed foods that are high in complex carbohydrates but low in fiber and fat, such as chips made with fat substitutes, are also in the red section of this group. They would be counted as just grain and starch swaps, but not fat swaps. They are not nutrient dense, and should not displace foods in the green and yellow subgroups.

## Summary Recommendations for the Grain & Starch Group

Three to twelve swaps of foods in the Grain & Starch Group are recommended for most people each day. This is a big range, because the number of swaps will vary widely depending on whether you are following a lower-carb, moderate-carb, or high-carb eating style. (Refer to Chapters 5, 6, 7, and 8 for a full description of each of these eating styles.) Your daily calorie level will also partially determine the number of swaps you have a day from this group. (Refer to Chapter 5 to pick a daily calorie level.) In order to meet your fiber needs and maximize your vitamin, mineral, and phytochemical intake for optimal health and well-being during weight loss, it is important to select as wide a variety of foods from the green inner subgroup as possible. It will most likely take a fair amount of time to learn how to identify these foods, and cook these foods according to your taste preferences. Adolescents and athletes may require about 20 swaps per day to provide enough energy and carbohydrates for growth, training, and competition. See Table 4-5 for a summary of important information regarding the Grain & Starch Group.

**Table 4-5.** Summary Information for the Grains & Starch Group

| Summary Nutrient Information for the Grains & Starch Group | |
|---|---|
| ◉ Calorie content per serving: 80 | ◉ Protein, grams per serving: 3 |
| ◉ Carbohydrate, grams per serving: 15 | ◉ Fat, grams per serving: 1 |
| **Serving Sizes for Selected Foods from the Grain & Starch Group** *(For more examples, refer to the Swap Lists beginning on page 263.)* | |
| ◉ 1 ounce of cold cereal | ◉ ½ cup of cooked grains, pasta, mashed potato |
| ◉ 1 very small (3 ounce) potato | ◉ ⅓ cup brown rice |
| ◉ ⅓ cup of starchy vegetables | ◉ 1 slice of bread or 4-6 crackers |
| **Recommended Number of Swaps per Day** *(See Chapters 6, 7, and 8 for specific recommendations.)* | |
| ◉ 3 to 12 servings for most individuals | ◉ About 20 servings per day for very active adults or adolescent athletes |

# Introduction—The Protein Group

The structure of the Protein Group emphasizes vegetarian protein sources and fish. This is because most Americans need to make a conscious effort to increase their fiber intake (found in vegetarian protein foods) and omega-3 polyunsaturated fatty acids (found predominantly in fish). You can, however, certainly include lean animal sources of protein from the yellow inner circle in the context of a healthy diet. Plant-based and animal-based high-protein foods provide different sets of nutrients. The main categories of high-protein foods and the nutrients they contain are as follows:

- Beans provide boron, iron, manganese, molybdenum, potassium, and folic acid.

- Eggs provide phosphorus, selenium, pantothenic acid, biotin, niacin, riboflavin, thiamin, vitamin A, vitamin $B_6$, and vitamin D.

- Fish provide chromium, copper, magnesium, phosphorus, potassium, selenium, zinc, niacin, vitamin A, vitamin $B_{12}$, and vitamin D.

- Poultry provides chromium, iron, phosphorus, potassium, niacin, pantothenic acid, vitamin $B_{12}$, and vitamin $B_6$.

- Meat provides chromium, iron, magnesium, phosphorus, potassium, selenium, zinc, niacin, pantothenic acid, thiamin, vitamin $B_{12}$, and vitamin $B_6$.

- Nuts provide boron, copper, iron, magnesium, manganese, molybdenum, potassium, vitamin E, and vitamin $B_6$.

- Cheese provides calcium, magnesium, phosphorus, zinc, riboflavin, thiamin, vitamin A and vitamin $B_{12}$.

- Soy-based products provide calcium (if calcium set), copper, iron, magnesium, phosphorus, zinc, folate, thiamin, vitamin $B_6$, vitamin C, and vitamin E.

There is a large body of research literature that supports the health-promoting effects of a vegetarian or predominantly plant-based diet, especially in combination with exercise and stress-reducing practices. Such a diet maximizes nutrient and phytochemical intake. However, you can certainly have a healthy diet if you select a variety of protein foods from the green inner circle and the yellow middle circle. The foods in the Bull's-Eye Food Guide are simply categorized in such a way as to encourage you to consider consuming vegetarian proteins and fish on a regular basis.

## The Green Inner Circle

The green inner subgroup of the Protein Group reflects the value of a plant-based, vegetarian-style diet. It also supports the beneficial role of omega-3 fatty acids. Although shown without division in the Bull's-Eye Food Guide graphic, there are five sections within the green inner subgroup: vegetable protein foods, egg whites or egg substitutes, fish, vegetable-starchy proteins, and vegetable-fatty protein. Most of the nonstarchy vegetable proteins are soy-based, such as tofu, soy patties, and textured soy protein (also called soy crumble). There is a growing body of literature that suggests that isoflavones in soy-based products protect against heart disease and possibly cancer. In addition, they are thought to reduce menopausal symptoms. Soybeans naturally provide a mix of high-quality proteins, healthy fats, and some carbohydrate. The carbohydrate content of soy-based meat substitute products varies, and those with around 10 to 15 grams of carbohydrate are counted as a Protein Group swap and a Grain & Starch Group swap. The vegetable-starchy proteins also require a Grain & Starch Group swap (i.e., ⅔ cup of cooked kidney beans counts as a Protein Group swap and a Grain & Starch Group swap). Legumes that are in this section (beans, lentils, and split peas) are also listed in the green subgroup of the Grain & Starch Group. One-third of a cup of beans has enough carbohydrates and calories to count as a Grain & Starch Group swap, but not enough protein to count as a swap from the Protein Group. In a ⅔ cup portion enough protein accumulates to count this amount as a Protein Group swap as well as a Grain & Starch Group swap.

Two animal-based protein sections are the egg whites section and the fish section. These foods are low in carbohydrate and high in protein with varying amounts of fat. Egg whites have virtually no fat and an extremely high-quality protein. Fish has omega-3 polyunsaturated fats, which can decrease blood stickiness (known as platelet aggregation) and inflammatory processes. Shellfish is very low in all fats, but some are high in dietary cholesterol. Although dietary cholesterol can have a negative effect on your blood cholesterol levels, it is really the saturated fat in your diet that increases your blood cholesterol the most. The potential effect is largely dependent on your genetic predisposition. Shellfish has almost no saturated fat.

Therefore, if you have high blood cholesterol, you can still have shellfish, but consider limiting it to about one meal per week—especially shrimp or crawfish. Some fish have higher mercury levels than other fish, and these fish (shark, swordfish, tilefish, golden bass, golden snapper, or king mackerel) should not be eaten on a regular basis.

The natural nut butters, such as natural peanut butter, comprise another section of the green subgroup of the Protein Group. They are high in protein and are a good source of monounsaturated fat, therefore they count as a swap from the Protein Group and a swap from the Fat Group.

### The Yellow Middle Circle

The middle yellow subgroup includes the lean animal sources of protein, such as white meat chicken, lean meats, and low-fat or fat-free cheeses. Cheeses are included in the Protein Group, rather than the Milk & Yogurt Group because cheese has protein and fat but virtually no carbohydrates, which is similar to other foods in the Protein Group. Foods in the Milk & Yogurt Group are very different in that they contain a lot of carbohydrate.

Eggs are also in the yellow middle circle, because their total fat content is similar to lean red meats. Similarly to shellfish, eggs have a lot of dietary cholesterol but not too much saturated fat. The fat and cholesterol is found in the yellow egg yolk and not in the white part of the egg, which is the source of the protein. If you have high blood cholesterol, you should consider limiting your intake of egg yolks to 3 eggs per week. Egg whites do not have to be limited at all.

On average, 35% of the calories provided by foods in the yellow middle circle subgroup are derived from fat, and much of this fat is saturated. White-meat poultry products without skin provide less than the average, with about 20% of calories derived from fat. Red meats, even many lean cuts, provide more than the average, with about 45% of calories derived from fat. When purchasing meat and poultry products, the information regarding the percentage of fat on the label can be confusing. This is because the packaging of fresh meat, poultry, and fish is not required to have nutrition information presented in the same format as "Nutrition Facts" labels on most other foods. Meat, such as ground beef, typically depicts the percentage of fat on the front of the package. This percentage reflects the percentage of fat in the product by weight, not by calories. This can be deceiving, because fat by weight is much lower than fat calculated by calories. See Table 4-6 for a comparison of percentages of fat calculated by percent weight and percent calories.

Percentages of fat in foods differ depending on whether you calculate by weight or by calories because water in the products adds weight but not calories. For example, in your mind, picture a glass of water on a scale. The water in the glass would weigh a fair amount, 237 grams, but have 0

**Table 4-6.** Percent of Calories and Weight Derived from Fat

| Food | Weight of Serving Size | Calories per Serving | Fat, Grams per Serving | Fat, by Weight | Fat, by Calories |
|------|------------------------|----------------------|------------------------|----------------|------------------|
| Ground beef, 80% lean | 3 ounces or 85 grams | 216 | 14 | 17% | 58% |
| Ground beef, 90% lean | 3 ounces or 85 grams | 182 | 9 | 11% | 45% |
| Ground turkey (may not always be lean) | 3 ounces or 85 grams | 193 | 11 | 13% | 51% |
| Turkey breast, no skin | 3 ounces 87 grams | 117 | 1 | 8% | 8% |
| Cheese | 3 ounces 84 grams | 342 | 27 | 32% | 71% |

calories and 0 grams of fat. (Remember as a frame of reference that a paperclip weighs 1 gram.) Now imagine that you pour in a tablespoon of oil, which is 100% fat. The weight indicated on the scale barely goes up—only 14 grams. Now the total weight of water and oil is 251 grams. The oil, therefore, accounts for only 6% of the total weight, and the water accounts for 94% of the weight. However, the 14 grams of fat also contributes 119 calories, which represents 100% of the calories in the glass of water. If the water and oil was packaged and labeled similarly to meat, the label would read "94% lean," which implies only 6% fat. However, this refers to percentage of fat by weight (or in other words the percentage of the total weight derived from the weight of the fat). If labeled as most other food products, there would be 119 total calories and 119 calories from fat, indicating 100% of total calories derived from fat. So as a rule of thumb, you should buy meat that is at least 90% lean, and therefore 10% fat by weight or less. Even ground beef that is labeled 90% lean has 45% of calories derived from fat. If not labeled 90% or 92% lean, ground turkey can have more calories derived from fat than very lean ground beef, with 51% of the calories in the turkey from fat. Turkey breast, white meat with no skin, is very lean with only 8% of weight and calories derived from fat. Ground turkey breast would also be lean, but other types of ground turkey have dark meat or high-fat skin ground into the mixture. Just for comparison, whole cheese is very high in calories and fat. In fact, cheddar cheese has 71% of its calories derived from fat. Leaner cuts of meat and turkey are certainly more expensive, however it is very important to buy these lower-fat versions—so look for these products on sale and cut back on portion sizes.

## The Red Outer Circle

The outer red subgroup includes three sections of higher-fat protein foods. Generally, these foods have an incredible 70% to 80% of their calories derived from fat. The fat in these foods is primarily unhealthy saturated or hydrogenated fats. Processed or hydrogenated nut butters also have added sugar and are in this outer subgroup as well. In addition to counting as a swap from the Protein Group, the foods in the red subgroup count as additional swaps from the Fat Group. To maintain an appropriate fat intake for the day, clients who choose to eat small to moderate amounts of these foods should save fat swaps to accommodate these foods. It is difficult to include many foods from this subgroup on a regular basis in a healthy diet. Foods in the outer subgroup are usually high in sodium and cholesterol as well as in saturated fats.

### Summary Recommendations for the Protein Group

Three to fifteen swaps of foods from the Protein Group are recommended for most people each day, although very tall people or athletes may need even more. This is a huge range, because the number of swaps will vary widely depending on if you are following a lower-carb, moderate-carb, or high-carb eating style. (Refer to Chapters 5, 6, 7, and 8 for a full description of each of these eating styles.) In addition, if you choose to follow a vegetarian-style diet, you will most likely follow a higher-carbohydrate and relatively lower-protein eating style, unless you supplement your food sources of protein with powder protein supplements. See Table 4-7 for a summary of important information regarding the Protein Group.

## Introduction—The Fat Group

The **Fat Group** includes foods that have insignificant amounts of protein and carbohydrate, and virtually all of their calories derived from fat. Depending on your selected eating style (refer to Chapter 5), the amount of fat in your diet will vary from 20% of your total calories up to around 35% of your total calories. As in other food groups, one swap from the inner circle provides the same amount of calories as one swap from the middle and outer circles. However, the nutritional quality of foods in the green inner circle is far superior to foods in the red outer circle. If you have a genetic predisposition for heart disease, the intake of fats in the red outer circle

**Table 4-7.** Summary Information for the Protein Group

| **Summary Nutrient Information for the Protein Group** | |
| --- | --- |
| ◉ Calorie content per serving: 55 | ◉ Protein, grams per serving: 7 |
| ◉ Carbohydrate, grams per serving: 0 | ◉ Fat, grams per serving: 3 |

**Serving Sizes for Selected Foods from the Protein Group**
*(For more examples, refer to the Swap Lists beginning on page 263.)*

| | |
| --- | --- |
| ◉ 3 ounces of tofu | ◉ ⅔ cup cooked beans (count as one Grain & Starch swap + 1 Protein swap) |
| ◉ 3 egg whites | ◉ 1 egg |
| ◉ 1 ounce chicken, fatty fish or lean meat* | ◉ 1 ounce cheese* |

**Recommended Number of Swaps per Day**
*(See Chapters 6, 7, and 8 for specific recommendations.)*

| | |
| --- | --- |
| ◉ 3 to 15 servings for most individuals | ◉ More for competitive athletes with high Calorie needs |

* Note: Depending on the fat content of selected cut or type, an additional ½ to 2 fat swaps may be required for each protein swap.

are likely to increase your risk for developing heart disease. When such fats are replaced with fats in the green inner circle, risks for heart disease, such as high LDL blood cholesterol levels, are decreased. See Chapter 3 for more details on this topic.

Including high-quality fats in your diet can add a lot of flavor. In addition, because fats take longer than carbohydrates and proteins to digest and pass through your digestive tract they help you to feel fuller longer. This may help you avoid unnecessary snacking. Healthy sources of fat also provide a lot of micronutrients, such as copper, magnesium, phosphorus, zinc, folate, niacin, vitamin $B_6$, and vitamin E.

## Green Inner Circle

Fats in the green section are primarily comprised of monounsaturated fatty acids or omega-3 polyunsaturated fatty acids. Monounsaturated fatty acids are a preferred source of fat, because when they replace saturated fats, they can actually decrease risk for heart disease. Monounsaturated fats can be added to the diet in an amount providing 20% of total calories without negative consequences. Using monounsaturated fats can help reduce carbohydrate intake for individuals deemed to be insulin resistant, such as those with type 2 diabetes or high triglycerides.

There are different types of polyunsaturated fatty acids. Two polyunsaturated fatty acids are necessary for good health but cannot be made by your body. Therefore, it is necessary to get them from your diet. These fatty acids are called linoleic acid (an omega-6 polyunsaturated fatty acid) and alpha-linolenic acid (an omega-3 polyunsaturated fatty acid). The required amounts of these fats are easily obtained by eating a variety of foods from the green inner subgroup. Three to six grams of linoleic acid meet the requirements of most adults. The necessary amount of alpha-linolenic acid has not yet been quantified.

Omega-3 polyunsaturated fatty acids are important for optimal health because they can reduce blood triglyceride levels, blood stickiness (platelet aggregation), and inflammatory processes. This is important because these three factors increase the risk of heart disease—the number one cause of death among American adults. Omega-3 polyunsaturated fats exert their maximal beneficial effects when they are found in the appropriate ratio with omega-6 polyunsaturated fats in your diet (estimates of the appropriate ratio range from 1 omega-3 to 4–10 omega-6s). It is not possible to try to calculate your dietary intake to this degree. Rather, you need to maximize your intake of foods known to be high in omega-3s while you decrease your intake of foods that provide a lot of omega-6s with not much omega-3s. Foods are arranged in the Bull's-Eye Food Guide to help you do this, because foods high in omega-3s are preferentially placed in the green inner circle. Foods high in omega-6 polyunsaturated fats are high in oils in the yellow subgroup and margarine in the red outer circle. Refer to Chapter 3 for a detailed discussion of fats.

Extracting oil from the plant is the first step in processing. The healthiest oils are extracted without chemical solvents. Cold pressing methods are the healthiest. This process simply involves mechanical extraction without heat, typically using hydraulic presses, and subsequent filtering. Virgin olive oil is prepared in this way. Expeller pressing is the next preferred process. Expeller presses use friction and pressure from a screw-type machine to squeeze oil out of seeds. The friction involved in this process produces some heat. Cold and expeller pressing methods do not extract all of the oil from the plant products. Therefore, these methods are not considered as efficient as solvent extraction, which is the cheapest, most efficient extraction method. During this method, the plant product (seed, nut, fruit) is ground first, and then washed with a solvent. The resulting product is subject to several additional treatments to remove the solvent, as well as to bleach, degum, and deodorize the product. These processing techniques remove nutrients, as well as flavor and color. Processing also increases the smoke point, meaning that the oil can be used in high-heat cooking methods, such as frying. All unrefined oils can become rancid over time, and this process is hastened with exposure to heat, light, and oxygen. Therefore, they should be stored in dark containers and in a cool place. Oil will also last longer if stored in the refrigerator. In summary, look for the following terms when selecting oils: cold pressed, mechanically extracted, or expeller pressed. Olive, canola, peanut, soybean, walnut, and flaxseed oils have health-promoting properties.

Healthy oils, nuts, seeds, olives, and avocados can be added when cooking to provide a lot of flavor to your meals. You can also find mixtures of olives and grilled vegetables in olive oil. Such mixtures can be spread onto tofu, chicken, fish, and lean meats to provide a lot of flavor to meals very quickly. Bruschetta—a mixture of olive oil, onion, olives, and tomatoes—is one rather common example of this type of mixture.

You may recall that natural peanut butter was listed in the inner circle of the Protein Group because in a peanut there is some protein, as well as fat. In this case 4 teaspoons of natural peanut butter is considered a Protein Group swap and a Fat Group swap. In a small amount of natural peanut butter, however, there is not enough protein to be counted as a Protein Group swap. Therefore, only 2 teaspoons of natural peanut butter is considered only a Fat Group swap.

## The Yellow Middle Circle

Fats in the yellow subgroup include oils with a high omega-6 polyunsaturated fatty acid content and a low omega-3 fatty acid content: corn, sunflower, safflower, and cottonseed oils. These oils have a better effect on blood cholesterol levels than saturated fats. However, because the goal is to increase the relative amount of omega-3 polyunsaturated fats in your diet relative to omega-6 polyunsaturated fats, it is helpful to decrease your intake of these oils. Therefore, use oils in the green inner subgroup, such as olive oil and cold-pressed or mechanically extracted canola oil, instead of vegetable oils in the yellow middle subgroup.

## The Red Outer Circle

Fatty foods in the red subgroup derive the majority of their calories from saturated fats or hydrogenated fats. In general, fats from animal products are high in saturated fats. High intakes of animal fats have been associated with an increased risk of some types of cancer. Hydrogenated fats, also known as trans fats, result from a manufacturing process in which hydrogen is added to the carbon chains of liquid oils to make them semisolid at room temperature. For example, liquid corn oil becomes semisolid margarine at room temperature. Trans fats have a more negative effect on blood cholesterol levels than saturated fats.

Both margarine and butter are found in the outer circle. However, because margarine is high in trans fats, butter is actually a somewhat better choice of bread spread. A variety of new bread spreads are being introduced that are based on a blend of nonhydrogenated vegetable oils. Such products are better choices than regular margarines.

Regular peanut butter—that is, peanut butter that is not labeled natural—is considered an outer circle fat. In this type of peanut butter the naturally occurring liquid peanut oil is hydrogenated and sweeteners are added. Therefore, this type of peanut butter is not considered healthy.

### Summary Recommendations for the Fat Group

Two to nine swaps from the Fat Group are recommended per day. With the higher number of fat swaps, however, it becomes increasingly important that the majority of swaps are selected from the green subgroup. Using the allotted number of fat swaps suggested each day is recommended. In other words, do not skip your fat swaps—the recommended amount of fat serves a purpose to promote optimal weight loss and health. See Table 4-8 for a summary of important information regarding the Fat Group.

## Introduction—The Milk & Yogurt Group

The Milk & Yogurt Group includes milk products that have substantial amounts of carbohydrate and protein, namely fluid milk and yogurt. Cheeses are located in the protein group, because they are high in protein and fat and have virtually no carbohydrate. This distinction allows you to plan diets that control for carbohydrate, as well as protein and calories. Milk and yogurt also provide the following micronutrients: calcium, magnesium, phosphorus, zinc, riboflavin, vitamin A, vitamin $B_{12}$, and vitamin D.

### The Green Inner Circle

The green inner subgroup includes nonfat milk products, as well as low-fat, low-sugar soy milk (less than 2.5 grams of fat and less than 12 grams of sugar). Some fat in soymilk is permitted because it is primarily essential

**Table 4-8.** Summary Information for the Fat Group

| **Summary Nutrient Information for the Fat Group** | |
| --- | --- |
| ◉ Calorie content per serving: 45 | ◉ Protein, grams per serving: 0 |
| ◉ Carbohydrate, grams per serving: 0 | ◉ Fat, grams per serving: 5 |

**Serving Sizes for Selected Foods from the Fat Group**
*(For more examples, refer to the Swap Lists beginning on page 263.)*

| | |
| --- | --- |
| ◉ 1 teaspoon oil | ◉ 2 teaspoons peanut butter |
| ◉ 10 peanuts | ◉ 6 almonds |
| ◉ 2 teaspoons salad dressing | ◉ 10 small green olives |
| ◉ 1 teaspoon butter | ◉ 1 tablespoon pumpkin seeds |
| ◉ ⅛ avocado | ◉ 1 teaspoon mayonnaise |

**Recommended Number of Swaps per Day***
*(See Chapters 6, 7, and 8 for specific recommendations.)*

◉ 2 to 9 servings for most individuals

* Remember: Foods in the Milk & Yogurt Group, Protein Group, and Grain & Starch Group may include fat swaps that need to be counted when planning total fat swaps for the day.

polyunsaturated fat with minimal saturated fat. When selecting soymilk, check to make sure that is fortified with calcium, riboflavin, vitamin A, and vitamin D. Although the absorption of calcium from soymilk is about 25% lower than the calcium absorption from cow's milk, it can still be a significant source of this mineral.

For those readers who choose to use aspartame, nonfat yogurts sweetened with aspartame are in this group as well. This is an effort to increase choices in this subgroup. However, it is highly recommended that over time you reduce your use of artificial sweeteners. This is partially because they perpetuate the desire for a sweet taste in all foods—not just dessert-type foods.

### The Yellow Inner Circle

One percent or low-fat milk, low-fat plain yogurt, and moderate-fat, moderate-sugar soymilk (less than 3 grams of fat and 18 grams of sugar) are in the yellow middle subgroup.

### The Red Outer Circle

Two percent and whole-fat milk are high in total fat and saturated fat, and are included in the red outer subgroup. Highly sweetened cow's milk and soymilk (greater than 20 grams of sugar) are in the red outer circle. Manufacturers and trade groups spend a lot of money on promotional campaigns to convince consumers and policy makers that these highly sweetened milk products are healthy, because of the calcium they provide. However, from a holistic perspective, the benefits of the calcium they provide are far outweighed by the negative effects of the sugar and calories they also provide. The net health effect is a negative one for those struggling to lose weight or maintain a healthy weight. Low-fat fruit-flavored yogurts sweetened with sugars or fruit juices are also in the red outer subgroup due to their high sugar content.

### Summary of Recommendations for the Milk & Yogurt Group

Two swaps per day from the Milk & Yogurt Group are recommended for adults, and three to four swaps are recommended for children and pregnant women. For those who choose not to include cow's milk in their diet, calcium, riboflavin, vitamin A, and vitamin D fortified soymilk is recommended as an appropriate substitute. See Table 4-9 for a summary of important information regarding the Milk & Yogurt Group.

**Table 4-9.** Summary Information for the Milk & Yogurt Group

| Summary Nutrient Information for the Milk & Yogurt Group | |
| --- | --- |
| ⦿ Calorie content per serving: 90 | ⦿ Protein, grams per serving: 8 |
| ⦿ Carbohydrate, grams per serving: 12 | ⦿ Fat, grams per serving: 0 |

**Serving Sizes for Selected Foods from the Milk & Yogurt Group**
*(For more examples, refer to the Swap Lists beginning on page 263.)*

⦿ 1, 8-ounce cup of low-fat milk*        ⦿ 1, 8-ounce cup of plain soy milk

⦿ 1, 8-ounce cup of plain low-fat yogurt*

**Recommended Number of Swaps per Day**
*(See Chapters 6, 7, and 8 for specific recommendations.)*

⦿ 2 servings for adults        ⦿ 3 to 4 servings for pregnant
                                women, and for children

* Note: Depending on the flavoring, amount of added sugar, and amount of fat, additional swaps from the Grain & Starch Group, Fruit Group, and Fat Group may be needed.

# Using Food Labels to Count Swaps

You probably eat some foods that you will not be able to find on the Swap Lists. In addition, some foods do not fit easily into one of the six major food groups. Some of these foods are listed on the page of swaps called Combo Foods. These foods count as one or more swaps from various food groups. Refer to the Swap Lists for this list.

As you are just starting your Bull's-Eye program, you may feel more comfortable selecting foods that you could find on the swap lists. Over time though, you may want to include foods that aren't on the swap lists. Therefore, it is helpful to be able to look at the Nutrition Facts section of a food label, and be able to estimate how to count a portion of the food in terms of swaps in the Bull's-Eye Food Guide system.

To determine the swaps for a new food, review the ingredient list and determine the food groups to which the primary ingredients belong. The primary ingredients are considered the first 10 ingredients or so. Keep in mind that the foods listed first in the ingredient list are present in greater amounts. Refer to the example in Table 4-10. In this example, the primary ingredients are summarized as follows: a variety of vegetables, grains (oats, wheat gluten, bulgur, brown rice), cheese, soy protein, and walnuts. Next, look at the number of calories, grams of carbohydrate, grams of protein, and grams of total fat in the amount of food defined on the label as a serving size. These numbers are circled in Table 4-10. A quick review of Table 4-1 indicates that 15 grams of carbohydrate is about equal to a swap from either the Grain & Starch Group, the Fruit Group, or the Milk & Yogurt Group. Three servings of vegetables would also equal 15 grams of carbohydrate. In addition, 7 grams of protein is needed for a swap from the Protein Group, and 5 grams of fat is equal to a swap from the Fat Group. Compare these numbers to the numbers circled on the food label in Figure 4-2: carbohydrate (15 compared to 20), protein (7 compared to 10), and fat (5 compared to 5). A rough estimate of swaps would be as follows: one Vegetable Group swap; one Grain & Starch Group swap; and one Protein Group swap. You may be wondering about the need for a Fat Group swap. Table 4-1 indicates that one swap from the Protein Group includes 3 grams of fat and one swap from the Grain & Starch Group includes 1 gram of fat. Therefore, in this example 4 of the 5 grams of fat shown on the label are accounted for by the Protein Group and Grain & Starch Group swaps. An additional Fat Group swap is not needed. To check your estimate add up the calories that would come from the swaps using the number of calories shown in Table 4-1: 25 calories (Vegetable Group swap) + 80 calories (Grain

& Starch Group swap) + 55 calories (Protein swap) = 160 calories. Then compare this number of calories to the calories shown on the food label, which in this example is also 160 calories. Keep in mind that the numbers often do not work out so precisely. That is okay, as long as the number of calories added up from the estimated swaps accounts for most of the total number of calories shown on the food label. In other words, just try to get close (plus or minus about 20 calories).

Some additional guidelines when reading food labels are as follows:

**Table 4-10.** Sample Combo Food—
Amy's Kitchen Chicago Burger (Vegetarian)

| | | |
|---|---|---|
| Serving Size (oz.) | 2.5 | **Ingredients:** Organic mushrooms, organic onions, organic celery, organic carrots, organic oats, wheat gluten, organic bulgur wheat, cheddar cheese (without animal enzymes or rennet), organic brown rice, organic walnuts, soy protein concentrate, filtered water, sea salt, organic potatoes, expeller pressed high oleic safflower oil, organic garlic |
| Calories: | 160 | |
| Calories from Fat: | 45 | |
| Total Fat (g): | 5 | |
| Saturated Fat (g): | 1.5 | |
| Cholesterol (mg): | 5 | |
| Sodium (mg): | 390 | |
| Total Carbohydrates (g): | 20 | |
| Dietary Fiber (g): | 3 | |
| Sugars (g): | 2 | |
| Protein (g): | 10 | |

◉ Most of the foods you eat each day should have less than 5 grams of sugar per serving size listed on the food label. Whole fruit products naturally have 15 grams of sugar per serving, milk naturally has 12 grams of sugar per cup, and yogurt naturally has about 15 grams of sugar per serving. These foods also provide a lot of nutrients. Therefore, the 5-gram rule does not apply to these foods. However, because these foods are high in sugar, you should not have more of these foods than suggested in the plans provided in later chapters.

◉ Most grain products you purchase, as well as fruit and vegetable products, should have a least 3 grams of fiber per serving size listed on the food label.

◉ Most products you buy should have less than 200 or 250 milligrams of sodium per serving size listed on the food label. This is especially true if you have high blood pressure or retain water easily.

## *Important Points To Remember from Chapter 4*

◉ You need to become familiar with the foods that are included in each food group and subgroup, as well as the unit of food that equals a swap.

◉ Eating a variety of foods from the green inner circle of each food group is important in meeting your nutritional needs, because each food group has a different set of nutrients, fibers, and phytochemicals. If you eliminate an entire food group for an extended period of time, you may be at risk for nutrient deficiencies.

◉ Food and beverage manufactures fortify foods with nutrients and promote foods in a way that makes it confusing to determine their overall nutritional quality. Therefore, consider the ingredients in the food you are considering and compare them to the foods placed in the Bull's-Eye Food Guide. Don't be fooled by highly fortified foods with poor quality ingredients!

⊚ A swap from a high-carbohydrate group (Grain & Starch Group, Fruit Group, and Milk & Yogurt Group) has about 15 grams of carbohydrate; a swap from a high-protein group (Protein Group and Milk & Yogurt Group) has about 7 grams of protein, and a swap from the Fat Group has about 5 grams of fat. If you know these numbers, you can estimate the types and numbers of swaps that would appropriately account for all of the calories in a portion of a given single food or multi-ingredient food.

# MAPPING YOUR JOURNEY

### *What You Will Discover in Chapter 5*

◉ To get started, you will select a calorie level and an eating style.

◉ The calorie level you select will be mostly based on your height and weight. There are five possible calorie levels.

◉ Eating style refers to the mix of carbohydrates, proteins, and fats that provides your calories. There are three possible eating styles—lower-carb, moderate-carb, and high-carb.

◉ Once you select a calorie level and an eating style, you can find appropriate sample menus in the Menus and Recipes section.

◉ It may be necessary to change your plan along your weight management journey.

## Creating Your Map and Planning Your Journey

When beginning your weight management journey, you need to create your map—the route you will take. There are two main components of your map or plan: (1) your calorie level and (2) your eating style. Research on weight management strategies indicates that the most important aspect of your plan is the first component—the number of calories you plan to eat each day relative to the number of calories you use each day. If you eat fewer calories than you use most days, you will lose weight. Depending on your genetic makeup and current lifestyle habits, the relative amount of calories you get from carbohydrates, proteins, and fats can matter. The right mix can make your appetite easier to control. In addition, the mix that is right for you may positively influence how your body stores and uses calories.

Scientists know that there are over 20 chemicals in our bodies that influence appetite, fat storage, calorie needs, and use of stored calories. Your genetics determines your potential to produce and use these chemicals. For example, your genes determine how much insulin you can produce, and how well the insulin can work. However, whether you actually do produce that amount or how well it actually does work is affected by the quality of your diet and your exercise habits. If you have unhealthy eating and exercise habits your body may not use the insulin as well as if you had healthy eating and exercise habits. Scientists are a long way from developing methods to determine whether a particular person makes appropriate amounts of the 20 or so chemicals needed for proper appetite and weight control, or if those chemicals are working well. Therefore, at this time, health care professionals cannot determine why any one person has difficulty keeping their weight at a healthy level. Early developments from this line of research are used later in the chapter to guide you in selecting the best eating style for you!

## Fuel (Calorie) Issues

When deciding on your dietary calorie level, you need to consider you calorie needs. In general, your body uses calories to maintain essential functions (such as breathing, heart pumping, and brain processing) and to support voluntary muscular function and physical activity. The calories you need to maintain essential functions are largely dependent on your height and muscle mass. Calories for these essential functions can come from the food you eat or from calories stored in your body. Most of the calories stored in your body are stored as body fat. If you eat 100 calories less than your body needs for these essential functions, your body will pull fat out of storage as an additional source of calories to meet your needs. The result, of course, is weight loss.

Your level of physical activity also affects the number of calories your body uses. The more physically active you are, the more calories you use. When trying to lose weight, the goal is to get those extra calories needed by pulling fat out of storage. (Refer to Chapter 11 for more information on physical activity.) Again, pulling fat out of storage causes weight loss.

Another factor that affects the amount of calories your body needs for essential functions is the amount of calories you are actually eating. If you are eating a lot more calories than your body needs, you will put more fat into storage and gain weight. However, after overeating for a while your body starts to waste some calories from the food you eat and not store all of it. Basically, your body becomes a less efficient machine, and loses energy as heat. You may actually feel warmer when overeating and gaining weight. On the other hand, when you eat fewer calories than your body needs, you pull fat out of storage to meet you calorie needs and you lose weight. However, after undereating for a while your body starts to save calories from the food you eat. Basically, you become a more-efficient machine, losing less energy as heat. When losing weight, you may be more likely to feel cold. In other words, the amount of calories you are eating when you first start a diet, can affect the amount of calories you need to eat to cause gradual weight loss.

## How Much Fuel Do You Need? Picking a Calorie Level

To begin the process of selecting a calorie level, refer to Table 5-1 if you are female and Table 5-2 if you are male. Once you have identified the suggested number of calories per day for someone of your height and weight,

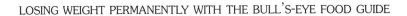

consider your own situation. Here are some factors that may allow you to eat more calories and still lose weight:

◉ You are younger than 30 years of age.

◉ You are very physically active (i.e., exercise for 30 minutes or more 5 or 6 days a week).

◉ You have been eating much more calories for a long period of time and your body has become like that less-efficient machine described above.

On the other hand, these factors may indicate that you have to eat fewer calories to lose weight:

◉ You are older than 50 years.

◉ You are very sedentary and don't participate in regular physical activity.

◉ You have experienced a big loss of muscle mass due to a prolonged illness or condition that was physiologically stressful (such as chemotherapy or radiation to treat cancer, a major surgical procedure, or a major orthopedic injury).

These factors will probably not require you to move up or down a whole level of suggested calories. You may, however, be able to add a 100 or 200 calories and still lose weight. Or, you may have to subtract 100 or 200 calories per day to start losing weight. Depending on your eating style, the guidelines for how to make these adjustments will be different. Therefore, these guidelines are given in Chapters 6, 7, and 8.

In reality everybody is unique, and the only way to be sure the selected number of calories will help you lose weight is to try following the menus at that calorie level in Menus and Recipes. Before you can pick the appropriate menus, however, you need to pick an eating style as guided in the next part of this chapter. If you are not losing about 1 pound a week on average, you can do one or both of the following: increase your level of physical activity or decrease your calorie intake. Refer to Chapter 11 for more information on physical activity. The chapter on your selected eating style will give more information on modifying calorie intake.

**Table 5-1.**

Estimated Calorie Needs for Women Based on Height and Weight

> **Directions:** *1st*—*Find your height within the categories shown along the top. In the example, the woman is 5'3", which is between 5'2" and 5'3¾". **2nd**—Follow down the column to find your weight within the categories given. In the example the woman weighs 210 pounds, which is between 161 and 290 pounds. **3rd**—Follow to the left along the row to find the recommended number of calories per day. In the example, 1500 calories/day would be suggested.*

| Recommended Calories/Day | **1st** Height, in inches | | | | | | |
|---|---|---|---|---|---|---|---|
| | 5'0"-5'1¾" | 5'2"-5'3¾" | 5'4"-5'5¾" | 5'6"-5'7¾" | 5'8"-5'9¾" | 5'10"-5'11¾" | ≥6'0" |
| 1200 Calories | wt.,lbs. <190 | wt., lbs. ≤160 **2nd** | | | | | |
| 1500 Calories **3rd** | wt., lbs. ≥190 | wt., lbs. 161-290 | wt., lbs. <260 | wt., lbs. <217 | wt., lbs. <180 | <178 | |
| 1800 Calories | | wt., lbs. ≥291 | wt., lbs. ≥260 | wt., lbs. ≥217 | wt., lbs. ≥180 | wt., lbs. ≥178-350 | wt., lbs. <320 |
| 2100 Calories | | | | | | wt., lbs. ≥350 | wt., lbs. ≥320 |
| 2400 Calories | | | | | | | |

**Table 5-2.**
Estimated Calorie Needs for Men Based on Height and Weight

> **Directions:** *1st*—*Find your height within the categories shown along the top. In the example, the man is 5'11", which is between 5'10" and 5'11¾". 2nd—Follow down the column to find your weight within the categories given. In the example the man weighs 210 pounds, which is less than 271 pounds. 3rd—Follow to the left along the row to find the recommended number of calories per day. In the example, 2100 calories/day would be suggested.*

| Recommended Calories/Day | Height, in inches | | | | | | |
|---|---|---|---|---|---|---|---|
| | 5'4"-5'5¾" | 5'6"-5'7¾" | 5'8"-5'9¾" | 5'10"-5'11¾" | 6'0"-6'1¾" | 6'2"-6'3¾" | ≥6'4" |
| 1200 Calories | | | **1st** | | | | |
| 1500 Calories | | | | | | | |
| 1800 Calories | wt., lbs. <266 | wt., lbs. <255 | wt., lbs. <180 | | | | |
| 2100 Calories | wt., lbs. ≥266 | wt., lbs. ≥255 | wt., lbs. ≥180-320 | wt., lbs. <271 **2nd** | wt., lbs. <240 | | |
| 2400 Calories | | | wt., lbs. ≥320 | wt., lbs. ≥271 | wt., lbs. ≥240 | wt., lbs. all weights | wt., lbs. all weights |

**3rd** (2100 Calories)

# Picking an Eating Style—
# What's behind the Big Debate

The best source or mix of calories when losing weight has been debated for a long time. Unfortunately, this debate has been clouded by a lot of misinformation and commercialism. There are more and more studies exploring the issue of relative amounts of dietary carbohydrates, proteins, and fats and their effects on weight and health. The biggest challenge to this type of research is the likelihood that there is no one right answer. The best mix, or eating style, depends on the individual. Remember, over 20 chemicals have been identified that effect appetite, fat storage, calorie needs, and use of stored calories. Depending on an individual's genetic makeup and activity level of these chemicals, the best mix of carbohydrates, proteins, and fats will vary.[1]

## The Three Eating Styles

There are three different eating styles that research indicates can support optimal health: lower-carb, moderate-carb, and high-carb. The best choice *for you* will be largely based on your suspected level of insulin resistance, as well as the results of a trial period. (Guidelines for evaluating your level of insulin resistance are in the next section.) Keep in mind that it is possible to transition from one style to another, depending on results. In all three eating styles the highest quality of carbohydrates, proteins, and fats are recommended—those found in foods that are in the green inner circle of the Bull's-Eye Food Guide. These different eating styles are defined by the percentage of total calories that come from carbohydrates, proteins, and fats. Refer to Table 5-3. In the lower-carb style, the lowest level of carbohydrates and the highest level of fats known to support good health are provided. In the high-carb style, the highest amount of carbohydrates and the lowest amount of fats shown to support good health are provided. The moderate-carb style provides carbohydrates and fats in between the other two styles. The contribution of protein to total calories varies from 20% to 25%.

**Table 5-3.** Eating Styles and Sources of Calories

| Source of Calories | Eating Style | | |
|---|---|---|---|
| | Lower-Carb | Moderate-Carb | High-Carb |
| Carbohydrates | 40% | 50% | 60% |
| Proteins | 25% | 20% | 20% |
| Fats | 35% | 30% | 20% |

## Guidelines for Evaluating Level of Insulin Resistance

At this time we do not have tests available to completely explore a person's mechanisms of appetite control and calorie balance. However, one main factor that is recognized to influence these processes is your body's ability to use a chemical called insulin. Insulin is produced in your pancreas. When you eat, the carbohydrates in your food are digested into sugars that are absorbed from your intestines into your blood. Your cells need sugar and have special "doorways" or receptors through which the sugar enters the cells. You can think of insulin as the "key" that opens the door, so the sugar can get into the cell. Some people produce many doors with broken locks. Therefore, the "insulin-key" doesn't always work, and the sugar can't get into the cells. This is called insulin resistance. The body senses the high sugar level, and produces more insulin-keys in hopes of getting more doors open. This may work for a while, allowing blood sugar levels to remain normal despite the insulin resistance. Unfortunately, high levels of insulin in the blood, as well as the high levels of sugar, can cause problems. The most common problems are high blood pressure, high blood fats called triglycerides, and low levels of health-promoting HDL cholesterol. High levels of insulin in the blood also *push dietary fat into fat stores* and may *increase appetite*. Your degree of resistance to insulin is the one well-known factor that determines the type of eating style that is most appropriate for weight loss.

Being overweight increases the likelihood that you will be insulin resistant, but not every overweight person is indeed insulin resistant. Your eating style will be largely determined by your suspected level of insulin resistance, based on the information in Table 5-4. Remember, there is no easy way to determine your level of insulin resistance, and therefore it is hard to know for sure. There are, however, signs that indicate an increased likelihood of insulin resistance. It is also important to note that insulin resistance is not a permanent condition. As you lose weight and increase your physical activity, your insulin resistance may decrease substantially. At that point you can try transitioning to a different eating style. After any change in your eating plan, monitor changes in your weight and health indicators (such as blood pressure and laboratory values) to determine whether the change will help you reach your destination—a healthy weight you can maintain.

There is an increased risk for insulin resistance when extra fat is stored in the abdominal area instead of the hips or legs. This is because the excess fat surrounds the liver and affects how the liver works. Your liver is a very busy manufacturing plant, and in addition to making sugar it can also make fats called triglycerides. When surrounded by fat, the liver makes more triglycerides, and in insulin resistance it also makes unnecessary sugar. It is not clear whether the abdominal obesity comes first, causing insulin resistance, or whether the insulin resistance comes first, causing the obesity. The order of occurrence may also depend on genetic predisposition, as well as on eating and exercise habits. Researchers have estimated that only 20% to 30% of overweight adults are insulin resistant.[2,3]

Insulin sensitivity is the opposite of insulin resistance. After a meal or snack, a person who is sensitive to insulin can clear blood of sugar fairly quickly. In addition, this person would not need to produce a lot of extra insulin. Therefore, after eating, the levels of insulin and sugar return to the pre-eating levels in a timely fashion—in about 2 hours. The insulin-sensitive person is not exposed to high levels of blood sugar and insulin for a prolonged period of time. If you are overweight and sensitive to insulin, then a higher-carbohydrate style of eating is best for weight loss and optimal health.

To determine your eating style, you need to consider the factors that would indicate your likelihood of insulin resistance.[4] These factors are listed in the first column of Table 5-4. Some of these factors you can observe

**Table 5-4.** How to Select an Eating Style

> **Directions:** Read each factor. In the corresponding row, circle the description of that factor that best describes your situation.

| Factor to consider when selecting your eating style | Suggested Eating Style | | |
|---|---|---|---|
| | **Indicators of High Insulin Resistance** Suggested: **Lower-Carb Style** | **Indicators of Lower Insulin Resistance** Suggested: **Moderate-Carb Style** | **Indicators of Insulin Sensitivity** Suggested: **High-Carb Style** |
| **Factor 1: Location of Excess Weight** | •Most excess weight around waist or abdomen<br>•Waist circumference: men—≥40 inches women—≥35 inches<br><br>•Waist-to-hip ratio: men—≥0.95 women—≥0.80 | •Excess weight equally dispersed<br>•Waist circumference: men—just under 40 inches women—just under 35 inches<br>•Waist-to-hip ratio: men—just under 0.95 women—just under 0.80 | •Most excess weight on hips, thighs, and/or legs<br>•Waist circumference: men—<40 inches women—≤35 inches<br><br>•Waist-to-hip ratio: men—<0.95 women—<0.80 |
| **Factor 2: Blood Sugar** | •Diagnosed type 2 diabetes (fasting blood sugar without medication ≥126 mg/dl) | •Normal<br>•Blood sugar just under 100 mg/dl | •Low normal<br>•Blood sugar <100 mg/dl<br><br>(continued on next page) |

Table 5-4. How to Select an Eating Style (continued)

| Factor to consider when selecting your eating style | Suggested Eating Style | | |
|---|---|---|---|
| | Indicators of High Insulin Resistance Suggested: Lower-Carb Style | Indicators of Lower Insulin Resistance Suggested: Moderate-Carb Style | Indicators of Insulin Sensitivity Suggested: High-Carb Style |
| **Factor 2: Blood Sugar** | • Impaired fasting glucose (fasting blood sugar 100-125 mg/dl) | | |
| **Factor 3: Blood Triglyceride Levels** | • High<br>• Triglycerides ≥150 mg/dl | • Normal<br>• Triglycerides just under 150 mg/dl | • Low normal<br>• Triglycerides <150 mg/dl |
| **Factor 4: Blood HDL Levels** | • Low<br>• Men <40 mg/dl<br>• Women <50 mg/dl | • Borderline<br>• Men 40-45<br>• Women 50-55 mg/dl | • High<br>• Men >45 mg/dl<br>• Women >55 mg/dl |
| **Factor 5: Blood Pressure** | • Diagnosed high blood pressure<br>• Blood pressure ≥130/85 mm Hg | • Normal blood pressure, but approaching defined high value of 130/85 mm Hg | • Normal blood pressure <120/80 mm Hg |
| **Factor 6: Level of Physical Activity** | • No regular physical activity | • Some regular physical activity (3 times a week or less) | • A lot of regular physical acitvity (more than 3 times a week) |

**Table 5-4.** How to Select an Eating Style (continued)

| Factor to consider when selecting your eating style | Suggested Eating Style | | |
|---|---|---|---|
| | Indicators of High Insulin Resistance Suggested: Lower-Carb Style | Indicators of Lower Insulin Resistance Suggested: Moderate-Carb Style | Indicators of Insulin Sensitivity Suggested: High-Carb Style |
| **Factor 7: Family History of Diabetes** | •More than one close relative (parent, sibling, grandparent, aunt, or uncle) | •One close relative (parent, sibling, grandparent, aunt, or uncle) | •No family history of diabetes |
| **Factor 8: For Women Only: Polycystic Ovary Syndrome** | •Diagnosed polycystic ovary syndrome | | |

yourself, such as your family history and where you carry your excess weight. Other factors require that you know particular laboratory values, and if you have specific illnesses or conditions. You should request this information from your health care provider if you do not already know. It is important that you understand these issues so you can take control of your health. The first five factors are considered the most important in assessing your likelihood of being insulin resistant. The last three factors are also suggestive of insulin resistance. For each factor, consider each of three descriptions. Determine which descriptions best fit your status regarding the given factor. The order in which the factors are listed is arbitrary. You may want to read through the following descriptions of the factors before considering your status. You may need to review this very important section more than once.

## Factor 1—Location of Excess Weight

The first factor is the location of excess body fat. Remember that excess abdominal fat is problematic. Waist circumference (the length around your waist) is easy to measure and a good indicator of abdominal fat. Using a tape measure, measure your waist at the level of your belly button. If you do not have a tape measure, use a string to determine the length. Then measure the length of the string using a ruler.

⦿ For men, a waist circumference greater than or equal to 40 inches is indicative of abdominal fat that would have the negative effect on the liver as described above.

⦿ For women a waist circumference of greater than or equal to 35 inches has the same effect.

Numbers close to these cutoff points may indicate a potential problem, whereas numbers much lower increase the likelihood of insulin sensitivity.

For those who are just marginally overweight, insulin resistance is still a potential problem—especially with a strong family history of diabetes. If your waist circumference is less than the numbers indicated above and you are only moderately overweight, you should compare your waist circumference with the circumference of your hips to see if you carry more of your excess weight around your waist/stomach or hips/thighs. To do this, measure your waist circumference as above. Then measure your hip circumference. Measure your hips at the widest level of your hips and buttocks area. Then divide your waist measurement by your hip measurement.

⦿ For men, a number equal to 0.95 or greater increases the likelihood of insulin resistance.

◉ For women, a number equal to 0.80 or greater increases the likelihood of insulin resistance.

Again, numbers approaching these cutoffs indicate insulin resistance may be an impending problem, and numbers significantly lower are more closely associated with insulin sensitivity.

## Factor 2—Blood Sugar Levels

Type 2 diabetes is a sure sign of insulin resistance. If it is well-treated, blood sugars may be normal, but the underlying insulin resistance is still a factor. Fasting blood sugar level (sugar measured in your blood 8 hours after eating or drinking) is an important measure considered by your health care provider to determine whether you have type 2 diabetes.

◉ Fasting blood sugar equal to or above 126 milligrams per deciliter is indicative of diabetes.

◉ Fasting blood sugar levels above 100 but less than 126 milligrams per deciliter indicate a decreased ability to use insulin well.

◉ Normal fasting blood sugar is less than 100 milligrams per deciliter. Fasting blood sugar that is in the higher end of the normal range may indicate an increasing insulin resistance, especially if there are other indicators of insulin resistance—but this is not a sure thing.

◉ Blood sugar well below the 100 cutoff mark is an indicator of insulin sensitivity.[5]

## Factor 3—Blood Triglyceride Levels

Triglycerides are a type of fat in your blood. They can come from the food you eat, or your body can make them from excess dietary carbohydrates or fatty acids. Triglyceride levels are an excellent indicator of insulin resistance.

- Triglyceride levels greater than 150 milligrams per deciliter indicate insulin resistance.

- Normal levels that are just under 150 milligrams per deciliter may indicate an increasing tendency towards insulin resistance.

- Triglyceride levels well under 150 milligrams per deciliter indicate the absence of insulin resistance, or insulin sensitivity.[4]

## Factor 4—Blood HDL Cholesterol Levels

There are two types of cholesterol that are routinely measured, HDL and LDL. Although HDL levels are always lower than LDL levels, the higher your HDL the less your risk for heart disease. Higher levels of LDLs increase your risk of heart disease. Insulin resistance does not increase your levels of LDL cholesterol, but it does cause changes in the LDL cholesterol. They become chemically changed in a way that makes it more likely for them to become incorporated into coronary artery plaque and increase your risk for heart disease. However, it is hard to measure these chemical changes, so LDL cholesterol is not considered a factor. HDL cholesterol levels are commonly measured.

- HDL less than 40 milligrams per deciliter for men and less than 50 milligrams per deciliter for women are indicative of insulin resistance.[4]

- For men, HDL levels between 40 and 45 milligrams per deciliter may be indicative of increasing insulin resistance. For women, HDL levels between 50 and 55 milligrams per deciliter may be indicative of increasing insulin resistance.

- High levels of HDL, greater than 45 milligrams per deciliter for men and 55 milligrams per deciliter for women, are indicative of insulin sensitivity.

## Factor 5—Blood Pressure

Insulin resistance, due to the resulting high insulin and high sugar levels, can cause high blood pressure.

- Blood pressure measurements greater than 130 over 85 millimeters of mercury are reflective of insulin resistance.[4]

- Blood pressure readings approaching 130 over 85 millimeters of mercury may indicate an increased risk for insulin resistance.

- Blood pressure readings well below 120 over 80 millimeters of mercury (which is considered normal blood pressure) do not support the presence of insulin resistance.

## Factors 6, 7, and 8—Physical Activity, Family History, PCOS

There are two other factors that also provide some information regarding your level of insulin resistance. Factor 6 is your level of physical activity, and Factor 7 is your family history of type 2 diabetes. If you are not physically active on a regular basis, you are at a higher risk of insulin resistance. On the other hand, regular physical activity is somewhat protective against insulin resistance. Having more than one close relative with insulin resistance increases the likelihood that you have a genetic predisposition for insulin resistance. Having no close relatives with insulin resistance means you have less chance of being genetically predisposed, unless these relatives suppress their predisposition with good eating and physical activity habits. Lastly, for women there is an eighth factor, polycystic ovary syndrome (PCOS), which is strongly indicative of insulin resistance.

## Making the Selection

As you consider each of these factors, consider which description best describes your situation. According to experts on the National Cholesterol Education Program panel, if your responses to three of the five first factors in the first column are yes, then you are most likely insulin resistant. The suggested eating style would be the lower-carb style. The experts who developed the National Cholesterol Education Program did not provide additional guidelines. However, based on the research literature, the following guidelines are reasonable for selecting an eating style (not necessarily for determining your level of insulin resistance).

- Select the lower-carb eating style if
  - You have three or more positive responses for the top five factors in the first column.
  - You have two positive responses for the top five factors in the first column plus one positive response in the first column for at least one factor in the shaded area.
  - You have PCOS (for women).

- Select the high-carb eating style if
  - You have all positive responses for the top five factors in the third column.
  - You have four positive responses for the top five factors in the third column, plus you accumulate at least 30 minutes of physical activity five or more times a week.

- Select the moderate-carbohydrate eating style in all situations not described above.

If you are insulin resistant, the research clearly indicates that a lower-carbohydrate eating style is necessary to correct the problem. However, eating styles with different carbohydrate contents have *not* been shown to have an effect on long-term weight loss. Therefore, if you are not insulin resistant, selecting a lower-carbohydrate style has no benefit for weight loss. Selecting the lower-carbohydrate eating style will lead to a lower intake of phytochemicals, and therefore should not be selected unless necessary to correct insulin resistance. Your taste preferences should also be taken into account. By picking the appropriate eating style, you are more likely to lose weight and keep the weight off.

## Ready, Set, Go

Once you have selected a calorie level and an eating style, refer to Menus and Recipes for sample menus to follow right away. Initially, you should try to follow the menus very closely. As you learn more about your Bull's-Eye Food Guide Program you will be able to use other tools and strategies to guide your food choices on a day-to-day basis. (Refer to Chapters 9 and 10 to learn about these other tools and strategies.)

The next step is to read the chapter on the eating style suggested for you, based on the information presented in Table 5-4. For detailed information on how to follow the lower-carb style, read Chapter 7. Read Chapter 8 for similar information on the moderate-carb eating style, and read Chapter 9 for the information on the high-carb eating style. As you lose weight and become more physically active you should see signs of improving insulin sensitivity, such as normalized blood sugar and triglyceride levels. Therefore, you may need to go back to Table 5-4 and reevaluate your level of insulin resistance, and you may need to switch to a different eating style. Therefore, after reading the chapter corresponding to the eating style you selected, you may also want to review the chapters on the other two eating styles.

After following the selected sample menu for 2 to 4 weeks, consider your results. You should lose about 1 pound a week, perhaps more during the first few weeks. The selected plan should not result in excessive hunger or very rapid weight loss. If this is the case, it will most likely not be sustainable. You may need to adjust your plan as you go, and reading Chapters 6, 7, or 8 will empower you with the knowledge you need to modify your plan so you continue to get results. Before you lose about 10 to 20 pounds, you need to read Chapter 11 to plan your pattern of weight loss to maximize your long-term success.

## Important Points To Remember from Chapter 5

◉ Insulin resistance causes high blood sugar, high triglycerides, low HDL cholesterol, and high blood pressure. Obesity and lack of physical activity increase the risk for insulin resistance.

◉ Your weight loss plan will be based on a calorie level and an eating style.

◉ The right mix of carbohydrates, proteins, and fats for you is based on your level of insulin resistance, which is reflected by your health indicators (blood sugar level, triglyceride level, HDL level, blood pressure, and location of excessive body fat).

◉ As you lose weight and improve your health you may need to change your eating style to continue to maximize your health while losing weight and keeping it off.

# THE LOWER-CARB ROUTE

### *What You Will Discover in Chapter 6*

⊚ You can decrease your insulin resistance by changing your diet, losing weight, and exercising.

⊚ You can decrease (and perhaps normalize) your blood sugar and insulin levels by (1) decreasing your intake of total carbohydrates, (2) eating higher quality carbohydrates, and (3) balancing those carbohydrates with healthy proteins and fats within your suggested calorie level.

⊚ For your selected calorie level you will find an eating plan that suggests the appropriate number of swaps from each food group for your meals and snack.

⊚ You may need to modify your plan for optimal benefits. Guidelines for doing so are provided in this chapter.

⊚ Timing of meals and snacks is important.

## How the Lower-Carb Route Can Get You to Your Destination

The lower-carb route is the best route—indeed the absolutely necessary route—if you have signs of insulin resistance. It has been estimated that about 24% of all American adults are insulin resistant. Among all over-weight adults, 40% are expected to be insulin resistant. Lastly, between 58% to 66% of overweight adults with conditions known to be associated with insulin resistance, such as high triglycerides, low HDL cholesterol levels, and high blood pressure are thought to be insulin resistant.[1,2] Refer to Chapter 5, especially Table 5-4, for a full explanation of insulin resistance. In summary, being insulin resistant means that your body makes the chemical insulin, but your cells cannot use it well. Your body requires insulin to push sugar that is in your blood into your cells, where it is needed. When insulin is not working well, the level of sugar in your blood increases. Your body tries to compensate for this by making more insulin. In some cases this works, and your blood sugar stays within the normal range. After a while your ability to compensate decreases, and blood sugar levels approach the high end of the normal range. When this compensation strategy fails, blood sugar levels become higher than normal even though the insulin levels are also high. When levels of sugar in your blood are high for a prolonged period of time, the sugar can damage organs such as eyes, kidneys, and nerves. High levels of insulin and insulin resistance cause other problems, such as high blood fats called triglycerides, high blood pressure, and an increased risk for heart disease. Therefore, decreasing blood sugar levels and insulin levels is important.[3,4]

Sugar in your blood can come from food you eat, or it can be made by your liver. Dietary sources of sugar result from the digestion of carbohydrates found in foods in the Grain & Starch Group, the Fruit Group, and the Milk & Yogurt Group. Less-refined or -processed foods that are high in fiber have a modest effect on blood sugar. To decrease your blood sugar, the following strategies are important: (1) eat high-quality carbohydrates from the green inner circle of the Bull's-Eye Food Guide, (2) decrease the amount of carbohydrates you eat, (3) eat carbohydrates with healthy foods from the Protein Group and/or the Fat Group, (4) participate in regular physical activity as described in Chapter 11, and (5) decrease your calorie intake enough to promote weight loss. The fourth and fifth strategies are very effective, because they decrease insulin resistance and allow your cells to use insulin to push sugar inside of them. Therefore, blood levels of insulin drop. Because the insulin is now far more effective, blood sugar enters cells readily and blood sugar levels normalize as well.[3,5,6]

When insulin and blood sugar levels approach normal levels, your body's ability to properly regulate appetite and fat storage improves. In addition, you can halt the negative physiological effects of high blood sugar and high blood insulin. After you have corrected the relatively high blood sugar and insulin levels, it is recommended that you maintain an exercise program and transition to the moderate-carb eating style.

The next section of this chapter provides detailed information on creating a very structured lower-carb plan. It is important for you to review and understand this information. For most people, it also helps to try to follow a detailed plan for some time before transitioning to a less-structured plan. However, everybody is unique and some people simply do not respond well to such a structured approach. For example, for some people the effort required to follow the structured plan leads them to think about food too much and be too restrictive. This can backfire and lead to more frequent overeating episodes. Be aware of this potential consequence. If this is the case for you, review the information below and keep a general sense of the structure in your mind. Then go to Chapters 9 and 10 for other strategies you can use to craft a more casual approach to the lower-carb eating style. In addition, refer to the menus in Menus and Recipes. A *less-structured or casual approach can work, but the results are typically slower. This is okay, as long as you prepare yourself for slower weight loss and adjust your expectations accordingly. Simply accept the slower weight loss as progress that is more likely to be permanent for many reasons discussed in Chapter 11.*

## The Detailed Map

The main issues with this approach are how low to reduce carbohydrate intake and how to balance carbohydrates, proteins, and fats. The following plan is designed to maximize the benefits of lowering carbohydrate intake, without exposing you to potential risks of bringing carbohydrates too low and, consequently, fats and proteins too high. See the section later in this chapter on disadvantages of taking this approach to the extreme.

On the lower-carb route, carbohydrates are limited to providing 40% of total calories. Fats provide 35% of total calories, and proteins provide 25%. It is essential that the majority of your carbohydrates come from high-fiber foods that are minimally processed and without added sweeteners (especially high-fructose corn syrup). Because the protein and fat content of this program is relatively high, it is also extremely important that you select the highest-quality foods from the green inner circle of these food groups most of the time. That does not mean that you can never have a favorite food from the red outer circle, but you have to plan to work some of these foods into your day. By working some of your favorite foods from the red outer circle into your plan, you increase the likelihood that you can sustain the program long enough to get to a healthy weight and then stay there. With the Bull's-Eye Food Guide system, you never have to count calories or grams of carbohydrates, proteins, or fats. All you have to do is simply keep track of the number of swaps you have from the six food groups each day. Review the food groups and the idea of "swapping" in Chapter 4 before finalizing your plan. For now, remember that a swap of food is the amount of a specific food that provides the number of calories assigned to the food group in which it is placed. It is not necessarily the amount of food you can eat at a meal or snack, because you may have more than one swap from a specific food group at a meal or snack. Consider a swap of food simply an assigned volume of food used as a counting unit to keep track of calories, carbohydrates, proteins, and fats.

First, note the calorie level you selected for yourself in Chapter 5 from Table 5-1 or 5-2. Then refer to Table 6-1, which indicates the number of swaps from the six different food groups suggested each day based on your calorie level. For example, reading down the column labeled "1500 Calories per Day" level, there are six Vegetable Group swaps, two Fruit Group swaps, four Grain & Starch Group swaps, eight Protein Group swaps, six Fat Group swaps, and two Milk & Yogurt Group swaps. If you cannot tolerate milk or yogurt, try soymilk products. If that does not work for you, trade in your two

**Table 6-1.** Lower-Carb Plans by Calorie Level

| Food Group | Swaps per Day from Each Food Group at Different Calorie Levels | | | | |
| --- | --- | --- | --- | --- | --- |
| | 1200 Calories/ Day | 1500 Calories/ Day | 1800 Calories/ Day | 2100 Calories/ Day | 2400 Calories/ Day |
| Vegetable | 4 | 6 | 6 | 6 | 8 |
| *For vegetables the numbers are minimums since vegetable group swaps are unlimited.* | | | | | |
| Fruit | 2 | 2 | 2 | 3 | 4 |
| Grain & Starch | 3 | 4 | 6 | 7 | 8 |
| Protein | 5 | 8 | 9 | 11 | 13 |
| Fat | 6 | 6 | 8 | 9 | 9 |
| Milk & Yogurt | 2 | 2 | 2 | 2 | 2 |

swaps from the Milk & Yogurt Group for one swap from the Protein Group and one swap from the Fruit Group. In addition, talk to your health care provider about taking a calcium supplement to ensure adequate calcium intake.

Remember, in the lower-carb style it is extremely important that the swaps from the Grain & Starch Group come from the green inner circle. One or at the most two swaps can be saved for a food in the yellow or red circles. All fruits should come from the green inner circle, and most vegetables should come from the green inner circle. If you select tomato sauce as a vegetable, check the ingredient list and make sure there are no added sweeteners. Protein selections can come from the green inner circle or the yellow middle circle, but selections from the red outer circle should be extremely limited. Also, keep in mind that if you do pick a food from the outer circle of the protein group you need to save fats for that food as well. Both of your swaps from the Milk & Yogurt Group should be from the green or yellow circles. All but one or two of your selections from the fat group should come from the green inner circle. If you have an elevated LDL cholesterol level, trans fats and saturated fats, such as the fats prevalent in foods in the outer red subgroup, should be carefully avoided. Fats found in foods in the outer circle of the Grain & Starch Group, the Protein Group, and the Milk & Yogurt Group are typically trans fats or saturated fats. Therefore, fat swaps that you save to put towards these foods should be limited as well.

The next step is to decide how to spread the swaps from the different food groups throughout the course of the day. Note that carbohydrates from food in the Grain & Starch Group or the Fruit Group should be balanced with a food from the Protein Group and/or the Fat Group. This is true for planning meals and snacks. In other words, you would avoid having something from the Grain & Starch Group or the Fruit Group alone. In Table 6-2 swaps from the different food groups at each calorie level are distributed into three meals and one snack. On the chart, highlight the calorie level that you have previously selected. Note how many swaps you have for each meal and snack. In Menus and Recipes, you will find daily menus to follow. You can also use the Swap Lists for each of the food groups to modify the menus or create new menus. See Tables 6-3 A and B for an example of selections made from the swap lists to create a lunch at the 1500-calorie-per-day level. If you do not like a particular item selected in these tables or in the daily menus, you can go to the Swap Lists to trade them in for swaps of different foods in the same group. For example, in Table 6-3A there is a note that you may not like grapes or may not have them available at the time. Therefore, the grapes can be traded in for one swap of a different fruit selected from the Fruit Group swap list in the Swap Lists, such as 1 apple, ½ a banana or 12 cherries. The sample daily menus demonstrate this point.

Many people's first response to menus such as the ones in Tables 6-3 A and B is that they think it looks like too much food. This is for a few reasons. First of all, many of the foods selected have a low caloric density. As described in Chapter 3, this means that there are only a small amount of calories for a given amount of food because the food is high in fiber or

**Table 6-2.** Swaps of Each Food Group by Calorie Level and Meal

| Meal | 1200 Calories/ Day | 1500 Calories/ Day | 1800 Calories/ Day | 2100 Calories/ Day | 2400 Calories/ Day |
|---|---|---|---|---|---|
| **Breakfast** | | | | | |
| Vegetable Group | | | | | |
| Fruit Group | | | | | |
| Grain & Starch Group | 1 | 1 | 1 | 1 | 2 |
| Protein Group | 1 | 1 | 1 | 2 | 2 |
| Fat Group | 1 | 1 | 1 | 2 | 2 |
| Milk & Yogurt Group | ½ | ½ | ½ | ½ | ½ |
| **Lunch** | | | | | |
| Vegetable Group | 2 | 2 | 2 | 2 | 3 |
| Fruit Group | 1 | 1 | 1 | 1 | 1 |
| Grain & Starch Group | 1 | 1 | 2 | 2 | 2 |
| Protein Group | 1 | 2 | 3 | 4 | 4 |
| Fat Group | 2 | 2 | 2 | 2 | 2 |
| Milk & Yogurt Group | ½ | ½ | ½ | ½ | ½ |
| **Dinner** | | | | | |
| Vegetable Group | 2 | 4 | 4 | 4 | 5 |
| Fruit Group | | | | | 1 |
| Grain & Starch Group | 1 | 2 | 3 | 3 | 3 |
| Protein Group | 3 | 4 | 4 | 4 | 6 |
| Fat Group | 2 | 2 | 3 | 3 | 3 |
| Milk & Yogurt Group | | | | | |
| **Snacks** | | | | | |
| Vegetable Group | | | | | |
| Fruit Group | 1 | 1 | 1 | 2 | 2 |
| Grain & Starch Group | | | | 1 | 1 |
| Protein Group | | 1 | 1 | 1 | 1 |
| Fat Group | 1 | 1 | 2 | 2 | 2 |
| Milk & Yogurt Group | 1 | 1 | 1 | 1 | 1 |

**Table 6-3A.**
A Sample Lunch from the 1500-Calorie Lower-Carb Plan **Sandwich** Option

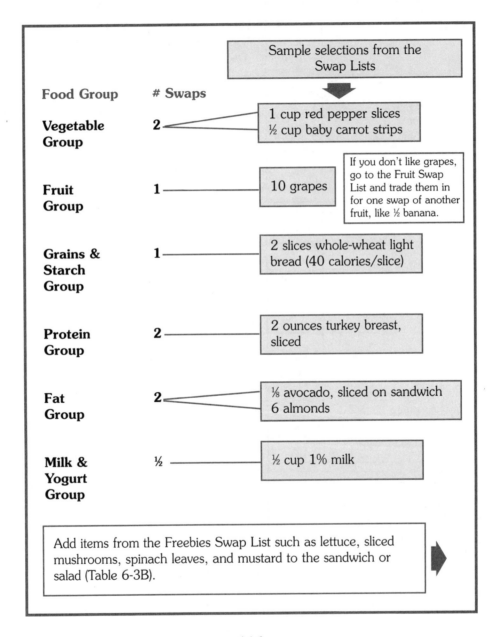

## Table 6-3B.

A Sample Lunch from the 1500-Calorie Lower-Carb Plan **Salad** Option

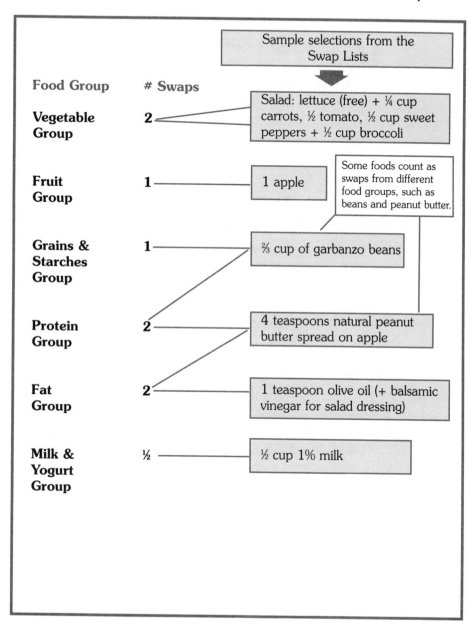

| Food Group | # Swaps | Sample selections from the Swap Lists |
|---|---|---|
| **Vegetable Group** | 2 | Salad: lettuce (free) + ¼ cup carrots, ½ tomato, ½ cup sweet peppers + ½ cup broccoli |
| **Fruit Group** | 1 | 1 apple |
| **Grains & Starches Group** | 1 | ⅔ cup of garbanzo beans |
| **Protein Group** | 2 | 4 teaspoons natural peanut butter spread on apple |
| **Fat Group** | 2 | 1 teaspoon olive oil (+ balsamic vinegar for salad dressing) |
| **Milk & Yogurt Group** | ½ | ½ cup 1% milk |

Some foods count as swaps from different food groups, such as beans and peanut butter.

water. Second, moderate amounts of many different types of foods are used in combinations in meals to best balance carbohydrates, proteins, and fats. Lastly, moderate amounts of many different foods are selected to provide a wide variety of nutrients, fibers, and phytochemicals. This also makes the display of food appear more satisfying and interesting. The lunch menus shown in Tables 6-3 A and B have about 490 calories. By comparison, a sandwich from a deli with no side dishes or drinks would provide at least 850 calories, and not nearly as many nutrients, fiber, or phytochemicals. Another common response to the swaps, meal patterns, and menus is frustration with the prospect of weighing and measuring foods and drinks. You may also be concerned about the portion sizes that are typically much smaller than what you were previously eating and drinking. To resolve these issues and barriers to moving forward, keep in mind that to start losing weight you simply have to eat less than you are currently eating until weight loss starts. Therefore, you may want to start off by determining how much you are currently eating. For a few days write down what you eat and figure out how many swaps from each food group you usually have at each meal and snack. Compare your usual number of swaps per meals and snacks to the numbers suggested. Then plan to gradually reduce the number of swaps you are currently eating to get closer to the suggested number of swaps. As you make each gradual reduction in swaps, monitor your weight for a few days. Reduce the number of swaps until weight loss starts. You are likely to find that you start to lose weight when you just get close to eating the suggested number of swaps.

You will soon develop a system of planning your meals, shopping, and cooking that allows you to put healthy, satisfying meals together quickly. At first this will probably require extra planning time as you develop your new habits and systems. After a while the new habits will come easily, and the time necessary to shop and cook will decrease.

## Considering Alcohol Intake

Alcohol needs to be limited for many health reasons, as well as because of the calories it provides. If you are already in the habit of having an alcoholic drink, you can continue to have one alcoholic drink a day—but no more. This should *not* be consumed on an empty stomach when it will have the most dramatic and negative effect on your liver's metabolic processes. Instead, have it with or immediately after dinner. One alcoholic drink is equivalent to 5 ounces of a dry wine, 12 ounces of beer, or 1½ ounces of 80-proof distilled spirits plain or with a noncaloric mixer. If you are not in the habit of drinking alcohol, you should not start now!

## Avoiding Getting Lost

The best way to avoid getting lost is to study your map before you start your journey. Using the menus is a good way to get started right away. While you are doing this, spend time learning the following: (1) the number of swaps from each of the food groups at your calorie level for each meal and snack as shown in Table 6-2, (2) the swap lists for each food group and subgroup of the Bull's-Eye Guides, (3) the concept of swapping as described in the beginning of Chapter 4, and (4) the description of each food group and subgroup as described in Chapter 4. Learning this information will allow you to modify the daily menus in Menus and Recipes and create an unlimited number of menus for meals and snacks.

In Chapters 9 and 10, you will learn many new strategies to help you develop new healthy eating and exercise habits. It will take you time to work with these strategies to change unhealthy habits and change your relationship with food. Most often, it is first necessary to become more aware of why and when you eat, and then to start to tease apart unhealthy habits in which eating is tied to emotions (such as stress, boredom, and anger) or specific behaviors (such as television viewing). For now, suffice it to say that along your journey you will at times lose your way—overeat, make many selections from the red outer circle, or stop exercising. *This is to be expected.* The biggest indicator of your overall progress and long-term success is how quickly you can get back on your planned route. This requires that you simply acknowledge your missteps and, without a lot of negativity, turn back on course. Permanent weight loss is a process that takes time, but the process is well worth the time and effort in terms of the permanence of the weight lost and the improvements in your overall health.

So what about the times when you really want a piece of cake or some other favorite dessert? You can add these items on occasion, but you have to plan ahead a bit. For example, imagine you are going to a birthday party and you know you will want a piece of cake. An average piece of cake counts as two swaps from the Grain & Starch Group and two swaps from the Fat Group. To save swaps for the cake, you would have a lot of vegetables and your protein swaps (three to six swaps of meat, fish, or chicken) for dinner. However, you would skip the starchy side dish and fats and save those swaps for the piece of cake. Of course this is not ideal, because you are having less-healthy foods from the red outer circle instead of healthy foods from the green inner circle. However, it is realistic, and allows you to have some of your favorite foods while staying on your plan.

You can take this idea of being flexible one step further by using the information in Chapter 4, Table 4-1. In this table you are given the calories and grams of carbohydrates, proteins, and fats provided by a swap of each of the food groups. If you are following the 1500 calorie per day, lower-carb route you would have the following swaps for snack: one Fruit Group swap, one Protein Group swap, one Fat Group swap, and one Milk & Yogurt Group swap. Table 6-4 shows how you could determine how many calories and grams of macronutrients these swaps provide. In this example, the swaps provide 250 calories. Therefore, when you are really craving a specific food you can read the food label (specifically the serving size and calories per serving information) and determine how much you could have of the given food for the 250 calories you have allotted. Ideally the new food would also have about the same number of grams of carbohydrates, proteins, and fats so it would be consistent with your lower-carb eating style. If it is a dessert-type food it should have at least some fats to balance the carbohydrates. Keeping in mind that the carbohydrates and fats in most dessert foods are not the high-quality health-promoting kinds, you would not want to do this too often. If the rest of your food selections for the day are of very high quality and this keeps you satisfied and on track, it is worth it! However, if you start to do this too often, the balance of carbohydrates, proteins, and fats will not be optimal, and your results will likely suffer.

**Table 6-4.**

Determining Calories Provided by Given Swaps for a Meal or Snack

*The example below is for the swaps provided for a snack on the 1500-calorie-per-day plan.*

| Food Groups & Number of Swaps | Calories per Swap | Carbohydrates (grams per swap) | Proteins (grams per swap) | Fats (grams per swap) |
|---|---|---|---|---|
| **1 Fruit** | 60 | 15 | 0 | 0 |
| **1 Protein** | 55 | 0 | 7 | 3 |
| **1 Fat** | 45 | 0 | 0 | 5 |
| **1 Milk** | 90 | 12 | 8 | 0 |
| **Totals** (Add the numbers in each column down) | **250 calories** | **27 grams of carbohydrate** | **15 grams` of protein** | **8 grams of fat** |

*This calculation indicates that 250 calories are available for the snack. As an alternative to using the swaps to create your snack, you could look on the food label of a favorite food and determine the amount you could have that would provide 250 calories. Ideally, that amount would provide roughly the same amount of carbohydrates, proteins, and fats.*

## Troubleshooting Along the Way

When planning a weight management journey, it is rare that you can map your whole trip from start to end perfectly from the very beginning. So far you have a great start—a calorie level, an eating style, menus, and swap lists. However, you may find that you need to adjust your map a bit.

## Dealing with Hunger Pangs

As you start to adjust your eating habits, you are likely to feel a bit hungry at times. However, being very hungry will make it difficult for you to stay on course and reach your destination. So hunger has to be thoughtfully considered. First you need to consider whether it is true "physiological hunger" or "psychological appetite." These two important concepts are further explained in Chapter 9.

If you are losing weight but feeling true physiological hunger throughout the day, think about when you are hungry. If you are hungry most of the day, you should add some swaps to your plan. You can add swaps to meals or snacks. First, try adding additional swaps from the Vegetable Group if possible. Then add swaps from the other food groups as suggested. Make one or two additions and monitor your weight and hunger. The goal is to add swaps until your hunger is manageable, and you are still losing weight (at least about 1 or 2 pounds a month but no more than an average of 1 to 1½ pounds a week). Add swaps in the following order to make sure the mix of carbohydrates, proteins, and fats is best for you: (1) two Vegetable Group swaps, (2) one or two additional Protein Group swaps from the green or yellow subgroups, (3) one Fat Group swap from the green subgroup, and lastly (4) one Fruit Group swap from the green subgroup.

If the weight loss is slow (less than 1 to 2 pounds a month) but you are experiencing hunger at a specific time of the day, try to save one or two swaps from meals to have as a snack at that difficult time. This is to avoid adding extra swaps, which may stop the weight loss altogether. Try to save a Fat Group swap from dinner to match with a swap from the Fruit Group or the Grain& Starch Group saved from lunch or dinner. This would allow for the following combinations:

⦿ Four dried apple rings (plain with no sugar or fats added) and six almonds (1 Fruit Group swap and 1 Fat Group swap)

⦿ Two teaspoons of natural peanut butter and ½ banana (one Fat Group swap and one Fruit Group swap)

⦿ Two teaspoons natural peanut butter and 4-6 whole-wheat crackers (one Fat Group swap and one Grain & Starch Group swap)

If the weight loss is slow and you are hungry, it is especially important to make sure you are doing adequate amounts of physical activity. Refer to Chapter 11 for information on types of physical activity and how to include physical activity into your day. By increasing your physical activity, you may be able to add additional swaps as noted in the second paragraph of this section and still lose weight.

## Timing of Meal and Snack Pit Stops

To minimize the negative effects of insulin resistance, which is high blood insulin and sugar levels, it is important to consider how often you eat during the day. Each time you eat, your blood sugar and insulin levels go up. If you are insulin resistant, they go up higher and take longer than usual to come back down to normal (or at least to pre-eating) levels. Therefore, if you are eating frequently throughout the day, your blood sugar and insulin levels will almost always be high. When levels of insulin and sugar are high for prolonged periods of time they can damage tissues and organs. Therefore, eating only three to four times a day is recommended—three meals and one snack. These events should be at least 4 hours apart. If you feel you have to have a second snack, try to keep it to one or two swaps saved from the Fat Group, such as 6–12 almonds or 10–20 peanuts. Fat in your diet does not cause an increase in blood sugar or insulin levels. However, adding extra fat swaps can make weight loss difficult because of the extra calories they provide, so portion control is critical.

In the morning, a variety of hormones are naturally released to help get you going. Many of these hormones cause your liver to produce sugar and increase the blood level of sugar. This helps provide energy for your body as it needs to start being more active. If you are insulin resistant, the morning is the most difficult time to keep blood sugar levels in or near the normal range, because your liver produces more sugar than it should produce. Therefore, your breakfast meal should not have too many carbohydrates, which when digested add to the problem. To limit carbohydrates at breakfast in the daily plans shown in Table 6-2, there are limited swaps from the

Grain & Starch Group, only half a swap from the Milk & Yogurt Group, and no swaps from the Fruit Group. Fruits are added later in the day. If you are hungry in the morning, you should add swaps from the Protein or Fat Groups.

### Artificial Sweeteners—Friends or Foes

Using artificially sweetened foods and drinks can have mixed results. In the short term, switching from sweetened drinks with hundreds of calories to artificially sweetened drinks with no calories may be helpful because you are taking in fewer calories. However, some research indicates that artificial sweeteners can trick you body into thinking it had real sugar and stimulate an insulin response. Because you are trying to decrease your blood levels of insulin, this is not favorable. In addition, artificially sweetened drinks and beverages can perpetuate your desire for sweet-tasting foods and encourage the consumption of extra desserts and sweets. They also can discourage you from developing preferences for unsweetened foods. Lastly, artificial sweeteners are often used in highly processed foods that are not generally recommended anyway. In summary, you may find it helpful to use artificially sweetened foods and beverages as a crutch in the beginning of your weight-loss journey. However, eventually you should aim to wean yourself off of them. Instead you will learn over time to change your eating habits and your relationship with food, so that you can save swaps to include a moderate serving of your favorite naturally sweetened food on occasion.

## Checking Your Progress

Of course, weight loss is one indicator of progress. However, there are other indicators of progress. Some are subjective and hard to measure, such as feeling better or being more energetic. Being able to wear some of your favorite clothes that had become too small can give you a sense of rejuvenation and progress. You may also feel a new sense of accomplishment and self-confidence as you start working with you new eating style and have success. There are other health indicators that you can ask your health care provider to monitor, such as blood sugar, triglycerides, HDLs, and blood pressure. These health indicators can significantly improve with just a 10% weight loss. (If your starting weight is around 150, 200, 250, or 300 pounds then this would equate to a 15, 20, 25, or 30 pound weight loss, respectively.) Blood sugar levels, blood triglyceride levels, and blood pressure typically respond the fastest. Changes in HDLs typically take longer to respond in a measurable way after you have changed your diet. If your signs of insulin resistance improve significantly and you have started an exercise program, you should consider transitioning to the moderate-carb route. If you do transition, you should continue to monitor your progress, changes in weight, and changes in laboratory values.

Recommended rates and patterns of weight loss are discussed in detail in Chapter 11. Make sure you read this chapter before you lose about 15 to 20 pounds. For now you just need to consider how you will monitor your weight loss. Before you think about how often you weigh yourself, you need to consider how the process of weighing yourself affects your emotional state. Some people can weigh themselves without judging themselves harshly. Many other people, however, experience a lot of negative emotions when weighing themselves. This is referred to as negative self-talk—unpleasant, negative, and often hurtful things you say to yourself. Chapter 10 presents different strategies to help you change your pattern of self-talk. Developing the ability to weigh yourself in an objective, unemotional fashion is very important for long-term success. Doing so will help you stay on course and catch problems early.

It is best to weigh yourself once a week, in the morning, without clothes. Keep in mind that your body weight normally fluctuates a few pounds a week—the taller and heavier you are the more your weight can fluctuate. This is due to changes in water weight, changes in fiber intake, timing of bowel movements, and changes in physical activity levels. In the beginning you will be learning how your weight fluctuates. It is absolutely normal to lose a few pounds, bounce back up a few pounds, and then lose them again. Sometimes you may feel that you are doing everything right, but your weight stays about the same for a few weeks, and then drops a few pounds all in one week. Basically, your weight is not something you can directly control. You can control what you eat and how much you exercise, and eventually your weight will respond. However, it usually does not respond in a very predictable and consistent manner. It is important to keep a record of your weight so that you can observe and learn from the trends. You are looking for a gradual decline over time, meaning over months. Along the way there will be bumps along the road, weight changes that are higher or lower than anticipated. Try not to overreact to these larger-than-normal jumps in your weight. The pattern over time is most important. This topic will be addressed again in Chapter 11.

## Advantages of the Lower-Carb Route

For those who are insulin resistant, the lower-carb route has the advantage of decreasing your blood sugar and blood insulin levels, and therefore reducing insulin resistance. As this occurs the negative effects caused by both high blood sugar and blood insulin will lessen. While you follow your plan, lose weight, and start to exercise, blood sugar levels and triglyceride levels will drop, HDL levels will increase, and blood pressure will drop.[5-8] If you have symptoms of polycystic ovarian syndrome (PCOS), these symptoms will improve as well. When this happens, it is recommended that you maintain your exercise program and transition to the moderate-carb eating style.

In addition, because of your high intake of fiber, antioxidants, phytochemicals, and micronutrients you will also be decreasing your overall risk for heart disease, gastrointestinal disorders, and many types of cancer. Since your intake of animal fats, saturated fats, trans fats, and omega-6 polyunsaturated fats are decreased and your intake of monounsaturated fats and omega-3 polyunsaturated fats are increased, you may also be able to reduce your baseline level of inflammatory processes. This may decrease your risk of heart disease and many other chronic conditions.[4,9-13]

In summary, the lower-carb route allows you to capture the benefits of reduced carbohydrate intake, popular among many diets, without exposing yourself to potential risks due to excessive intakes of animal proteins and saturated or trans fatty acids.[4,14]

## Disadvantages of the Lower-Carb Route
## Taken to the Extreme

*There are no disadvantages to following the lower-carb route as described in this chapter.* However, there are no long-term studies indicating that staying on such a program after you improve your insulin resistance is beneficial. Therefore, it is strongly recommended that you transition to the moderate-carb eating style when your insulin resistance improves. If you select high-quality foods from the green inner circle and continue to exercise, you are likely to maintain your improved insulin sensitivity on the moderate-carb program.

Problems may occur when this approach is taken to the extreme— bringing carbohydrate intake to about 50 grams a day or less and eating excessive amounts of animal protein and saturated or trans fats. This is especially true if you are older than 50 years and if you follow an extremely-low-carbohydrate diet for an extended period of time.[15] An extreme approach has two consequences. First of all, it promotes an excessive intake of animal protein and saturated fat, and to a lesser degree trans fat. A few studies examining very-low-carbohydrate diets that are high in animal protein and fats demonstrated worsening of risk factors for heart disease and decreased blood flow through coronary arteries.[16,17] Second, it severely limits the intake of fiber, antioxidants, and phytochemicals to such a degree that supplementation (as recommended by popular low-carbohydrate diets) cannot meaningfully compensate. Fruits, vegetables, legumes (dried beans, peas, and lentils), and whole grains have hundreds of different phytochemicals that act synergistically to promote optimal health and prevent disease. It is not possible at this time to create supplements that contain meaningful amounts of these nutrients in forms that are easily absorbed. In addition, the relative amounts of nutrients and phytochemicals necessary to support their synergistic effects and promote optimal health are not known. All studies examining the effects of high intakes of *dietary* phytochemicals and antioxidants have shown strongly positive results. However, studies examining the effects of *supplemental* intakes of phytochemicals and antioxidants have often not found positive results. In summary, scientists have gathered a large body of research literature over decades that indicates diets high in animal proteins and saturated fats and low in fiber and phytochemicals increase the risk of heart disease and cancer over time.[4,9,10,12,14,15,18,19]

Bone loss is another issue of concern on very-low-carbohydrate diets. Very-low-carbohydrate diets, those with about 50 grams of carbohydrate a day or less, promote a condition called ketosis. (In some people less than 100 grams of carbohydrates a day can cause ketosis.) Extended periods of ketosis and the need to excrete ketones in urine is associated with loss of calcium in urine as well. Therefore, calcium is leached from bones. Most very-low-carbohydrate diets also limit or exclude milk because of its 12 grams of carbohydrate per cup. This combination of increased calcium losses and limited calcium intake will likely lead to bone loss. The problem is intensified by most people's limited physical activity levels. Physical activity strengthens bones. However, even if you exercise ½ to 1 hour a day, you are likely to be rather sedentary the other 23 hours of the day—or at least most of them.[20]

Kidney damage is often brought up to be a risk for those following a high-protein diet. However, there is limited research to substantiate this claim. Some studies indicate that high-protein diets can accelerate loss of kidney function (or kidney damage) in people who have a preexisting mild loss of kidney function. This is especially true if the dietary protein is from nondairy animal protein sources (such as meat). However, in people with normal kidney function, it does not appear that short-term high-protein diets have a negative effect on kidney function. The problem is that there are no signs or symptoms of early kidney problems. You may have some decline in kidney function and not know it yet. The following factors can increase your risk for kidney problems: high blood pressure, diabetes, and age over 65 years. In other words, many people who are insulin resistant are at increased risk. Therefore, following a very-low-carbohydrate diet with a very-high-protein content is not recommended, especially for those who are insulin resistant and have high blood pressure or diabetes.[21,22]

Relatively short-term studies examining the effects of extremely-low-carbohydrate diets compared to low-fat diets have been conducted. Such studies have not shown negative changes in some markers of disease risk when following low-carbohydrate diets for just 1 year. However, there are some limitations to how the studies were conducted. No studies have been conducted long enough to examine resulting rates of disease occurrence. Studies exploring the effects of diet on rates of heart disease or cancer would require following patients eating different diets for at least 10 years. Researchers would then compare the rates of diseases among the groups eating different diets. The 1-year study that has been completed compared weight lost by subjects following a very-low-carbohydrate diet and those following a low-fat diet. Researchers found that those following the extremely-low-carbohydrate diet lost more weight in the first 3 months. However, after following subjects for 1 year, they found that participants following the lower-carbohydrate diet gained weight back more quickly so that by the end of the study there was no significant difference in weight lost between the two groups. Therefore, participants on the extremely-low-carbohydrate diet did not lose more weight at the end of a year, yet sacrificed the known benefits of a diet high in phytochemicals and fiber.[5-7]

The lower-carb approach explained in this chapter gives you the benefits of decreased carbohydrate intake (especially refined carbohydrates and sweeteners), as well as the benefits of a diet high in natural food-based phytochemicals, fibers, and micronutrients. Why take the risk of potentially increasing your risk for heart disease, cancer, osteoporosis, and kidney problems when research has shown that your weight loss will not be greater after 1 year on such an extreme approach?

You can read Chapters 7 and 8 for a detailed description of the moderate-carb and high-carb route. Over time, consider transitioning to one of these styles as many years of research confirm the benefits of such eating styles in the long run. However, for more practical information on changing your eating and exercise habits and planning your weight management journey, skip to Chapters 9, 10, and 11.

### *Nitty-Gritty Details Regarding Insulin Resistance*

A further explanation of insulin resistance will help you understand why a lower-carbohydrate diet will help you lose weight and be healthy. However, it is not necessary to understand all of this information to get started. If you are interested, read this section as you are starting to change your diet and follow your map. The process by which insulin resistance and the resulting high insulin levels cause problems is described in this section. First of all, there are documented relationships among obesity, proinflammation states, prothrombolytic states, and insulin resistance. However, which comes first and how one causes another has not been fully worked out. Inflammation is a function of the immune system and is part of the process of heart disease. Thrombosis refers to clot formation, which is part of plaque formation and heart disease. What is becoming increasingly clear is that fat cells, especially those in the abdominal region, secrete many powerful chemicals that increase inflammation and thrombosis. Obesity and inflammation in turn increase insulin resistance. The result is a vicious self-perpetuating cycle, which can be broken with decreased calorie and carbohydrate intake, increased physical activity, and weight loss.[23–28]

Fat cells also store fat and normally release fatty acids into the blood only when they are needed. However, with insulin resistance fat cells release too many fatty acids into the blood too often throughout the day. These fatty acids are picked up by your liver, and in response the liver makes triglycerides and a type of cholesterol package called VLDLs. Triglycerides get packaged inside VLDLs, which carry triglycerides around your blood. There are many types of cholesterol packages that carry cholesterol and triglycerides. The ones you might be more familiar with are LDLs and HDLs. High LDL levels increase your risk for heart disease, because they tend to get incorporated into plaque in one or more of your coronary arteries. This makes plaque thicker, which reduces blood flow through the vessel and to the heart muscle. Eventually the plaque gets so thick that one or more blood vessels get completely closed off. This causes a heart attack.

## *Nitty-Gritty Details Regarding Insulin Resistance (continued)*

HDLs protect against heart disease, because they pick up extra cholesterol in the body and bring it back to the liver. The liver can get rid of cholesterol by making necessary products, such as hormones, from it. The liver also makes bile from cholesterol. Bile is needed to digest fats. Once made in the liver bile is stored in the gallbladder until needed. When you eat fat, the gallbladder squirts bile into your digestive tract. If you have a lot of fiber in your diet, the bile gets dragged out of your body when you have a bowel movement. This is the best way to get cholesterol out of your body. Therefore, a combination of high HDLs and a high fiber diet decreases your risk for heart disease. If you do not have a lot of fiber in your diet the bile gets absorbed back into your body, and the cholesterol gets recycled.

When insulin-resistant fat cells release fatty acids, the liver makes more triglycerides and VLDLs. In the blood, increased VLDLs have a negative effect on the metabolism of HDLs, and ultimately cause their breakdown. Therefore, high triglycerides and VLDLs are almost always associated with low HDLs. High VLDLs can also negatively impact LDLs. Although the VLDLs do not change the number of LDLs, they cause the LDLs to become chemically changed. This change makes the LDLs denser and more likely to be incorporated into artery plaque. The combination of high triglycerides and VLDLs, low HDLs, and dense LDLs dramatically increases the risk for heart disease.[3,4,19,29–31]

Insulin resistance also leads to increases in blood pressure through a few different processes. Insulin normally leads the kidneys to conserve sodium and water. The kidneys have mechanisms to detect fluid volume, and can limit the ability of insulin to cause retention of sodium and water. With insulin resistance, the kidneys do not get the message when fluid volume is adequate, and sodium and water continue to be retained. The resulting increased blood volume increase blood pressure. Insulin also helps to keep blood vessels dilated or open. With insulin resistance, the vessels do not respond to this action of insulin, and as a result blood vessels are constricted or partially closed. Therefore, insulin resistance causes more blood to try to flow through more narrow vessels, leading to increased pressure within the vessels. This is measured as an increase in blood pressure.[21,22,32]

***Nitty-Gritty Details Regarding Insulin Resistance*** *(continued)*

In women, insulin is thought to encourage the normal development of ovarian follicles so that each month one follicle becomes dominant and ovulates. With insulin resistance, this selection process is not effective, and dysfunctional follicles result. This leads to multiple small cysts, which contain viable eggs inside dysfunctional cysts. With weight loss and improved insulin sensitivity symptoms improve.[33]

Insulin resistance almost always leads to type 2 diabetes over time. Initially, the high levels of insulin produced successfully compensate for the cells' inability to use it well. However, eventually your pancreas (the organ responsible for making insulin) can no longer keep up the high production rate. The amount of insulin produced is no longer adequate to compensate sufficiently. When this happens, blood sugar levels increase and ultimately exceed the limit set as diagnostic criteria for type 2 diabetes.

As described above, advanced insulin resistance syndrome is a cluster of disorders related to the body's inability to use insulin effectively: type 2 diabetes, hypertension, dyslipidemia, PCOS (in women only), and central obesity.

## *Important Points To Remember from Chapter 6*

- You can lower your blood levels of sugar and insulin by doing the following: decrease the carbohydrates in your diet, improve the quality of those carbohydrates, and balance the carbohydrates with healthy proteins and fats. This leads to decreased insulin resistance, and a decreased risk for associated conditions, such as heart disease and type 2 diabetes.

- Structured lower-carb eating plans at the appropriate calorie level will start you off on your weight management journey.

◉ Learn how to modify your plan and include favorite foods to help you stay on course and reach your destination.

◉ Expect to stumble or lose your way along your journey—but get back on course quickly by objectively recognizing your missteps and not over-reacting.

◉ Begin to consider your strategy to monitor your weight and check your progress. More detail about this is given in Chapter 10.

◉ The lower-carb route presented allows you to benefit from decreased carbohydrate intake, as well as from high intakes of phytochemicals, fibers, and micronutrients. It also allows you to avoid the potential risks of excessive protein or saturated/trans fat intake.

# THE MODERATE-CARB ROUTE

### *What You Will Discover in Chapter 7*

◉ The moderate-carb plan provides the known benefits of a plant-based, high-fiber diet with moderate amounts of healthy fats for those with uncertain insulin sensitivity.

◉ For your selected calorie level, you will find an eating plan with the appropriate number of swaps from each food group for your meals and snack.

◉ You may need to modify your plan for optimal benefits. Guidelines for doing so are provided in this chapter.

◉ Guidelines for modifying this approach for a higher protein trial are provided. During this trial, fats are kept at 30% of total calories.

◉ Timing of meals and snacks is important.

## How the Moderate-Carb Route Can Get You to Your Destination

The moderate-carb route is the best route if you are not clearly insulin resistant or very insulin sensitive. It is also a good choice if you have been following the lower-carb plan with resulting weight loss and improvements in blood sugar, blood triglyercide, and blood pressure measurements. At this point your insulin resistance will have decreased, especially if you have increased your physical activity. You can then benefit from the known health-promoting effects of a more plant-based diet higher in fiber and phytochemicals than the lower-carb plan.[1-7]

Refer to Chapter 5, especially Table 5-4, for a full explanation of the factors used to determine your status regarding insulin resistance or sensitivity. In summary, if you are insulin resistant, your body makes appropriate amounts of insulin, but your cells cannot use it to usher blood sugar into your cells. If you are sensitive to insulin, then your body makes insulin in appropriate amounts, and your cells use it well. Your body needs insulin to push sugar that is in your blood into your cells, where it is used for energy. The carbohydrates in foods (such as foods from the Grain & Starch Group, the Fruit Group, and the Milk & Yogurt Group) are broken down into sugar and absorbed into your blood. Insulin is secreted in response to this. Within a few hours the sugar is normally transported into your cells, and your blood sugar levels go back down to pre-eating levels. Your laboratory values will indicate whether you are sensitive or resistant to insulin, as shown in Table 5-4.

Your sensitivity to insulin determines the effect sugar has on your body. Sugar in your diet causes an increase in blood sugar and a subsequent increase in insulin levels. If you are sensitive to insulin, it works to bring the blood sugar levels down. However, highly sweetened foods and drinks (including fruit drinks, fruit juices, and flavored milks), especially those low in fiber and fat, make this rise and drop in blood sugar more dramatic. For some people, these drops in blood sugar can happen quickly and are associated with feeling very hungry, shaky, or sluggish shortly after eating. The increased hunger can lead to subsequent overeating. Individuals diagnosed with hypoglycemia will recognize these symptoms. A moderate-carb eating style is appropriate in this case. If you are not very sensitive to insulin, your body compensates by producing extra insulin in order to increase effectiveness. These higher-than-normal insulin levels and insulin resistance cause serious problems, such as high triglycerides, high blood pressure, and type 2 diabetes. For more information on this, read the section called the "Nitty-Gritty Details Regarding Insulin Resistance" at the end of Chapter 6. Whether you are insulin resistant or sensitive, you should reduce the amount of sugar in your diet to avoid negative consequences. In the moderate-carb eating style, you should select most of your Grain & Starch swaps and Fruit swaps from the green inner subgroup to avoid added sweeteners. It is important to know the amount of sugars in the foods you typically eat.

Common sweeteners are high-fructose corn syrup, corn syrup, and sugar. Refined grains and starches that are in low in fiber, such as white bread, white rice, or pasta, can also result in rapid increases in blood sugar levels. Therefore, high-fiber, unprocessed grains and starches, and whole fruits are highly recommended. The fiber in these foods slows down the digestion and absorption of sugar and promotes a more stable blood sugar level. This in turn makes you feel full and more satisfied for a longer period. Many Americans eat three to five times the recommended amount of sugar without even realizing it, because food manufacturers add sweeteners to almost all processed foods. As a rough rule of thumb, you should eat less than 25 grams of added sugars or other sweeteners per 1,000 calories. For the eating plans in this book the added sugar and sweetener limits would be as follows: 30 grams of sugar in the 1200-calorie plan; 38 grams in the 1500-calorie plan; 45 grams in the 1800-calorie plan; 53 grams in the 2100-calorie plan; and 60 grams in the 2400-calorie plan. Remember, these limits are for *added sugar* and do not include the sugar that naturally occurs in fruit (about 15 grams of sugar per swap), some types of vegetables (5 grams of sugar per swap of some vegetables like carrots and beets), and milk or yogurt (12 grams of sugar per swap). These naturally occurring sugars are already accounted for in the eating plans in this book.

It is important to become more aware of how much added sugar you eat and drink, because hidden sugars are a big source of calories. You can track your sugar intake by looking on food labels and noting the grams of sugar listed just under the grams of total carbohydrate. This number, however, includes sugars naturally found in milk and fruit as well as added sugars. So when you eat or drink milk- or fruit-based products, you need to do a little extra math. You can estimate the added sugars in a milk-based food or drink by subtracting 12 from the grams of sugar in a cup of the milk or yogurt product. For example, if a cup of flavored milk has 26 grams of sugar, you would subtract 12 grams from 26 grams. There would be an estimated 14 grams of added sugar per cup of the flavored milk. For comparison, there are 4 grams of sugar in a paper packet of sugar. Therefore, a cup of the flavored milk would have 3½ packets of sugar added to it. On the food label it is also important to notice the number of servings in a container, because many seemingly single-use containers really have 2 servings per container. Therefore, if the bottle of the flavored milk was 16 ounces and you drank the whole bottle, it would provide 28 grams of added sugar, or 7 packets of sugar. This is about the same amount of added sugar as in one 8-ounce glass of soda.

Fruit-based products have to be considered in a similar fashion. For example, applesauce is typically sweetened and has about 24 grams of sugar per ½ cup. You can assume 15 grams is natural sugar in the fruit, and subtract 15 grams from 24 grams. Nine grams would be the estimated amount of added sugar, or a little bit more than two packets of sugar. Choosing unsweetened natural applesauce allows you to avoid the intake of these added sugars. You can see how easily the grams of added sugar can add up over the course of a day.

The next section of this chapter provides detailed information on creating a very structured moderate-carb plan. It is important to review and understand this information. For most people, it is also helpful to try to follow a detailed plan for some time before transitioning to a less-structured plan. However, everybody is unique and some people simply do not respond well to such a structured approach. For example, for some people the effort required to follow the structured plan leads them to think about food too much and be too restrictive. This can backfire and lead to more frequent overeating episodes. Be aware of this potential consequence. If this is the case for you, review the information below and keep a general sense of the structure in your mind. Then go to Chapters 9 and 10 for other strategies you can use to craft a more casual approach to the moderate-carb eating style. Also refer to the menus in Menus and Recipes.

A *less structured or casual approach can work, but the results are typically slower. This is okay, as long as you prepare yourself for slower weight loss, and adjust your expectations accordingly.* Simply accept the slower weight loss as progress that is more likely to be permanent, for many reasons discussed in Chapter 11.

## The Detailed Map

On the moderate-carb route, carbohydrates provide 50% of total calories. Fats provide 30% of total calories, and proteins provide 20% of total calories. It is essential that the majority of your carbohydrates come from high-fiber foods that are minimally processed and do not contain added sweeteners (especially high-fructose corn syrup). These foods tend to have a lower glycemic index as well. (For more on the topic of glycemic index refer to Chapter 3.) Choosing the best foods is easy to do with the Bull's-Eye Food Guide system, because you simply have to select most of your foods from all of the food groups from the green inner circle. If you have high LDL cholesterol, making your selections from the Protein Group and the Fat Group from the green inner circle will help to decrease them. To lower LDL cholesterol levels, also check the ingredient lists on packaged foods and avoid partially hydrogenated and hydrogenated oils. This does not mean that you can never have a favorite food from the red outer circle, but you have to plan to work some of these foods into your day. By working some of your favorite foods from the red outer circle into your plan, you increase the likelihood that you can stay on the program long enough to get to a healthy weight and then *stay there*. With the Bull's-Eye Food Guide system, you never have to count calories or grams of carbohydrates, proteins, or fats. All you have to do is simply keep track of the number of swaps you have from the six food groups each day and make most of your selections from the green inner circle. Review the food groups and the idea of swapping in Chapter 4 before finalizing your plan. For now, remember that a swap of food is the amount of a specific food that provides the number of calories assigned to the food group in which it is placed. A swap is not necessarily the amount of food you can eat at a meal or snack, because you may have more than one swap from a specific food group at a meal or snack. Consider a swap of food simply as an assigned volume of food used as a counting unit to keep track of calories, carbohydrates, proteins, and fats.

First, note the calorie level you selected for yourself in Chapter 5, Table 5-1 or 5-2. Then refer to Table 7-1. Table 7-1 indicates the number of swaps from the six different food groups suggested each day based on your calorie level. For example, reading down the column labeled "1500 Calories/Day," there are six Vegetable Group swaps, three Fruit Group swaps, six Grain & Starch Group swaps, five Protein Group swaps, five Fat Group swaps, and two Milk & Yogurt Group swaps. If you cannot tolerate milk or yogurt, try soymilk products (the soymilk should be low-fat with less than 12 grams of sugar per serving, making it comparable to cow's milk). If that does not work for you, trade in your two swaps from the Milk & Yogurt Group for one swap from the Protein Group and one swap from the Fruit Group. In addition, talk to your health care provider about taking a calcium supplement to ensure adequate calcium intake.

Remember, it is extremely important that most swaps from the Grain & Starch group come from the green inner circle. One, or at the most two, swaps can be saved for a food in the yellow or red circles. All fruits should come from the green inner circle, and most vegetables should come from the green inner circle. Protein selections can come from the green inner circle or the yellow middle circle, but selections from the red outer circle should be extremely limited. Also, keep in mind that if you do pick a food from the outer circle of the protein group you need to save fats for that food as well. Both of your swaps from the Milk & Yogurt Group should be from the green inner or yellow middle circles. If possible, all of your selections from the Fat Group should come from the green inner circle. If you need to use a bread spread, try one from the middle yellow group that is made from liquid vegetable oils that are not partially hydrogenated. As an alternative, you can try natural peanut butter on your bread or dip bread into a teaspoon of olive oil flavored with herbs. Another option would be to make homemade yogurt cheese. To make yogurt cheese simply do the following: (1) measure a cup of plain fat-free yogurt, (2) line a strainer with

**Table 7-1.**
The Moderate-Carb Plans by Calorie Level

| Food Group | Swaps per Day from Each Food Group at Different Calorie Levels | | | | |
|---|---|---|---|---|---|
| | 1200 Calories per Day | 1500 Calories per Day | 1800 Calories per Day | 2100 Calories per Day | 2400 Calories per Day |
| Vegetable* | 6 | 6 | 6 | 6 | 6 |
| Fruit | 2 | 3 | 3 | 4 | 4 |
| Grain & Starch | 4 | 6 | 8 | 10 | 12 |
| Protein | 4 | 5 | 7 | 8 | 9 |
| Fat | 4 | 5 | 6 | 6 | 8 |
| Milk & Yogurt | 2 | 2 | 2 | 2 | 2 |

*For vegetables, these numbers are minimums because Vegetable Group swaps are unlimited.

a coffee filter and place the strainer over a bowl, (3) scoop the yogurt into the coffee filter and cover with plastic wrap or foil, (4) refrigerate for 24 hours, (5) drain liquid that collects in the bowl, (6) refrigerate for an additional 12 to 24 hours, and (7) remove thickened yogurt and place in a resealable tub. You can flavor the yogurt according to your taste preferences. For example, you can use scallions and a minced olive, or you can use vanilla extract and cinnamon. The possibilities are endless. After flavoring the yogurt, you can use it on crackers, toast, or sandwiches, and you can use it as a vegetable dip. Made in this way, 8 tablespoons of the yogurt cheese count as one Milk & Yogurt swap, therefore, 4 tablespoons would only count as half of a Milk & Yogurt Group swap.

Fats found in foods in the outer circle of the Grain & Starch Group, the Protein Group, and the Milk & Yogurt Group are typically high in trans fats or saturated fats. Therefore, fat swaps that you save to put toward these foods should be limited as well, because these fats are known to increase LDL cholesterol levels in genetically susceptible people.

The next step is to decide how to distribute the swaps from the different food groups throughout the course of the day. Whenever possible, balance carbohydrates from food in the Grain & Starch Group or the Fruit Group with a food from the Protein Group, the Fat Group, or the Milk & Yogurt Group. This applies to planning meals and snacks. In Table 7-2 swaps from the different food groups at each calorie level are distributed into three meals and one snack. On the chart, highlight the calorie level that you have previously selected. Note how many swaps you have for each meal and snack. In Menus and Recipes, you will find daily menus to follow. You can also use the Swap Lists for each of the food groups to modify the menus or create new menus. See Tables 7-3 A and B for an example of selections made from the Swap Lsts to create a lunch at the 1500-calorie per day level. If you do not like a particular item selected in these tables or in the menus in Menus and Recipes, you can go to the Swap Lists to trade them in for swaps of different foods in the same group. For example, in Table 7-3A there is a note that you may not like grapes, or may not have them available at the time. Therefore, the grapes can be traded in for one swap of a different fruit selected from the Fruit Group Swap List, such as 1 apple, ½ banana, or 12 cherries. The sample daily menus in Menus and Recipes demonstrate this point.

Many people's first response to menus like the ones in Tables 7-3A and B is that they think it looks like too much food. This may be for a few reasons. First of all, many of the foods selected have a low caloric density. As described in Chapter 3, this means that there are only a small amount of calories for a given amount of food because the food is high in fiber or water. Second, moderate amounts of many types of foods are used in combinations in meals to best balance carbohydrates, proteins, and fats. Finally, different types of foods are selected to provide a wide variety of nutrients, fibers, and phytochemicals. This also makes the display of food appear more satisfying and interesting. The lunch menus shown in Tables 7-3A and B have about 370 calories. By comparison, a typical sandwich from a deli with no side dishes or drinks would provide at least 850 calories, and not nearly as many nutrients, fiber, or phytochemicals.

## Table 7-2.
### Swaps of Each Food Group by Calorie Level and Meal

| Meal | 1200 Calories per Day | 1500 Calories per Day | 1800 Calories per Day | 2100 Calories per Day | 2400 Calories per Day |
|---|---|---|---|---|---|
| **Breakfast** | | | | | |
| Vegetable Group | | | | | |
| Fruit Group | 1 | 1 | 1 | 1 | 1 |
| Grain & Starch Group | 1 | 2 | 2 | 2 | 3 |
| Protein Group | 1 | 1 | 1 | 1 | 1 |
| Fat Group | 1 | 1 | 1 | 1 | 1 |
| Milk & Yogurt Group | 1 | 1 | 1 | 1 | 1 |
| **Lunch** | | | | | |
| Vegetable Group | 2 | 2 | 2 | 2 | 2 |
| Fruit Group | | 1 | 1 | 1 | 1 |
| Grain & Starch Group | 1 | 2 | 2 | 2 | 3 |
| Protein Group | 1 | 1 | 2 | 2 | 2 |
| Fat Group | 1 | 1 | 2 | 2 | 2 |
| Milk & Yogurt Group | | | | | |
| **Dinner** | | | | | |
| Vegetable Group | 4 | 4 | 4 | 4 | 4 |
| Fruit Group | | | | | |
| Grain & Starch Group | 2 | 2 | 2 | 4 | 4 |
| Protein Group | 2 | 3 | 4 | 4 | 5 |
| Fat Group | 1 | 2 | 2 | 2 | 3 |
| Milk & Yogurt Group | | | | | |
| **Snacks** | | | | | |
| Vegetable Group | | | | | |
| Fruit Group | 1 | 1 | 1 | 2 | 2 |
| Grain & Starch Group | | | 2 | 2 | 2 |
| Protein Group | | | | 1 | 1 |
| Fat Group | 1 | 1 | 1 | 1 | 2 |
| Milk & Yogurt Group | 1 | 1 | 1 | 1 | 1 |

**Table 7-3A.**
A Sample Lunch from the 1500 Calorie Moderate-Carb Plan **Sandwich** Option

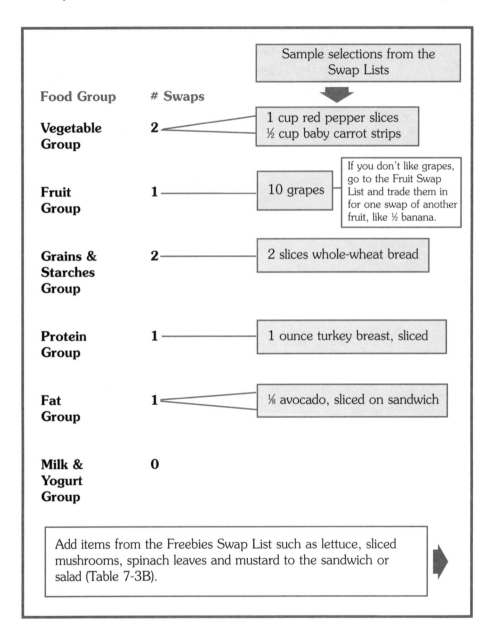

| Food Group | # Swaps | Sample selections from the Swap Lists |
|---|---|---|
| **Vegetable Group** | 2 | 1 cup red pepper slices / ½ cup baby carrot strips |
| **Fruit Group** | 1 | 10 grapes — If you don't like grapes, go to the Fruit Swap List and trade them in for one swap of another fruit, like ½ banana. |
| **Grains & Starches Group** | 2 | 2 slices whole-wheat bread |
| **Protein Group** | 1 | 1 ounce turkey breast, sliced |
| **Fat Group** | 1 | ⅛ avocado, sliced on sandwich |
| **Milk & Yogurt Group** | 0 | |

Add items from the Freebies Swap List such as lettuce, sliced mushrooms, spinach leaves and mustard to the sandwich or salad (Table 7-3B).

## Table 7-3B.
A Sample Lunch from the 1500 Calorie Moderate-Carb Plan **Salad** Option

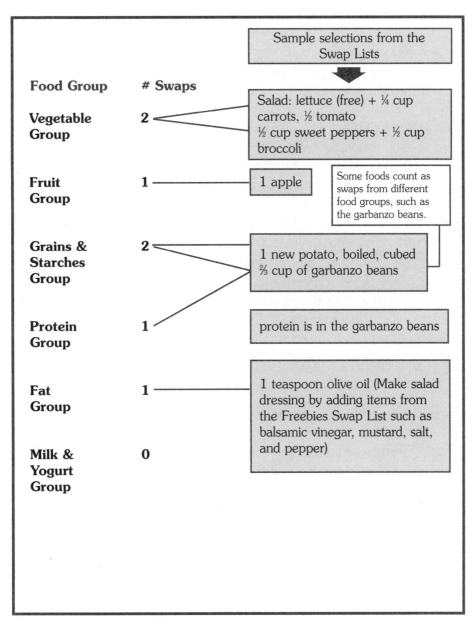

| Food Group | # Swaps | Sample selections from the Swap Lists |
|---|---|---|
| **Vegetable Group** | **2** | Salad: lettuce (free) + ¼ cup carrots, ½ tomato<br>½ cup sweet peppers + ½ cup broccoli |
| **Fruit Group** | **1** | 1 apple |
| **Grains & Starches Group** | **2** | 1 new potato, boiled, cubed<br>⅔ cup of garbanzo beans |
| **Protein Group** | **1** | protein is in the garbanzo beans |
| **Fat Group** | **1** | 1 teaspoon olive oil (Make salad dressing by adding items from the Freebies Swap List such as balsamic vinegar, mustard, salt, and pepper) |
| **Milk & Yogurt Group** | **0** | |

Some foods count as swaps from different food groups, such as the garbanzo beans.

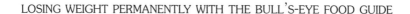

Another common response to the swaps, meal patterns, and menus is frustration with the prospect of weighing and measuring foods and drinks. You may also be concerned about the portion sizes, which are typically much smaller than what you were previously eating and drinking. To resolve these issues and barriers to moving forward, keep in mind that to start losing weight, you simply have to eat less than you are currently eating until weight loss starts. Therefore, you may want to start off by determining how much you are currently eating. For a few days write down what you eat and figure out how many swaps from each food group you usually have at each meal and snack. Compare your usual number of swaps per meals and snacks to the numbers suggested. Next, plan to gradually reduce the number of swaps you are currently eating to get closer to the suggested number of swaps. As you make each gradual reduction in swaps, monitor your weight for a few days. Reduce the number of swaps until weight loss starts. You are likely to find that you start to lose weight when you just get close to eating the suggested number of swaps.

You will soon develop a system of planning your meals, food shopping, and cooking that allows you to put healthy, satisfying meals together quickly. At first this will probably require extra planning time as you develop your new habits and systems. After a while the new habits will come easily, and the time necessary to shop and cook will decrease.

### Considering Alcohol Intake

Alcohol needs to be limited for many health reasons, as well as because of the calories it provides. If you are already in the habit of having an alcoholic drink, you can continue to have one alcoholic drink a day—but no more. This should *not* be consumed on an empty stomach when it will have the most dramatic and negative effect on your liver's metabolic processes. Instead, have it with or immediately after dinner. One alcoholic drink is equivalent to 5 ounces of a dry wine, 12 ounces of beer, or 1½ ounces of 80-proof distilled spirits plain or with a noncaloric mixer. If you are not in the habit of drinking alcohol, you should not start now!

## Avoiding Getting Lost

The best way to avoid getting lost is to study your map before you start your journey. Using the menus is a good way to get started right away. While you are doing this, spend time learning the following: (1) the number of swaps from each of the food groups at your calorie level for each meal and snack as shown in Table 7-2; (2) the swap lists for each food group and subgroup of the Bull's-Eye Guide; (3) the concept of swapping as described in the beginning of Chapter 4; and (4) the description of each food group and subgroup as described in Chapter 4. Learning this information will allow you to modify the daily menus in Menus and Recipes and create an unlimited number of menus for meals and snacks.

In Chapters 9 and 10, you will learn many new strategies to help you develop new healthy eating and exercise habits. It will take you time to work with these strategies to change unhealthy habits and change your relationship with food. Most often, it is first necessary to become more aware of why and when you eat, and then to start to tease apart unhealthy habits in which eating is tied to emotions (such as stress, boredom, or anger) or specific behaviors (such as television viewing). For now, suffice it to say that along your journey you will at times lose your way—overeat, make many selections from the red outer circle, or stop exercising. *This is to be expected.* The biggest indicator of your overall progress and long-term success is how quickly you can get back on your planned route. This requires that you simply acknowledge your missteps and, without a lot of negativity, turn back on course. Permanent weight loss is a process that takes time, but the process is well worth the time and effort in terms of the permanence of the weight lost and the improvements in your overall health.

So what about the times when you really want a piece of cake or some other favorite dessert? You can add these items on occasion, but you have to plan ahead a bit. For example, imagine you are going to a birthday party and you know you will want a piece of cake. An average piece of birthday cake counts as two swaps from the Grain & Starch Group and two swaps from the Fat Group. To save swaps for the cake, you would have a lot of vegetables and your protein swaps (two to five swaps of meat, fish, or chicken) for dinner. However, you would skip the starchy side dish and fats and save those swaps for the piece of cake. Of course this is not ideal, because you are having less-healthy foods from the outer circle instead of healthy foods from the green inner circle. However, it is realistic and allows you to have some of your favorite foods while staying on your plan.

You can take this idea of being flexible one step further by using the information in Chapter 4, Table 4-1. In Table 4-1 you are given the calories and grams of carbohydrates, proteins, and fats provided by a swap of each of the food groups. If you are following the 1500-calorie per day, moderate-carb route you would have the following swaps for snack: one Fruit Group swap, one Fat Group swap, and one Milk & Yogurt Group swap. Table 7-4 shows how you could determine how many calories and grams of macronutrients these swaps provide. In this example, the swaps provide 195 calories. Therefore, when you are really craving a specific food you can read the food label (specifically the serving size and calories per serving information) and determine how much you could have of the given food for the 195 calories you have allotted. Ideally the new food would also have about the same number of grams of carbohydrates, proteins, and fats so it would be consistent with your moderate-carb eating style. If it is a dessert-type food, it should have at least some fats to balance the carbohydrates. Keeping in mind that the carbohydrates and fats in most dessert foods are not the high-quality, health-promoting kinds, you would not want to do this too often. If the rest of your food selections for the day are of very high quality and this keeps you satisfied and on track, it is worth it! However, if you start to do this too often, the balance of carbohydrates, proteins, and fats will not be optimal and your results will likely suffer.

## *Troubleshooting Along the Way*

When planning a weight management journey, it is rare that you can map your whole trip from start to end perfectly from the very beginning. So far you have a great start—a calorie level, an eating style, menus, and swap lists. However, you may find that you need to adjust your map a bit.

**Table 7-4.**

Determining Calories Provided by Given Swaps for a Meal or Snack

The example below is for the swaps provided for snack on the 1500-calorie per day plan.

| Food Groups & Number of Swaps | Calories per Swap | Carbohydrates (grams per swap) | Proteins (grams per swap) | Fats (grams per swap) |
|---|---|---|---|---|
| **1 Fruit** | 60 | 15 | 0 | 0 |
| **1 Fat** | 45 | 0 | 0 | 5 |
| **1 Milk** | 90 | 12 | 8 | 0 |
| **Totals** (Add the numbers in each column down.) | **195 Calories** | **27 grams of carbohydrate** | **8 grams of protein** | **5 grams of fat** |

This calculation indicates that 195 calories are available for the snack. As an alternative to using the swaps to create your snack, you could look on the food label of a favorite food and determine the amount you could have that would provide 195 calories. Ideally, that amount would provide roughly the same amount of carbohydrates, proteins, and fats as well.

## Dealing with Hunger Pangs

As you start to adjust your eating habits, you are likely to feel a bit hungry at times. Being very hungry, however, will make it difficult for you to stay on course and reach your destination, so hunger has to be thoughtfully considered. First you need to consider whether it is true "physiological hunger" or "psychological appetite." These important topics are explained in detail in Chapter 9.

If you are losing weight but feeling true physiological hunger throughout the day, think about when you are hungry. If you are hungry most of the day, you should add some swaps to your plan. You can add swaps to meals or snacks. First, try adding additional swaps from the Vegetable Group if possible. Then add swaps from the other food groups as suggested. Make one or two additions and monitor your weight and hunger. The goal is to add swaps until your hunger is manageable, and you are still losing weight (at least about 1 or 2 pounds a month but no more than an average of 1 to 1½ pounds a week). Add swaps in the following order to make sure the mix of carbohydrates, proteins, and fats is best for you: (1) two Vegetable Group swaps, (2) one or two additional Protein Group swaps from the green or yellow subgroups, (3) one Grain & Starch Group swap from the green subgroup, and lastly (4) one Fruit Group swap from the green subgroup.

If the weight loss is slow (less than 1 to 2 pounds a month), but you are experiencing hunger at a specific time of the day, try to save one or two swaps from meals to have as a snack at that difficult time. This is to avoid adding extra swaps, which may stop the weight loss altogether. Try to save a half of a swap from the Milk & Yogurt Group from breakfast to match with a full or a half of a swap from the Fruit Group or a full or half of a swap from the Grain & Starch Group saved from lunch or dinner. This would allow for the following combinations:

- A smoothie made with ½ cup skim milk (half of a Milk & Yogurt Group swap) and ¼ banana or ½ peach (half of a Fruit Group swap) blended with ice (You can also add freebies like a sprinkle of cinnamon and a dash of vanilla.)

- A yogurt parfait with ½ cup plain nonfat yogurt (half of a Milk & Yogurt Group swap) layered with ¼ banana thinly sliced (half of a Fruit Group swap) and 1½ tablespoons of Grape-Nuts (half of a Grain & Starch Group swap)

- ¾ cup puffed rice cereal (half of a Grain & Starch Group swap), ½ cup of 1% milk (half of a Milk & Yogurt Group swap), and 1 tablespoon raisins (half of a Fruit Group swap)

If the weight loss is slow and you are hungry, it is especially important to make sure you are doing adequate amounts of physical activity. Refer to Chapter 11 for guidelines regarding the types and amounts of physical activity recommended. By increasing your physical activity, you may be able to add additional swaps as noted in the second paragraph of this section and still lose weight.

## Timing of Meal and Snack Pit Stops

In general, eating three to four times a day is recommended—three meals and one snack. However, as much as possible the timing of your meals and snacks should be guided by your level of hunger. This is fully discussed in Chapter 9. For now, it is important to understand that going long periods of time without eating may lead to the unnecessary breakdown of muscle tissue. An adequate level of blood sugar (between 60 and 100 milligrams per deciliter of blood) is necessary for your body to function best. As time passes since your last eating event, your blood sugar decreases. As this happens your liver is signaled to make sugar. Your liver has some stored carbohydrate called glycogen that it easily breaks down into sugar molecules. However, after following a diet low enough in calories to promote weight loss for some time, these stores may be low. Therefore, your liver has to make glucose from scratch. Unfortunately, your body cannot make glucose from fats, but it can make glucose from amino acids, the building blocks of protein and muscle tissue. When you go long periods of time without eating, your body is more likely to turn to muscle tissue as a source of amino acids to make glucose. Over time, this could lead to the loss of excessive amounts of muscle tissue, which makes further weight loss more difficult. To avoid this, you should not skip breakfast. Other meals and a snack should not be much more than 4 to 6 hours apart, especially if you are susceptible to low blood sugar as indicated by feelings of shakiness and headaches after not eating for a prolonged time. If you are susceptible to these feelings, it might be helpful to divide your lunch swaps into a smaller lunch and a snack. For example, you may want to save your fat swap and a fruit swap if possible. You can use these swaps for 2 teaspoons of natural peanut butter on an apple, or 6 almonds and 2 tablespoons of raisins for a snack a few hours after lunch.

### *Experimenting with Protein*

Research on the potential role of dietary protein in weight control is in its infancy. This moderate-carb meal plan provides a springboard for you to experiment with increasing levels of protein to help with weight loss and appetite control *if you want to try something different*. This approach is different than the lower-carb approach, because the fat content remains at about 30% of total calories. Protein is increased by taking away carbohydrates from the Grain & Starch Group. Because there is only a little research on this approach, it was not considered as a primary eating style. However, it may be worth a try if a higher-protein eating style is consistent with your general food preferences.[8–12] In order to try this approach without exposing yourself to potential negative effects of saturated fats, the vast majority of protein swaps need to come from the green inner circle, or from chicken, turkey, or very lean meat. Before you consider these changes, have your health care provider check your kidney function. Diabetics are at a higher risk for kidney problems, so if you are diabetic you should not try increasing your protein intake to this extent. Instead try the lower-carb plan presented in Chapter 6, which reduces carbohydrates by increasing healthy fats, not just protein. Healthy fats, in the amounts suggested, will not have a negative effect on kidneys.

The primary potential benefit of increased dietary protein, within reason, is the potential for the dietary protein to minimize losses of muscle tissue during weight loss. Therefore, for the same amount of total weight lost, more of the loss is fat as opposed to muscle. The potential for this beneficial effect is greater if you are participating in regular physical activity, as discussed in Chapter 11. Researchers have proposed a variety of different mechanisms that could explain how dietary protein can be protective of muscle tissue, but more research is needed.[13] In the meantime, if you find you are struggling with hunger at the suggested calorie level, you can try the higher-protein approach by changing swaps as noted below. The changes noted will increase your dietary protein to 30% of your total calories. Carbohydrates are decreased to about 40% of total calories, and dietary fats are kept to 30% of total calories. As you change swaps, determine whether there are changes in your level of hunger and weight.

Remember that you need to be participating in a regular exercise program to truly benefit from this approach, and to limit your loss of muscle tissue. Here are the specific guidelines based on your suggested calorie level:

- ◉ 1200 calories
  - Increase Protein Group swaps to seven per day
  - Decrease Grain & Starch Group swaps to three and decrease Fat Group swaps to three per day

- ◉ 1500 calories
  - Increase Protein Group swaps to eight and Milk & Yogurt Group swaps to three per day
  - Decrease Grain & Starch Group swaps to four, Fruit Group swaps to two, and Fat Group swaps to four per day

- ◉ 1800 calories
  - Increase Protein Group swaps to 10 and Milk & Yogurt Group swaps to 3 per day
  - Decrease Grain & Starch Group swaps to five and Fat Group swaps to five per day

- ◉ 2100 calories
  - Increase Protein Group swaps to 12 and Milk & Yogurt Group swaps to 3 per day
  - Decrease Grain & Starch Group swaps to seven, Fruit Group swaps to three, and Fat Group swaps to five per day

- ◉ 2400 calories
  - Increase protein swaps to 14 and Milk & Yogurt Group swaps to 4 per day
  - Decrease Grain & Starch Group swaps to seven and Fat Group swaps to five per day
  - At this level of protein intake, it is very important that most of your selections are from the green inner circle, or poultry or very lean meats from the yellow middle circle.

Follow the same guidelines as noted previously to modestly increase swaps to deal with hunger pangs, if necessary. After you reach your weight goals, you should gradually transition back to a lower protein intake by reversing the changes noted above.

### *Artificial Sweeteners—Friends or Foes*

Using artificially sweetened foods and drinks can have mixed results. In the short term, switching from sweetened drinks with hundreds of calories to artificially sweetened drinks with no calories may be helpful because you are taking in fewer calories. However, some research shows artificial sweeteners can trick your body into thinking it had real sugar and stimulate an insulin response, which is generally not favorable. In addition, artificially sweetened foods and beverages can perpetuate your desire for sweet-tasting foods and encourage the consumption of extra desserts and sweets. They also can discourage you from developing preferences for unsweetened foods. Lastly, artificial sweeteners are often used in highly processed foods that are not generally recommended anyway. In summary, you may find it helpful to use artificially sweetened foods and beverages as a crutch in the beginning of your weight-loss journey. However, eventually you should aim to wean yourself off of them. Instead you will learn over time to change your eating habits and your relationship with food, so that you can save swaps to include a moderate serving of your favorite naturally sweetened food on occasion.

## Checking Your Progress

Of course, weight loss is one indicator of progress. However, there are other indicators of progress. Some are subjective and hard to measure, such as feeling better or being more energetic. Being able to wear some of your favorite clothes that had become too small can give you a sense of rejuvenation and progress. You may also feel a new sense of accomplishment and self-confidence as you start to have success working with your new eating style. There are other health indicators that you can ask your health care provider to monitor, such as LDL cholesterol levels and blood pressure. These health indicators can significantly improve with just a 10% weight loss. (If your starting weight is around 150, 200, 250, or 300 pounds then this would equate to a 15, 20, 25, or 30 pound weight-loss, respectively.) Changes in blood cholesterol and triglyceride levels typically take 3 months to respond in a measurable way after you have changed your diet.

Recommended rates and patterns of weight loss are discussed in detail in Chapter 11. Make sure you read this chapter before you lose about 15 to 20 pounds. For now you just need to consider how you will monitor your weight loss. Before you think about how often you weigh yourself, you need to consider how the process of weighing yourself affects your emotional state. Some people can weigh themselves without judging themselves harshly. Many other people, however, experience a lot of negative emotions when weighing themselves. This is referred to as negative self-talk—unpleasant, negative, and often hurtful things you say to yourself. Chapter 10 presents different strategies to help you change your pattern of self-talk. Developing the ability to weigh yourself in an objective, unemotional fashion is very important for long-term success. Doing so will help you stay on course and catch problems early.

It is best to weigh yourself once a week, in the morning, without clothes. Keep in mind that your body weight normally fluctuates a few pounds a week—the taller and heavier you are the more your weight can fluctuate. This is due to changes in water weight, changes in fiber intake, timing of bowel movements, and changes in physical activity levels. In the beginning you will be learning how your weight fluctuates. It is absolutely normal to lose a few pounds, bounce back up a few pounds, and then lose them again. Sometimes you may feel that you are doing everything right, but your weight stays about the same for a few weeks, and then drops a few pounds all in one week. Basically, your weight is not something you can directly control. You can control what you eat and how much you exercise, and eventually your weight will respond. However, it usually does not respond in a very predictable and consistent manner. It is important to keep a record of your weight, so that you can observe and learn from the trends. You are looking for a gradual decline over time, meaning over months. Along the way there will be bumps along the road, weight changes that are higher or lower than anticipated. Try not to overreact to these larger-than-normal jumps in your weight. The pattern over time is most important. This topic will be addressed again in Chapter 11.

## Advantages of the Moderate-Carb Route

If you are not clearly insulin resistant or insulin sensitive, an eating plan with moderate amounts of carbohydrates and fats is best. The total calories consumed a day, as well as the *quality* of the foods providing those calories is most important. Researchers who have examined the effects of an eating plan similar to the one described in this chapter have demonstrated successful weight loss and an improvement in HDL cholesterol and triglyceride levels.[14,15] If such an eating plan consists of foods selected primarily from the green inner circle of the Bull's-Eye Guide, then the nutrient, phytochemical, antioxidant, and fiber contents of the diet will be high. Research indicates that such a diet can prevent cancer and heart disease. Dietary antioxidants help prevent oxidative reactions that lead to the production of free radicals, which damage your body's cells and tissues. Your body has natural defenses against these free radicals; however, dietary antioxidants boost these defense mechanisms and help prevent potential damage. Excessive oxidative damage is associated with an increased risk for cancer, heart disease, cataracts, and general aging. Therefore, having a lot of antioxidants in your diet can prevent or slow down these processes.[1-3,7,16]

A diet high in fiber (30 to 50 grams a day) can reduce your risk for heart disease. As fully explained in Chapter 3, here is a brief explanation of how this occurs. The liver can make hormones and other products, such as bile, from cholesterol. Bile is needed to digest fats. When you eat fat, bile is excreted into your digestive tract. Fiber in your diet traps the bile and drags it out of your body when you have a bowel movement. This is the best way to get cholesterol out of your body. If you do not have a lot of fiber, the bile gets back into your body through your colon and gets recycled. As you increase your fiber intake, it is also important to increase your water intake to at least 8 cups a day. If you would like to maximize the heart disease prevention power of this diet, ask your health care provider about adding 1 to 3 grams of long-chain omega-3 fatty acid (fish oil) supplements.

A diet similar to the one presented in this chapter has been shown in many studies to lower blood pressure measurements. Similar to the moderate-carb plan described in this chapter, the diet in these studies had the following characteristics: (1) high in fiber; (2) lots of vegetables; (3) a few servings of whole fruits; (4) two servings of low-fat, unsweetened milk and yogurt; (5) moderate protein content; and (6) low saturated fat content. This type of eating style provides a wide array of nutrients, such as calcium, magnesium, and potassium, which are known to help control blood pressure. In addition, the plan provides a diet with a low glycemic index and a low sodium content by emphasizing foods from the green inner circle of the Bull's-Eye Guide.[17,18]

If you try increasing the protein content of your eating plan, there may be some important benefits related to the type of weight lost. By increasing your protein intake to about 30% of your total calories (or about 0.68 grams of protein per pound of body weight), you may be able to hold onto more of your muscle mass as you lose weight. Therefore, at your lower weight you will have retained muscle mass and, preferentially, lost more fat. This makes it easier to keep the weight off, because muscle tissues use more energy than fat tissue. Having more muscle makes you use more calories every minute of every day without even knowing it. Therefore, having more muscle tissue helps you burn more of the calories you eat.[8,12]

A moderate-carb eating style with a lot of fiber can also support a healthy gastrointestinal tract, which is essential for optimal health. The average person has about 2 pounds of bacteria (comprised of over 400 different species) living in his or her gastrointestinal tract, which is referred to as the microflora. The microflora is made up of friendly bacteria that promote health (probiotics) and unfriendly or pathogenic bacteria that can cause illness if able to multiply unchecked. An unhealthy balance of microflora can result from poor diet, illness, and some medications. A variety of different dietary fibers and phytochemicals in plant-based foods encourage the growth and activity of a healthy mix of microflora. Diet plays a determining role in the kinds and number of microorganisms in your gastrointestinal tract. A healthy gastrointestinal system with adequate probiotics is thought to optimize health (making nutrients such as vitamin K and vitamin $B_{12}$), prevent disease (especially some types of cancer), and reverse some illnesses (chronic diarrhea). Your body's immune function is dependent on interactions among the microflora, the lining of your intestinal tract, and the part of your immune system active in your gut. The gastrointestinal tract needs regular immune stimulation by probiotics to start and regulate appropriate immune responses to pathogens and antigens, as well as to not overrespond and cause allergies and autoimmune diseases.[19–22]

## Disadvantages of the Moderate-Carb Route

*There are no disadvantages to following the basic moderate-carb route or the higher-protein version as described in this chapter.* However, you may experience problems if you select many foods from the red outer circle. This is especially true if you try increasing your protein intake and select a lot of protein foods from the red outer circle. These foods are high in saturated fat, which increases your risk for heart disease and cancer. Selecting a lot of foods from the red outer circle of the Grain & Starch Group and the Fruit Group will increase your intake of sugars, sweeteners, and refined grains, especially refined-grain products with added trans fats (partially hydrogenated oils). During the time when high-carbohydrate diets were popular, sugar intake among Americans increased 28%—up to 1¼ pounds of added sweeteners per person per week. Part of the reason for this was the lack of clear nutrition recommendations from public health officials, the trend for food manufacturers to add corn syrup sweeteners to the majority of processed foods, and confusion among the public. This type of a high-sugar, high-carbohydrate eating plan has been shown by researchers to increase appetite and total calorie intake. In addition, diets with a high glycemic index (diets high in sweeteners and refined starches) have been shown to increase the risk for coronary artery disease, insulin resistance and type 2 diabetes. Therefore, you need to carefully read food labels and avoid added sweeteners and trans/hydrogenated fats.[3,5,23–25]

The moderate-carb eating plan in this book and the Bull's-Eye Guide will clearly guide you in developing the healthiest moderate-carb plan that can facilitate weight loss and prevent chronic illnesses, as well as promote optimal health and well-being. You have the option of a moderate-protein or a higher-protein version. As you lose weight and increase your level of physical activity, you may markedly improve your level of insulin sensitivity. At this point, you may consider transitioning to the high-carb plan. Alternatively, if your health status changes, and you believe you have become more insulin resistant, you may consider transitioning to the lower-carb plan. In any case, it is most important that you create an eating style that is close to the recommended number of calories, and includes mostly high-quality foods from the inner circle of the Bull's-Eye Guide. For more practical information on changing your eating and exercise habits and planning your weight management journey, skip to Chapters 9, 10, and 11.

## Important Points To Remember from Chapter 7

- ◉ You can lower your risk of heart disease and cancer and optimize your health with a diet that is high in phytochemicals and fiber, as well as low in saturated fats and trans fats.

- ◉ Structured moderate-carb eating plans at the appropriate calorie level will start you off on your weight-management journey.

- ◉ You can, and should, modify your plan and include favorite foods to help you stay on course and reach your destination.

- ◉ Expect to stumble or lose your way along your journey—but get back on course quickly by objectively recognizing your missteps and not overreacting.

- ◉ Begin to consider your strategy to monitor your weight and check your progress. (Refer to Chapter 10 for more information.)

- ◉ The moderate-carb route presented empowers you to take a moderate dietary approach and craft a higher-protein style to potentially maximize your muscle mass while losing weight.

# THE HIGH-CARB ROUTE

### *What You Will Discover in Chapter 8*

◉ The high-carb plan provides the known benefits of a plant-based, high-fiber diet for those who are sensitive to the action of insulin.

◉ For your selected calorie level, you will find an eating plan with the appropriate number of swaps from each food group for your meals and snack.

◉ You may need to modify your plan for optimal benefits. Guidelines for doing so are provided in this chapter.

◉ Timing of meals and snacks is important.

## How the High-Carb Route Can Get You to
## Your Destination

The high-carb route is the best route if you are not insulin resistant, as described in Table 5-4. It has been estimated that *only* about 24% of all American adults are insulin resistant. Among all overweight adults, 40% are expected to be insulin resistant.[1,2] Those who are insulin resistant will benefit from the lower-carb plan to reverse the insulin resistance, and then should gradually transition to the moderate-carb or high-carb plan. Refer to Chapter 5 for a full explanation of the factors used to determine whether you are insulin resistant or sensitive.

To summarize, being insulin sensitive means that your body makes the chemical insulin in appropriate amounts, and your cells use it well. Your body requires insulin to push sugar that is in your blood into your cells, where it is needed. The carbohydrates in foods (such as foods from the Grain & Starch Group, the Fruit Group, and the Milk & Yogurt Group) are broken down into sugar and absorbed into your blood. Insulin is secreted in response to this. Within a few hours the sugar is transported into your cells, and your blood sugar levels go back down to pre-eating levels. Your laboratory values will indicate whether you are sensitive to insulin as shown in Table 5-4. If you are very sensitive, the sugar in your blood goes into your cells fairly quickly. Sweetened foods and drinks (including fruit drinks, fruit juices, and flavored milks), especially those low in fiber and fat, make this drop in blood sugar more dramatic. These drops can be associated with feeling very hungry, shaky, or sluggish shortly after eating. The increased hunger can lead to subsequent overeating. If symptoms such as these are bothersome, you may want to try the moderate-carb plan to see if it helps lessen the symptoms.

Research over decades has shown that a higher-carb, lower-fat diet comprised of whole foods naturally high in fiber and low in sugar, trans fats, and saturated fats is the healthiest diet to follow for many people.[3–5] In response to research in this area, food manufactures developed an array of low-fat foods. Unfortunately, the majority of these foods are highly processed carbohydrate foods in which the fiber has been removed and sweeteners have been added. White pasta, white rice, white breads, refined sweetened cereals, bagels, crackers, low-fat cakes, low-fat cookies, low-fat frozen desserts, sweetened yogurts, flavored milks, juice drinks, and sodas characterize this style of eating. These types of foods have been stripped of their fibers, many nutrients, and phytochemicals. In addition, they tend to lead to excessive increases in blood levels of sugar and insulin. Consumers were lead to believe that all low-fat foods were healthy. Whole foods naturally high in fibers, nutrients, and phytochemicals have not been adequately emphasized. In addition, a perception developed that portion sizes of low-fat high-carbohydrate foods are not that important because carbohydrates are not as calorically dense as fats. However, refined and sweetened high-carbohydrate foods have a higher caloric density than their whole food counterparts—they provide more calories for the same amount of food. Low-fiber foods are also less filling, generally leading to larger intakes. High-carbohydrate, low-fat styles of eating can be very healthy, if the sources of carbohydrates are whole foods, such as those in the green inner circle of the Bull's-Eye Food Guide.[3–5]

High-carbohydrate diets are increasingly being blamed for the obesity epidemic, because the percentage of calories coming from carbohydrates in the diets of Americans increased through the 1980s and 1990s. However, the trends are more complex than this simple explanation. Over the last two decades Americans have increased their daily calorie intake—men by 168 calories per day and women by 335 calories per day. The amount of grams of fat per day also increased. However, because carbohydrate intake increased more than fat, the relative percent of total calories coming from fat decreased and the percentage of total calories coming from carbohydrates increased. In other words, the obesity epidemic cannot be blamed on increased carbohydrate intake, as the creators of low-carbohydrate diets would have you believe, but on increased overall calorie intake.[6–8]

Evidence that diets high in carbohydrates can lead to weight loss and improved health is plentiful, even overwhelming. Such research includes well-controlled studies on tens of thousands of subjects by hundreds of researchers looking at the effect of high-carbohydrate, low-fat diets on weight management, diabetes, high blood pressure, heart disease, and cancer.[3,9–20] This type of evidence cannot be ignored. Additional evidence in support of high-carbohydrate, low-fat diets comes from a study in which researchers are following 438 individuals who lost an average of 30 pounds and successful maintained that loss for 5 years. These subjects report following a low-calorie, low-fat diet to lose weight and keep the weight off. Participants in the study limit fat to about 24% of total calories, which is similar to the eating style presented in this chapter.[21]

As noted above, sweeteners are increasingly being added to foods during manufacturing, as opposed to at the kitchen table. Common sweeteners are high-fructose corn syrup, corn syrup, and sugar. Refined grains and starches, such as white bread, white rice or pasta, can have the same effect even without added sweeteners. Therefore, high-fiber, unprocessed grains and starches and whole fruits are highly recommended. The fiber in these foods slows down the digestion and absorption of sugar and promotes a more stable blood sugar level. This, in turn, makes you feel full and more satisfied for a longer period. Many Americans eat three to five times the recommended amount of sugar without even realizing it, because food manufacturers add sweeteners to almost all processed foods. As a rough rule of thumb, you should eat less than 25 grams of added sugars or other sweeteners per 1000 calories. You can determine this by looking on food labels and noting the grams of sugar listed just under the grams of total carbohydrate. For the eating plans in this book, the added sugar and sweetener limits would be as follows: 30 grams of sugar in the 1200-calorie plan; 38 grams in the 1500-calorie plan; 45 grams in the 1800-calorie plan; 53 grams in the 2100-calorie plan; and 60 grams in the 2400-calorie per day plan. Remember, these limits are for added sugar and do not include the sugar naturally occurring in fruit (about 15 grams of sugar per swap), some vegetables (5 grams of sugar per swap of some vegetables like carrots and beets), and milk or yogurt (12 to 15 grams of sugar per swap). These naturally occurring sugars are already accounted for in the eating plans in this book.

It is important to become more aware of how much added sugar you eat and drink, because hidden sugars are a big source of unnecessary calories. You can track your sugar intake by looking at the number on food labels; be aware, however, that this number includes sugars naturally found in milk and fruit as well as added sugars. So when you eat or drink milk- or fruit-based products, you need to do a little extra math. You can estimate the added sugars in a milk-based food or drink by subtracting 12 from the grams of sugar in a cup of the milk or yogurt product. For example, if a cup of flavored milk has 26 grams of sugar, you would subtract 12 grams from 26 grams. There would be an estimated 14 grams of added sugar per cup of the flavored milk. As a frame of reference, there are 4 grams of sugar in a paper packet of sugar. Therefore, a cup of the flavored milk would have 3½ packets of sugar added to it. On the food label it is also important to notice the number of servings in a container, because many seemingly single-use containers really have 2 servings per container. Therefore, if the bottle of the flavored milk was 16 ounces and you drank the whole bottle, it would provide 28 grams of added sugar, or 7 packets of sugar. This is about the same amount of added sugar as in one 8-ounce glass of soda.

Fruit-based products have to be considered in a similar fashion. For example, applesauce is typically sweetened and has about 24 grams of sugar per ½ cup. You can assume 15 grams is natural sugar in the fruit, and subtract 15 grams from 24 grams. Nine grams would be the estimated amount of added sugar, or a little bit more than 2 packets of sugar. Choosing unsweetened natural applesauce allows you to avoid the intake of these added sugars. You can see how easily the grams of added sugar can add up over the course of a day.

The next section of this chapter provides detailed information on creating a very structured high-carb plan. It is important to review and understand this information. For most people, it is also helpful to try to follow a detailed plan for some time before transitioning to a less-structured action plan. However, everybody is unique and some people simply do not respond well to such a structured approach. For example, for some people the effort required to follow the structured plan leads them to think too much about food and be too restrictive. This can backfire and lead to more frequent overeating episodes. Be aware of this potential consequence. If this is the case for you, review the information below and keep a general sense of the structure in your mind. Then go to Chapters 9 and 10 for other strategies you can use to craft a more casual approach to the high-carb eating style. Also refer to the menus in the Menus and Recipes section.

*A less structured or casual approach can work, but the results are typically slower. This is okay, as long as you prepare yourself for slower weight loss, and lower your expectations accordingly.* Simply accept the slower weight loss as progress that is more likely to be permanent, for many reasons discussed in Chapter 11.

## The Detailed Map

On the higher-carb route, carbohydrates provide 60% of total calories. Fats provide 20% of total calories, and proteins provide 20% of total calories. It is essential that the majority of your carbohydrates come from high-fiber foods that are minimally processed and do not contain added sweeteners (especially high-fructose corn syrup). These foods tend to have a lower glycemic index as well. Choosing the best foods is easy and consistent with the Bull's-Eye Food Guide system, because you simply have to select most of your foods from all of the food groups from the green inner circle. If you have high LDL cholesterol, making your selections from the Protein Group and the Fat Group from the green inner circle will help to decrease them. To lower LDL cholesterol levels, also check the ingredient lists on packaged foods and avoid partially hydrogenated and hydrogenated oils. This does not mean that you can never have a favorite food from the red outer circle, but you have to plan to work some of these foods into your day. By working some of your favorite foods from the red outer circle into your plan, you increase the likelihood that you can stay on the program long enough to get to a healthy weight and then stay there. With the Bull's-Eye Food Guide system, you never have to count calories or grams of carbohydrates, proteins, or fats. All you have to do is simply keep track of the number of swaps you have from the six food groups each day and make most of your selections from the green inner circle. Review the food groups and the idea of swapping in Chapter 4 before finalizing your plan. For now, remember that a swap of food is the amount of a specific food that provides the number of calories assigned to the food group in which it is placed. It is not necessarily the amount of food you can eat at a meal or snack, since you may have more than one swap from a specific food group at a meal or snack. Consider a swap of food simply an assigned volume of food used as a counting unit to keep track of calories, carbohydrates, proteins, and fats.

First, note the calorie level you selected for yourself in Chapter 5 from Table 5-1 or 5-2. Then refer to Table 8-1. Table 8-1 indicates the number of swaps from the six different food groups suggested each day based on your calorie level. For example, reading down the column labeled "1500 Calories/Day," there are six Vegetable Group swaps, four Fruit Group swaps, seven Grain & Starch Group swaps, five Protein Group swaps, two Fat Group swaps, and two Milk & Yogurt Group swaps. If you cannot tolerate milk or yogurt, try soymilk products (the soymilk should be low-fat with less than 12 grams of sugar per serving, making it comparable to cow's milk). If that does not work for you, trade in your two swaps from the Milk & Yogurt Group for one swap from the Protein Group and one swap from

**Table 8-1.**
The Higher-Carb Plans by Calorie Level

| Food Group | Swaps per Day from Each Food Group at Different Calorie Levels | | | | |
|---|---|---|---|---|---|
| | 1200 Calories per Day | 1500 Calories per Day | 1800 Calories per Day | 2100 Calories per Day | 2400 Calories per Day |
| Vegetable* | 6 | 6 | 6 | 6 | 6 |
| Fruit | 3 | 4 | 4 | 5 | 5 |
| Grain & Starch | 5 | 7 | 10 | 12 | 14 |
| Protein | 3 | 5 | 5 | 6 | 7 |
| Fat | 2 | 2 | 3 | 3 | 3 |
| Milk & Yogurt | 2 | 2 | 2 | 2 | 3 |

*For vegetables, these numbers are minimums because Vegetable Group swaps are unlimited.

the Fruit Group. In addition, talk to your health care provider about taking a calcium supplement to ensure adequate calcium intake.

Remember, it is extremely important that most swaps from the Grain & Starch Group come from the green inner circle. One or at the most two swaps can be saved for a food in the yellow or red circles. All fruits should come from the green inner circle, and most vegetables should come from the green inner circle. Protein selections can come from the green inner circle or the yellow middle circle, but selections from the red outer circle should be kept to a minimum. Also, keep in mind that if you do pick a food from the outer circle of the protein group you need to save fats for that food as well. These fat swaps would be considered red outer circle fat swaps. Both of your swaps from the Milk & Yogurt Group should be from the green inner or yellow middle circle. If possible, all of your selections from the Fat Group should come from the green inner circle. If you need to use a bread spread, try one from the middle yellow group that is made from liquid vegetable oils that are not partially hydrogenated. As an alternative, you can try natural peanut butter on your bread or dip bread into a teaspoon of olive oil flavored with herbs. Another option would be to make homemade yogurt cheese. To make yogurt cheese simply do the following: (1) measure a cup of plain fat-free yogurt, (2) line a strainer with a coffee filter and place the strainer over a bowl, (3) scoop the yogurt into the coffee filter and cover with plastic wrap or foil, (4) refrigerate for 24 hours, (5) drain liquid that collects in the bowl, (6) refrigerate for an additional 12 to 24 hours, and (7) remove thickened yogurt and place in a resealable tub. You can flavor the yogurt according to your taste preferences. For example, you can use scallions and a minced olive, or you can use vanilla extract and cinnamon. The possibilities are endless. After flavoring the yogurt, you can use it on crackers, toast, or sandwiches, and you can use it as a vegetable dip. Made in this way, 8 tablespoons of the yogurt cheese count as one Milk & Yogurt Group swap; therefore, 4 tablespoons would only count as half of a Milk & Yogurt Group swap.

Fats found in foods in the outer circle of the Grain & Starch Group, the Protein Group, and the Milk & Yogurt Group are typically trans fats or saturated fats. Therefore, fat swaps that you save to put towards these foods should be limited as well, because these fats are known to increase LDL cholesterol levels in genetically susceptible people.

The next step is to decide how to distribute the swaps from the different food groups throughout the course of the day. Whenever possible, balance carbohydrates from food in the Grain & Starch Group or the Fruit Group with a food from the Protein Group, the Fat Group, or the Milk & Yogurt Group. This applies to planning meals and snacks. In Table 8-2 swaps from the different food groups at each calorie level are distributed into three meals and one snack. On the chart, highlight the calorie level that you have previously selected. Note how many swaps you have for each meal and snack. In Menus and Recipes, you will find daily menus to follow. You can also use the Swap Lists for each of the food groups to modify the menus or create new menus. See Tables 8-3A and B for examples of selections made from the swap lists to create a lunch at the 1500-calorie per day level. If you do not like a particular item selected in these tables or in the daily menus in Menus and Recipes, you can go the Swap Lists to trade them in for swaps of different foods in the same group. For example, in Table 8-3A there is a note that you may not like grapes, or may not have them available at the time. Therefore, the grapes can be traded in for one swap of a different fruit selected from the Fruit Group Swap List, such as 1 apple, ½ banana, or 12 cherries. Reviewing the sample daily menus and associated notes in Menus and Recipes will help demonstrate this.

Many people's first response to menus like the ones in Tables 8-3A and B is that they think it looks like too much food. This may be for a few reasons. First of all, many of the foods selected have a low caloric density. As described in Chapter 3, this means that there are only a small amount of calories for a given amount of food because the food is high in fiber and/or water. Secondly, moderate amounts of many different types of foods are used in combinations in meals to best balance carbohydrates, proteins, and fats. Lastly, moderate amounts of many different foods are selected to provide a wide variety of nutrients, fibers, and phytochemicals. This also makes the display of food appear more satisfying and interesting. The lunch menus shown in Tables 8-3A and B have about 425 calories. By comparison, a typical sandwich from a deli with no side dishes or drinks would provide at least 850 calories, and not nearly as many nutrients, fiber, or phytochemicals.

**Table 8-2.**
Swaps of Each Food Group by Calorie Level and Meal

| Meal | 1200 Calories per Day | 1500 Calories per Day | 1800 Calories per Day | 2100 Calories per Day | 2400 Calories per Day |
|---|---|---|---|---|---|
| **Breakfast** | | | | | |
| Vegetable Group | | | | | |
| Fruit Group | 1 | 1 | 1 | 1 | 1 |
| Grain & Starch Group | 1 | 2 | 3 | 3 | 3 |
| Protein Group | | | | 1 | 1 |
| Fat Group | | | | | |
| Milk & Yogurt Group | 1 | 1 | 1 | 1 | 1 |
| **Lunch** | | | | | |
| Vegetable Group | 2 | 2 | 2 | 2 | 2 |
| Fruit Group | 1 | 1 | 1 | 1 | 1 |
| Grain & Starch Group | 1 | 2 | 2 | 3 | 3 |
| Protein Group | 1 | 2 | 2 | 2 | 2 |
| Fat Group | 1 | 1 | 1 | 1 | 1 |
| Milk & Yogurt Group | | | | | 1 |
| **Dinner** | | | | | |
| Vegetable Group | 4 | 4 | 4 | 4 | 4 |
| Fruit Group | | | | 1 | 1 |
| Grain & Starch Group | 2 | 2 | 3 | 4 | 5 |
| Protein Group | 2 | 3 | 3 | 3 | 4 |
| Fat Group | 1 | 1 | 1 | 1 | 1 |
| Milk & Yogurt Group | | | | | |
| **Snacks** | | | | | |
| Vegetable Group | | | | | |
| Fruit Group | 1 | 2 | 2 | 2 | 2 |
| Grain & Starch Group | 1 | 1 | 2 | 2 | 3 |
| Protein Group | | | | | |
| Fat Group | | | 1 | 1 | 1 |
| Milk & Yogurt Group | 1 | 1 | 1 | 1 | 1 |

Another common response to the swaps, meal patterns, and menus is frustration with the prospect of weighing and measuring foods and drinks. You may also be concerned about the portion sizes, which are typically much smaller than what you were previously eating and drinking. To resolve these issues and barriers to moving forward, keep in mind that to start losing weight, you simply have to eat less than you are currently eating until weight loss starts. Therefore, you may want to start off by determining how much you are currently eating. For a few days write down what you eat and figure out how many swaps from each food group you usually have at each meal and snack. Compare your usual number of swaps per meals and snacks to the numbers suggested. Then plan to gradually reduce the number of swaps you are currently eating to get closer to the suggested number of swaps. As you make each gradual reduction in swaps, monitor your weight for a few days. Reduce the number of swaps until weight loss starts. You are likely to find that you start to lose weight when you just get close to eating the suggested number of swaps.

You will soon develop a system of shopping and cooking that allows you to put healthy, satisfying meals together quickly. At first this will probably require extra planning time as you develop your new habits and systems. After a while the new habits will come easily, and the time necessary to shop and cook will decrease.

## Considering Alcohol Intake

Alcohol needs to be limited for many health reasons, as well as because of the calories it provides. If you are already in the habit of having an alcoholic drink, you can continue to have one alcoholic drink a day—but no more. This should *not* be consumed on an empty stomach when it will have the most dramatic and negative effect on your liver's metabolic processes. Instead, have it with or immediately after dinner. One alcoholic drink is equivalent to 5 ounces of a dry wine, 12 ounces of beer, or 1½ ounces of 80-proof distilled spirits plain or with a noncaloric mixer. If you are not in the habit of drinking alcohol, you should not start now!

**Table 8-3A.**
A Sample Lunch from the 1500 Calorie High-Carb Plan **Sandwich** Option

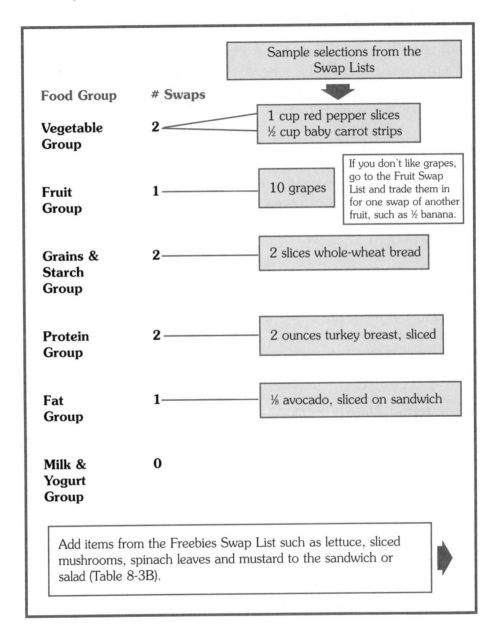

| Food Group | # Swaps | Sample selections from the Swap Lists |
|---|---|---|
| **Vegetable Group** | 2 | 1 cup red pepper slices / ½ cup baby carrot strips |
| **Fruit Group** | 1 | 10 grapes (If you don't like grapes, go to the Fruit Swap List and trade them in for one swap of another fruit, such as ½ banana.) |
| **Grains & Starch Group** | 2 | 2 slices whole-wheat bread |
| **Protein Group** | 2 | 2 ounces turkey breast, sliced |
| **Fat Group** | 1 | ⅛ avocado, sliced on sandwich |
| **Milk & Yogurt Group** | 0 | |

Add items from the Freebies Swap List such as lettuce, sliced mushrooms, spinach leaves and mustard to the sandwich or salad (Table 8-3B).

**Table 8-3B.**
A Sample Lunch from the 1500 Calorie High-Carb Plan **Salad** Option

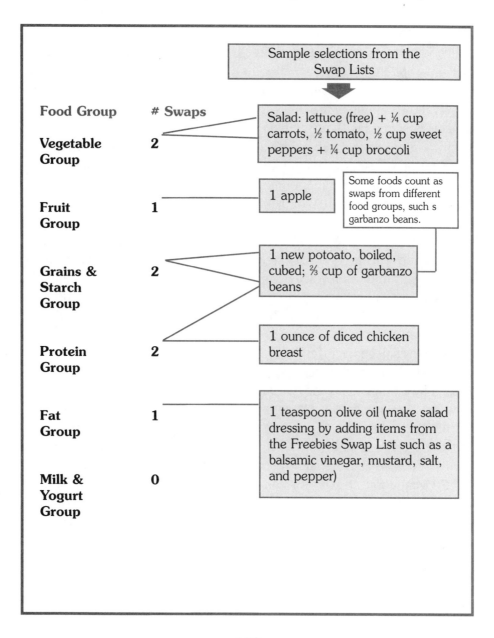

| Food Group | # Swaps | Sample selections from the Swap Lists |
|---|---|---|
| **Vegetable Group** | 2 | Salad: lettuce (free) + ¼ cup carrots, ½ tomato, ½ cup sweet peppers + ¼ cup broccoli |
| **Fruit Group** | 1 | 1 apple |
| **Grains & Starch Group** | 2 | 1 new potoato, boiled, cubed; ⅔ cup of garbanzo beans |
| **Protein Group** | 2 | 1 ounce of diced chicken breast |
| **Fat Group** | 1 | 1 teaspoon olive oil (make salad dressing by adding items from the Freebies Swap List such as a balsamic vinegar, mustard, salt, and pepper) |
| **Milk & Yogurt Group** | 0 | |

Some foods count as swaps from different food groups, such s garbanzo beans.

## Avoiding Getting Lost

The best way to avoid getting lost is to study your map before you start your journey. Using the menus is a good way to get started right away. While you are doing this, spend time learning the following: (1) the number of swaps from each of the food groups at your calorie level for each meal and snack as shown in Table 8-2; (2) the swap lists for each food group and subgroup of the Bull's-Eye Food Guide; (3) the concept of swapping as described in the beginning of Chapter 4; and (4) the description of each food group and subgroup as described in Chapter 4. Learning this information will allow you to modify the menus in Menus and Recipes and create an unlimited number of menus for meals and snacks.

In Chapters 9 and 10, you will learn many new strategies to help you develop new healthy eating and exercise habits. It will take you time to work with these strategies to change unhealthy habits and change your relationship with food. Most often, it is first necessary to become more aware of why and when you eat, and then to start to tease apart unhealthy habits in which eating is tied to emotions (such as stress, boredom, or anger) or specific behaviors (such as television viewing). For now, suffice it to say that along your journey you will at times lose your way—overeat, make many selections from the red outer circle, or stop exercising. *This is to be expected.* The biggest indicator of your overall progress and long-term success is how quickly you can get back on your planned route. This requires that you simply acknowledge your missteps and, without a lot of negativity, turn back on course. Permanent weight loss is a process that takes time, but the process is well worth the time and effort in terms of the permanence of the weight loss and the improvements in overall health.

So what about the times when you really want a piece of cake or some other favorite dessert? You can add these items on occasion, but you have to plan ahead a bit. For example, imagine you are going to a birthday party and you know you will want a piece of cake. An average piece of birthday cake counts as two swaps from the Grain & Starch Group and two swaps from the Fat Group. To save swaps for the cake, you would have a lot of vegetables and your protein swaps (two to four swaps of meat, fish, or chicken) for dinner. However, you would skip the starchy side dish and fats and save those swaps for the piece of cake. Of course this is not ideal, because you are having less-healthy foods from the outer circle instead of healthy foods from the green inner circle. However, it is realistic and allows you to have some of your favorite foods while staying on your plan.

You can take this idea of being flexible one step further by using the information in Chapter 4, Table 4-1. In Table 4-1 you are given the calories and grams of carbohydrates, proteins, and fats provided by a swap of each of the food groups. If you are following the 1500-calorie per day, lower-carb route you would have the following swaps for snack: two Fruit Group swaps, one Grain & Starch Group swap, and one Milk & Yogurt Group swap. Table 8-4 shows how you could determine how many calories and grams of macronutrients these swaps provide. In this example, the swaps provide 290 calories. Therefore, when you are really craving a specific food, you can read the food label (specifically the serving size and calories per serving information) and determine how much you could have of the given food for the 290 calories you have allotted. Ideally the new food would also have about the same number of grams of carbohydrates, proteins, and fats so it would be consistent with your higher-carb eating style. If it is a dessert-type food it should have at least some fats to balance the carbohydrates. Keeping in mind that the carbohydrates and fats in most dessert foods are not the high-quality, health-promoting kinds, you would not want to do this too often. If the rest of your food selections for the day are of very high quality and this keeps you satisfied and on track, it is worth it! However, if you start to do this too often, the balance of carbohydrates, proteins, and fats will not be optimal, and your results will likely suffer.

## Troubleshooting Along the Way

When planning a weight management journey, it is rare that you can map your whole trip from start to end perfectly from the very beginning. So far you have a great start—a calorie level, an eating style, menus, and swap lists. However, you may find that you need to adjust your map a bit.

**Table 8-4.**

Determining Calories Provided by Given Swaps for a Meal or Snack

The example below is for the swaps provided for snack on the 1500-calorie per day plan.

| Food Groups & Number of Swaps | Calories per Swap | Carbohydrates (grams per swap) | Proteins (grams per swap) | Fats (grams per swap) |
|---|---|---|---|---|
| **2 Fruits** | 120 | 30 | 0 | 0 |
| **1 Grain & Starch** | 80 | 15 | 3 | 1 |
| **1 Milk** | 90 | 12 | 8 | 0 |
| **Totals** (Add the numbers in each column down.) | **290 Calories** | **57 grams of carbohydrate** | **11 grams of protein** | **1 gram of fat** |

This calculation indicates that 290 calories are available for the snack. As an alternative to using the swaps to create your snack, you could look on the food label of a favorite food and determine the amount you could have that would provide 290 calories. Ideally, that amount would provide roughly the same amount of carbohydrates, proteins, and fats.

## Dealing with Hunger Pangs

As you start to adjust your eating habits, you are likely to feel a bit hungry at times. Being very hungry, however, will make it difficult for you to stay on course and reach your destination, so hunger has to be thoughtfully considered. First you need to consider whether it is true "physiological hunger" or "psychological appetite." For more details about this important topic refer to Chapter 9.

If you are losing weight but feeling true physiological hunger throughout the day, think about when you are hungry. If you are hungry most of the day, you should add some swaps to your plan. You can add swaps to meals or snacks. First, try adding additional swaps from the Vegetable Group if possible. Then add swaps from the other food groups as suggested. Make one or two additions and monitor your weight and hunger. The goal is to add swaps until your hunger is manageable and you are still losing weight (at least about 1 or 2 pounds a month but no more than an average of 1 to 1½ pounds a week). Add swaps in the following order to make sure the mix of carbohydrates, proteins, and fats is best for you: (1) two Vegetable Group swaps, (2) one or two additional Protein Group swaps from the green or yellow subgroups, (3) one Grain & Starch Group swap from the green subgroup, and finally (4) one Fruit Group swap from the green subgroup.

If the weight loss is slow (less than 1 to 2 pounds a month) but you are experiencing hunger at a specific time of the day, try to save one or two swaps from meals to have as a snack at that difficult time. This is to avoid adding extra swaps, which may stop the weight loss altogether. Try to save a half of a swap from the Milk & Yogurt Group from breakfast to match with a full or a half of a swap from the Fruit Group or a full or half of a swap from the Grain & Starch Group saved from lunch or dinner. This would allow for the following combinations:

- A smoothie made with ½ cup skim milk (half of a Milk & Yogurt Group swap) and ¼ banana or ½ peach (half of a Fruit Group swap) blended with ice. (You can also add freebies like a sprinkle of cinnamon and a dash of vanilla.)

- A yogurt parfait with ½ cup plain nonfat yogurt (half of a Milk & Yogurt Group swap) layered with ¼ banana thinly sliced (half of a Fruit Group swap) and 1½ tablespoons Grape-Nuts (half of a Grain & Starch Group swap)

- About ¾ cup puffed rice cereal (half of a Grain & Starch Group swap), ½ cup of skim milk (half of a Milk & Yogurt Group swap) and 1 tablespoon of raisins (half of a Fruit Group swap)

If the weight loss is slow and you are hungry, it is especially important to make sure you are doing adequate amounts of physical activity. Refer to

Chapter 11 for more details about physical activity. By increasing your physical activity, you may be able to add additional swaps as noted in the second paragraph of this section and still lose weight.

## Timing of Meal and Snack Pit Stops

In general, eating three to four times a day is recommended—three meals and one snack. However, as much as possible, the timing of your meals and snacks should be guided by your level of hunger. This is fully discussed in Chapter 9. For now, it is important to understand that going long periods of time without eating may lead to the unnecessary breakdown of muscle tissue. An adequate level of blood sugar (between 60 and 100 milligrams per deciliter of blood) is necessary for your body to function best. As time passes since your last eating event, your blood sugar decreases. As this happens your liver is signaled to make sugar. Your liver has some stored carbohydrate called glycogen that it easily breaks down into sugar molecules. However, after following a diet low enough in calories to promote weight loss for some time, these stores are low. Therefore, your liver has to make glucose from scratch. Unfortunately, your body cannot make glucose from fats, but it can make glucose from amino acids, the building blocks of protein and muscle tissue. When you go long periods of time without eating, you are more likely to turn to muscle tissue as a source of amino acids to make glucose. Over time, this could lead to the loss of excessive amounts of muscle tissue, which makes further weight loss more difficult. To avoid this, you should not skip breakfast. Other meals and a snack should be not much more than 4 to 6 hours apart, especially if you are susceptible to low blood sugar, as indicated by feelings of shakiness and headaches after not eating for a prolonged time. If you are susceptible to these feelings, it might be helpful to divide your lunch swaps into a smaller lunch and a snack. For example, you may want to save your fat swap and a fruit swap if possible. You can use these swaps for 2 teaspoons of natural peanut butter on an apple, or six almonds and 2 tablespoons of raisins.

## Experimenting with Decreasing Fat Further

If you have been having success on the higher-carbohydrate plan described so far in this chapter, you may want to take this approach a step farther. This is especially true if you have high LDL cholesterol that has been responding to this lower-carbohydrate approach, and you are interested in reducing it further. There are a series of studies that have demonstrated a greater reduction of dietary fat to 10% of total calories, while maintaining a high-nutritional-quality diet, can reverse existing heart disease. This is only possible if you are also participating in regular physical activity and selecting foods of high nutritional quality. This means that you select most of your foods from the green inner circle of the Bull's-Eye Food Guide.

Here are the specific guidelines to modify your swaps to decrease the percent fat to 10% to 15% of total calories and to increase the percentage of carbohydrate to about 65% of total calories. You would also be striving to increase your dietary fiber to 50 grams per day. Make sure you increase your water intake to 8 to 12 cups a day, because the extra fiber needs to be able to draw water into your gastrointestinal tract in order to be passed easily. This is very important! The guidelines are based on your suggested calorie level:

- 1200 calories
  - Increase Grain & Starch Group swaps to six per day
  - Decrease Fat Group swaps to one per day

- 1500 calories
  - Increase Grain & Starch Group swaps to nine per day
  - Decrease Fat Group swaps to one and Protein Group swaps to three per day

- 1800 calories
  - Increase Grain & Starch Group swaps to 12 per day
  - Decrease Fat Group swaps to one and Protein Group swaps to three per day

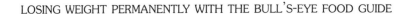

- 2100 calories
  - Increase Grain & Starch Group swaps to 15 per day
  - Decrease Fat Group swaps to one and Protein Group swaps to four per day

- 2400 calories
  - Increase Grain & Starch Group swaps to 16, Fruit Group swaps to 6, and Vegetable Group swaps to 8 per day
  - Decrease Fat Group swaps to two, Protein Group swaps to five, and Milk & Yogurt Group swaps to two per day

You should make these changes in your swaps gradually, and monitor your weight, feelings of hunger/fullness, and your overall health with your health care provider. You may end up crafting an eating style that is somewhere in between the basic guidelines in this chapter and the lower-fat style described above. Follow the same guidelines as noted above to modestly increase swaps to deal with hunger pangs, if necessary.

## Artificial Sweeteners—Friends or Foes

Using artificially sweetened foods and drinks can have mixed results. In the short-term, switching from sweetened drinks with hundreds of calories to artificially sweetened drinks with no calories may be helpful, because you are taking in fewer calories. However, some research indicates that artificial sweeteners can trick your body into thinking it had real sugar and stimulate an insulin response, which is generally not favorable. In addition, artificially sweetened foods and beverages perpetuate your desire for sweet-tasting foods and encourage the consumption of extra desserts and sweets. They also can discourage you from developing preferences for unsweetened foods. Lastly, artificial sweeteners are often used in highly processed foods that are not generally recommended anyway. In summary, you may find it helpful to use artificially sweetened foods and beverages as a crutch in the beginning of your weight loss journey; however, eventually, you should aim to wean yourself off of them. Instead you will learn over time to change your eating habits and your relationship with food, so that you can save swaps to include a moderate serving of your favorite natural-ly sweetened food on occasion.

## Checking Your Progress

Of course, weight loss is one indicator of progress. However, there are other indicators of progress. Some are subjective and hard to measure, such as feeling better or being more energetic. Being able to wear some of your favorite clothes that had become too small can give you a sense of rejuve-nation and progress. You may also feel a new sense of accomplishment and self-confidence as you start working with you new eating style and have success. There are other health indicators that you can ask your health care provider to monitor, such as LDL cholesterol levels and blood pressure. These health indicators can significantly improve with just a 10% weight loss. (If your starting weight is around 150, 200, 250, or 300 pounds then this would equate to a 15-, 20-, 25-, or 30-pound weight loss, respec-tively.) Changes in blood cholesterol and triglyceride levels typically take 3 months to respond in a measurable way after you have changed your diet.

Recommended rates and patterns of weight loss are discussed in detail in Chapter 11. Make sure you read that chapter before you lose about 15 to 20 pounds. For now you just need to consider how you will monitor your weight loss. Before you think about how often you weigh yourself, you need to consider how the process of weighing yourself affects your emo-tional state. Some people can weigh themselves without judging them-selves harshly. Many other people, however, experience a lot of negative emotions when weighing themselves. This is referred to as negative self-talk—unpleasant, negative, and often hurtful things you say to yourself. Chapter 10 presents different strategies to help you change your pattern of self-talk. Developing the ability to weigh yourself in an objective, unemo-tional fashion is very important for long-term success. Doing so will help you stay on course, and catch problems early.

It is best to weigh yourself once a week, in the morning, without clothes. Keep in mind that your body weight normally fluctuates a few pounds a week—the taller and heavier you are, the more your weight can fluctuate. This is because of changes in water weight, changes in fiber intake, timing of bowel movements, and changes in physical activity levels. In the beginning you will be learning how your weight fluctuates. It is absolutely normal to lose a few pounds, bounce back up a few pounds, and then lose again. Sometimes you may feel that you are doing everything right, but your weight stays about the same for a few weeks, and then drops a few pounds all in 1 week. Basically, your weight is not something you can directly control. You can control what you eat and how much you exercise, and eventually your weight will respond. However, it usually does not respond in a very predictable and consistent manner. It is important to keep a record of your weight so that you can observe and learn from the trends. You are looking for a gradual decline over time, meaning over months. Along the way there will be bumps along the road, weight changes that are higher or lower than anticipated. Try not to overreact to these larger than normal jumps in your weight. The pattern over time is most important. This topic will be addressed again in Chapter 11.

If your progress stalls or you would like to include more healthy proteins and fats in your diet, you can transition to the moderate-carb route at the same calorie level.

## Advantages of the High-Carb Route

Decades of research indicate that those that are not insulin resistant will greatly benefit from following a largely plant-based diet that is high in carbohydrates and fiber and low in saturated fats. Such a diet has a very-low-calorie density, meaning that you can enjoy a greater quantity of food without a lot of calories, because most of the foods have a high water and fiber content.[3,9–20,21,22,23] The high-carb, plant-based eating style described in this chapter is very high in antioxidants and phytochemicals, which researchers have shown can prevent cancer and heart disease. Dietary antioxidants help prevent oxidative reactions that lead to the production of free radicals, which damage your body's cells and tissues. Your body has natural defenses against these free radicals; however, dietary antioxidants boost these defense mechanisms and help prevent potential damage. Excessive oxidative damage is associated with increased risk for cancer, heart disease, cataracts, and general aging. Therefore, having a lot of antioxidants in your diet can prevent or slow down these processes.[22,24–30]

In addition, a diet similar to the high-carb plan described in this chapter in combination with regular physical activity and stress reduction strategies has been shown to cause a regression in coronary artery plaque. In other words, patients who were known to have moderate-to-severe amounts of plaque in their arteries were able to significantly reduce the amount of plaque and therefore increase blood flow to their hearts by following a diet similar to this eating plan. As fully explained in Chapter 3, here is one explanation of how this occurs. The liver can make hormones and other products, such as bile, from cholesterol. Bile is needed to digest fats. When you eat fat, your body excretes bile into your digestive tract. Fiber in your diet traps the bile and drags it out of your body when you have a bowel movement. This is the best way to get cholesterol out of your body. If you do not have a lot of fiber, the bile gets back into your body through your colon and gets recycled. There are also many other mechanisms at work to explain why a very-low-fat diet can decrease your risk or severity of heart disease. If you would like to maximize the heart disease prevention power of this diet, discuss adding 1 to 3 grams of long-chain omega-3 fatty acid (fish oil) supplements with your health care provider.[3,18–20,31,32]

A high-carbohydrate diet like the one presented in this chapter has been shown in many studies to lower blood pressure. Similar to the high-carb plan described in this chapter, the diet in these studies had the following characteristics: (1) high in fiber; (2) lots of vegetables; (3) a few servings of whole fruits; (4) 2 servings of low-fat, unsweetened milk, and yogurt; (5) moderate protein content; and (6) low saturated fat content. These foods provide important nutrients such as calcium, magnesium, and potassium that are known to help control blood pressure.[11,12] In addition, the plan provides a diet with a low glycemic index and a low sodium content by emphasizing foods from the green inner circle of the Bull's-Eye Food Guide.

A high-carb eating style with a lot of fiber can also support a healthy gastrointestinal tract, which is essential for optimal health. The average person has about 2 pounds of bacteria (comprised of over 400 different species) living in their gastrointestinal tract, which is referred to as the microflora. The microflora is made up of friendly bacteria that promote health (probiotics), and unfriendly or pathogenic bacteria that can cause illness if able to multiply unchecked. An unhealthy balance of microflora can result from poor diet, illness, and some medications. A variety of different dietary fibers and phytochemicals in plant-based foods encourage the growth and activity of a healthy mix of microflora. Diet plays a determining role in the kinds and number of microorganisms in your gastrointestinal tract. A healthy gastrointestinal system with adequate probiotics is thought to optimize health (making nutrients such as vitamin K and vitamin $B_{12}$), prevent disease (especially some types of cancer), and reverse some illnesses (e.g., chronic diarrhea). Your body's immune function is dependent on interactions among the microflora, the lining of your intestinal tract, and the part of your immune system active in your gut. The gastrointestinal tract needs regular immune stimulation by probiotics to start and regulate appropriate immune responses to pathogens and antigens, as well as to not overrespond and cause allergies and autoimmune diseases.[33–36]

## Disadvantages of the High-Carb Route

*There are no disadvantages to following the high-carb route as described in this chapter.* For those that are insulin resistant, however, it should not be your first choice. For anybody selecting this eating style, problems may occur if a large amount of the carbohydrates come from sugars and refined grains, especially refined grain products with added trans fats (partially hydrogenated oils). The high-carb plan presented in this chapter should be thought of as a very high-fiber eating style with lots of whole grains, vegetables, legumes, and whole or dried fruits. In the past, when Americans have tried to follow high-carbohydrate, low-fat diets, they have selected highly processed and refined grains (such as bagels, pasta, refined and sweetened cereals, white rice, white bread, and pretzels), and highly sweetened products (such as fat-free frozen desserts like frozen yogurt and sherbet, fat-free cakes and cookies, and highly sweetened fruit drinks). Between

1970 and 1995, when high-carbohydrate, low-fat diets were popular, sugar intake among Americans increased by 28 pounds per person per year (22%). In 2003, the intake of sweeteners per person per year was 142 pounds.[36] Part of the reason for this was the lack of clear nutrition recommendations from public health officials, the trend for food manufacturers to add corn sweeteners to the majority of processed foods, and general confusion among the public. This type of a high-sugar, high-carbohydrate eating plan has been shown by researchers to increase appetite, total calorie intake, and the risk for many chronic illnesses, such as heart disease and type 2 diabetes.[5,13,15,38]

The high-carb eating plan presented in this chapter and the Bull's-Eye Food Guide will clearly guide you in developing the healthiest high-carb plan that can facilitate weight loss and prevent chronic illnesses, as well as promote optimal health and well-being. For more practical information on changing your eating and exercise habits, and planning your weight management journey, read Chapters 9, 10, and 11.

## *Important Points To Remember from Chapter 8*

◉ You can lower your risk of heart disease and cancer and optimize your health with a plant-based diet that is high in phytochemicals and fiber, as well as low in animal fats and trans fats.

◉ Structured high-carb eating plans at the appropriate calorie level will start you off on your weight management journey.

◉ You can, and should, modify your plan and include favorite foods to help you stay on course and reach your destination.

◉ Expect to stumble or lose your way along your journey—but get back on course quickly by objectively recognizing your missteps and not overreacting.

◉ Begin to consider your strategy to monitor your weight and check your progress. (More about this in Chapter 10.)

◉ The high-carb route presented allows you to get the maximum benefit from a high intake of phytochemicals, fibers, and micronutrients. It also allows you to avoid the potential risks of excessive protein or saturated/trans fat intake.

# GETTING A BETTER
# SENSE OF DIRECTION

## What You Will Discover in Chapter 9

⦿ The Bull's-Eye Food Guide is an excellent tool to plan for high-quality foods. The swapping system is a structured method of planning appropriate amounts of food to eat, but this system is not connected to your internal signals of hunger and fullness.

⦿ To maximize long-term success, it is helpful to transition to the hunger-fullness scaling system to determine how much to eat based on your internal signals of hunger and fullness.

⦿ To plan meals and snacks that are consistent with the eating style you selected (high-carb, moderate-carb, or lower-carb), you need to consider the relative amounts of foods from each food group, especially the Grain & Starch Group, the Protein Group, and the Fat Group. You can use common household items to estimate relative portions.

The Bull's-Eye Food Guide and swapping system provides an initial sense of direction for travel on your weight management journey. Selecting foods primarily from the green inner circle points you in the direction of a high-quality eating style. Using the swapping system and recommended eating plan points you in the direction of the right mix and amount of calories.

Now it is time to look at other complementary tools that will empower you along your lifelong journey towards optimal health and weight. Keep in mind that eating fewer calories than you use is key to weight loss. If you eat fewer calories but most of your food choices are in the red outer circle, you will lose weight but not achieve optimal health. Eating fewer calories from *healthy* foods is key to *long-term healthy* weight loss. After all, you want to be healthier—not just smaller. There are a few ways to approach the process of cutting back on calories. The two *least* healthy ways are as follows: (1) completely avoiding a whole category of foods, such as all grains and starches, and (2) eating only a few specified foods, such as cabbage soup or grapefruits. These methods are easy at first, because they require less planning or thought on a day-to-day basis. By avoiding whole groups of foods, you actually just end up eating fewer calories, which of course leads to weight loss. However, few people are able to follow such an approach for a few months or more, so temporary weight loss is followed by weight gain. Emotionally, this is a very frustrating and stressful process. In addition, such diets are likely to provide inadequate amounts of some vitamins, minerals, fibers, or phytochemicals, and therefore have negative effects on long-term overall health. Such negative effects are typically subtle, and associated problems (such as heart disease, cancer, or osteoporosis) take a long time to develop. This makes it easy to ignore the possibility of these problems.

The two *healthiest* ways to cut back on calorie intake are as follows: (1) using a system that allows for a variety of healthy foods and makes counting calories easy, such as the Bull's-Eye Food Guide system, or (2) learning how to eat in a way that is connected to your true physical hunger and fullness, rather than in response to emotions or external cues. So far, the materials in this book have helped you with the first method to get started on your weight management journey. This method is largely dependent on learning the suggested eating style and eating approximately the amount or swaps of food recommended. This method is a great teaching tool, but it does not empower you to understand your current eating habits, your relationship with food, or strategies to change this relationship.

This chapter will focus on the second of the healthiest methods: eating high-quality foods in response to true physiological hunger and stopping eating when you are just comfortably full. The next chapter will introduce tools to explore your relationship with food and deal with emotional and psychological aspects of eating. These tools and strategies empower you to address your old unhealthy eating habits deeply and comprehensively. Therefore, they require a lot of thought and practice over an extended period of time. The time and effort you put into this process will enable you to successfully reach your destination—long-term maintenance of a healthy weight. It will be important for you to keep an open mind, try and retry different tools and strategies, and have patience. While you are practicing with these tools, you can rely on the menus and swapping system to plan meals and snacks. Consider the menus and swapping system as crutches that you can use for a short time while you relearn hunger-related eating. As you get more skilled at using these new tools, you will rely less on use of the swapping system in a way that requires weighing and measuring. You will continue to use the Bull's-Eye Food Guide to help you make high-quality, healthy food choices.

## The Bull's-Eye Swapping System— A Crutch for the Beginning of Your Journey

The Bull's-Eye Food Guide swapping system helps your track calories indirectly. Once you pick a calorie level and eating style, you are given a number of swaps from six different food groups to use each day and get started with weight loss. By eating the suggested number of servings from each of the food groups you are really counting calories, as well as balancing your carbohydrates, proteins, and fats. To follow your plan closely, you need to weigh or measure the amount of foods you eat and beverages you drink—

at least most of the time. After doing so for a while, you will be able to visually estimate (or "eyeball") the appropriate number of swaps for meals and snacks throughout the day. If weight loss slows down too much or stops, it is helpful to go back to weighing and measuring swaps of food. This is because after estimating for an extended period of time, your estimations tend to get much larger than the measured amounts. You may also generally become less aware of what you are eating during meals and between meals. So weighing and measuring foods again, helps you increase your awareness and estimate more accurately.

Another approach to estimating portion sizes is using the dimensions of your hands. The size of your hands is proportional to your body size, which is the main determinant of your calorie needs. Therefore, selecting serving sizes of foods by comparing the serving of food to the dimensions of your hand can be quite helpful at home and when eating out or traveling. In this approach use the following guidelines:

- Combined servings of all starchy foods in a meal (including any combination of cereals, pasta, rice, beans, corn, peas, or potatoes) should be equal to a pile no bigger than the size of one of your fists.

- Combined servings of high-protein foods (such as meat, fish, or chicken) should be about the size of the palm of one of your hands—the same length, width, and thickness (no fingers included).

- Combined servings of all fatty foods in a meal (such as olive oil or butter) should be equal to the amount that would fill a hole created by your thumbprint.

- In addition to the foods mentioned here, have mountains of hot and cold vegetables at the very beginning and during your meals—especially lunch and dinner. This is essential because vegetables take the edge off your appetite and make it possible to stick to the serving sizes of starches, proteins, and fats noted above.

- As a general rule all beverages should be noncaloric, except for one or two servings of low-fat milk a day. Try noncaloric flavored seltzers, iced herbal teas, or water with a slice of citrus fruit.

Most people find it difficult to weigh and measure foods and beverages they eat and drink for extended periods of time. It is recommended that you do so for about 4 weeks, or if you get stuck and can't seem to lose additional weight. However, you need to move on to a more self-empowering way of monitoring food intake that is based more on your internal signals of hunger and fullness rather than restrictions arbitrarily imposed by a diet program. Doing so is the basis of a realistic healthy eating style and weight management plan. In this chapter you will practice such a method—hunger-fullness scaling. You will need to learn and practice tools explained in Chapter 10 to successfully and completely adopt hunger-fullness scaling as your primary tool of managing your calorie intake and your weight. That process will come next.

## Hunger-Fullness Scaling—
## A Strategy for Long-Term Travel

Hunger-fullness scaling is a realistic strategy for long-term weight management. The process involves the following: (1) becoming very aware of how physically hungry or full you are before, during and after eating; (2) becoming very sensitive to subtle differences in hunger and fullness; and (3) responding appropriately to different levels of hunger and fullness. To measure your level of hunger or fullness, use the 0 to 10 scale described in Table 9-1.

### The Hunger-Fullness Scale

On the hunger-fullness scale, 5 is noted to be comfortable, neither hungry nor full. As time passes, you would get increasingly hungry if you did not eat. Increasing hunger is represented by increasingly lower numbers on the scale. A 4 on the scale is when you first become aware that you are less than comfortably full, but you are still comfortable. Next hunger cues begin to kick in and your stomach begins to feel empty. At 2 you are very

## Table 9-1. Hunger Fullness Scale

| 0 | 1 | 2 | 3 | 4 | 5 | 6 | 7 | 8 | 9 | 10 |
|---|---|---|---|---|---|---|---|---|---|---|
| Faint, weak Headache | Slight headache Feeling fatigued | Stomach feels emptier and may growl | Stomach begins to feel empty | Begin to feel hungry, but still comfortable | Comfortable | Begin to feel full but still have room | Feeling comfortably full | Clothes begin to feel tight | Feel uncomfortably full, sleepy | Completely stuffed; may have reflux |

| | Breakfast | Lunch | Dinner | Snack |
|---|---|---|---|---|
| **Planned Food Intake** | | | | |
| **Actual Intake** | | | | |
| **Notes** | | | | |

• 192 •

hungry, your stomach feels empty and may be growling. A 1 on the scale may be associated with a headache, feeling fatigued, or shaky hands. Finally at 0, you are starving, and feelings of fatigue, light-headedness, and shakiness are more intense. Higher numbers are associated with fullness. Fullness is a bit trickier to judge than hunger. This is because your stomach has to send chemical signals to your brain so that you recognize fullness. These chemical signals need about 20 to 30 minutes to travel through your bloodstream to your brain. Therefore, for about a half hour after you stop eating you continue to feel increasingly full. Just above comfortable, 6 on the hunger-fullness scale indicates that you are just beginning to feel full. A 7 represents being comfortably full. Eight is when your clothes start to feel tight, and 9 is when you feel uncomfortably full. At 10 you are completely stuffed, and may experience burping or reflux from your stomach up your esophagus. Everybody experiences hunger and fullness differently, so you should consider the descriptors above as guidelines. Modify the scale to reflect you personal signals of hunger and fullness.

## Using the Hunger-Fullness Scale

Now, to start becoming aware of your own levels of hunger and fullness, as well as of subtle differences in levels of hunger and fullness, use the hunger-fullness scaling worksheet presented in Table 9-1. In the first row, you are encouraged to generally plan to have healthy foods available for meals and snacks. Typically, it is most efficient to do this type of planning on a weekly basis by creating a shopping list and making one major food shopping trip for the week. Use the daily menus in Menus and Recipes for ideas. Then each night, plan more specifically for the next day. In the beginning it is best to write your plan down on a worksheet similar to Table 9-1. For example, if you go to bed with the idea that you will have whole-wheat bread, natural peanut butter, and banana for breakfast, it is easier to complete the plan and make the breakfast sandwich than to start thinking from scratch. If you are hungry you can eat it before you leave in the morning. If you aren't hungry, you can wrap it up and take it with you. This will prevent stopping off at the deli or the hot truck when hunger cues begin and you do not have a plan or easy access to healthy foods. Following your plan saves hundreds of calories. When and how much of your breakfast sandwich you eat will depend on your level of hunger in the morning. Similarly, if you know you will be out of the house or at work when you get hungry in the afternoon, give some thought as to what choices you will have for lunch. Will there be a place with a healthy salad bar—lean meat, fish, or chicken, beans, lots of vegetables, olive oil-based salad dressing, and whole grains? Or will your only choices be a high-fat deli sandwich, burgers, hot dogs, pizza, or fries? If healthy options will be limited, plan to bring lunch.

Dinner often seems the most overwhelming to pull together due to busy work and home schedules. Plan to have healthy leftovers from the weekend. When you make salad or vegetables, plan leftovers so you do not need to make these items every night. Perhaps you can cook whole-wheat pasta or brown rice while you are getting ready in the morning, rinse with cold water and refrigerate for easy reheating when you get home. Do whatever you can the night before or in the morning to commit yourself to eating at home rather than eating out or taking in on a regular basis. The calories in menu items when you eat out or take-in are almost always excessively high—way beyond what you would estimate them to be due to hidden fats and sweeteners. Involve all family members in pulling the day's meals together. When advancing to this internally guided system, you do not plan amounts of food you will eat. You are simply planning to have high-quality foods accessible, so you can put healthy meals together according to the timing and level of your hunger.

Sometimes you will not follow through on your plan. Therefore, in the next row of the worksheet shown in Table 9-1, write in the foods you actually do eat at each meal and snack soon after eating. Take time to reflect how often and under what circumstances you deviate from your plan. Does it happen more often when you are stressed or with certain people? How about when you are tired or lonely? Increasing your awareness of these types of patterns is the first step to exploring your relationship with food and improving your eating habits. Chapter 10 provides more tools to help you deal with these issues. For now, you are trying to notice patterns and trends in your levels of physiological hunger and fullness and how closely the amount of food you eat is related to your hunger and fullness. You will also be evaluating the quality of foods in your diet—meaning how many foods are from the green inner circle.

Although you are not recording amounts of food, you will be recording levels of hunger and fullness as a means to reconnect the amount of food you eat to internal physiological signals. As an infant, this connection was intact, and you ate when you were hungry and stopped eating when you were full. However, as you grew you were probably encouraged to finish bottles, take one more bite, or clean your plate. As you grew even older, you were increasingly exposed to advertisements luring you to eat, eat, eat! You were also likely exposed to vending machines and snack stands at schools and community sites, as well as instructed to sell candy to raise funds for your school, team, or club. These cues prompted you to eat, and disconnected eating from physiological hunger and fullness. Reestablishing this connection takes practice and effort. On the hunger-fullness worksheet, there are gray bubbles in the actual intake row. In the first bubble highest in the box record your level of hunger before you start eating, and in the second bubble record your level of fullness after you are done eating. At first you may find it difficult to assign a number to your level of hunger and fullness, but as you practice you will become increasingly confident in your ability to do so. Finally, in the notes cell, write how you were feeling, whom you ate with, and where you ate, as well as other factors that may affect what or how much you eat. The goal is to stay between a 2 or 3 on the hunger side and 7 on the fullness side. When your hunger gets to a level 2 or 3, you should begin to eat. If you let yourself get too hungry, such as a level 0 or 1, you are more likely to make poor choices, eat quickly, and eat too much in response. You should stop eating at a level 7, and about a half hour after eating you may bounce up to an 8. If you eat beyond this level, you are eating for reasons other than physiological hunger. You should keep hunger-fullness records for a few days or weeks and look for patterns and trends.

There are two common patterns that are problematic. First, you may find that you rarely let yourself get lower than a 4 on the hunger scale, because you are not comfortable with initial signs of hunger or because you get in the habit of picking frequently in response to external cues without much thought of hunger. You may also be using eating as a coping strategy to deal with emotions, such as anger, frustration, boredom, loneliness, or stress. (Chapter 10 helps you develop alternative coping strategies.) Over time you get used to high levels of fullness—an 8 or 9 on the scale starts to feel normal, and 5 starts to feel like hunger. Another problematic pattern is when you diet and ignore initial signs of hunger, and let yourself get too hungry. Such intense levels of hunger make it more likely that you will select a high-fat or -sugar food when you do eat. It also makes it more likely that you will eat quickly, overshoot initial signs of fullness, and overeat. In response to guilt associated with overeating, you are more likely to try to delay eating until a 0 or 1 again. Therefore, you bounce between 0 and 1 on the hunger scale and 9 or 10 on the fullness scale. This pattern is typically associated with a lot of negative feelings about eating choices and decisions.

As you complete the worksheets, you will become more aware of your internal hunger and fullness throughout the whole day. The next step is to work on appropriate responses—eating when you are hungry and delaying nonhunger eating until you are truly hungry. Resist trying to withhold eating too long in efforts to lose weight. Plan to have high-quality foods available when you typically get hungry. This usually means bringing foods from home. When you are eating, eat slowly and be aware of your increasing level of fullness. If you typically eat to 9 or 10 on the fullness scale, try to stop eating at 8 or 9 instead. When this feels more comfortable, then try stopping at an 8 consistently, and then at a 7.

To successfully retrain your body to interpret hunger and fullness, you need to tease apart habits tying eating to other activities, such as watching television. You may need to develop alternative strategies to cope with feelings, such as stress or loneliness. In addition, you may need to find other ways to reward yourself and fill your "down time" or your "me time." As noted above, such strategies are presented in Chapter 10. For now, consider one simple tool of developing a personalized "Top10 List" of things to do to delay non-hunger-related eating until you are truly hungry. To do this, consider what is realistic to do in different environments and at different times of the day. For example, you may put on your list some activities that are realistic to do at work, at home with the kids around, or at night when you are alone. Some examples might include the following: taking a walk; writing a letter; meditative breathing; calling a friend; participating in a hobby such as woodworking, knitting, making a scrapbook; taking a bath; doing stretching exercises; filing or polishing your nails; taking a nap or going to sleep; reading a book or magazine; doing yoga or tai chi; or listening to a guided-imagery tape.

When you are tempted to eat while you are not hungry, make a commitment to do one thing on your list for 15 minutes and then to recheck your hunger. If you are truly hungry after 15 minutes, then eat. If you are not below a 4 on the hunger scale, pick another thing to do on your list for another 15 minutes and then recheck your hunger again. Continue this process until the urge to eat dissipates or until you become legitimately hungry and eat. At first it may be difficult to delay eating, but by practicing this process you will be increasingly aware of your hunger and fullness and of subtle differences in the level of hunger and fullness. You will also become increasingly confident in your ability to respond appropriately—to delay nonhunger eating and to eat when you are hungry. Mastering the hunger-fullness scaling process is one of the keys to long-term success. Skills and strategies you learn in Chapter 10 will help you with this process. Although the concept is simple, it may take months or years to master this strategy and fully transition from the Bull's-Eye Food Guide swapping system to this internally guided system as your automatic, habitual mode of operating.

## Considering Your Selected Eating Style

When using this worksheet you are moving away from the very structured planning of meals and snacks and the practice of weighing and measuring your food intake. After initially following the suggested structured pattern for a few weeks, you should have a general feel for how to combine foods from the different food groups for your eating style—high-carb, moderate-carb, or lower-carb. To get an idea of the relative amount of food from the Grain & Starch Group to pair up with foods from the Protein Group and the Fat Group see Table 9-2. For example, on the lower-carb plan you would have *about* one Grain & Starch Group swap with every one and a half swaps from the Protein Group and every one and a half swaps from the Fat Group. If you were having dinner, the *relative* amounts of starch, protein, and fat you would strive for would be about ⅓ cup of brown rice to 1½ ounces of chicken and 1½ teaspoons of olive oil with at least 2 cups of vegetables. Although when you eat the total amount of food you eat should be guided by your hunger or fullness, you should strive to get close to the relative proportion of foods that is appropriate for your eating style. For moderate hunger, you might have ⅔ cups of brown rice to 3 ounces of chicken, and 3 teaspoons of olive oil to sauté 2 to 3 cups of vegetables. If you were even hungrier, you may have 1 cup of brown rice and 4½ ounces of chicken. At this point, you may not want to use all of your fat swaps on olive oil. You may use 3 teaspoons to sauté at least 2 cups of vegetables, and use the other 1½ fat swaps for nine almonds on the side. If you are still hungry, try more vegetables or try using one of your fruit swaps before adding more swaps from the other foods groups. If you are following the moderate-carb or high-carb plan, you use the same general principles. Strive to follow the guidelines for the relative amounts of Grain & Starch Group swaps, Protein Group swaps, and Fat Group swaps when planning the quality of foods on the hunger-fullness scaling worksheet, but whether you halve, double, or triple the baseline number of swaps would depend on your level of hunger. At this point you should just be estimating, not measuring, portion sizes. Keep in mind the following when estimating food amounts:

- One cup of a food would look like a tennis ball

- One ounce of a food from the Protein Group would be about the size of a lipstick or Chapstick tube

- Four ounces of protein looks like a deck of cards

- A teaspoon of fat looks like a stack of five quarters

**Table 9-2.**

Three Different Eating Styles and Relative Amounts of Swaps
from the Six Food Groups in the Bull's-Eye Food Guide

| Food Group | Lower-Carb | Moderate-Carb | High-Carb |
|---|---|---|---|
| Grain & Starch Group | 1 | 1 | 1 |
| Protein Group | 1½ | 1 | ½ |
| Fat Group | 1½ | 1 | ¼ |

There are no limits on nonstarchy vegetables. Have at least 3 cups a day. Most people should also have 2 cups of low-fat milk or yogurt a day. For information on fruits refer to the text.

| *Food Examples to Indicate Relative Amounts* | ⅓ cup brown rice for every 1½ ounces of salmon and every 1½ teaspoons of olive oil to sauté vegetables | ⅓ cup brown rice for every 1 ounce of salmon and every 1 teaspoon of olive oil to sauté vegetables | ⅓ cup brown rice for every ½ ounce of salmon and every ¼ teaspoon of olive oil to sauté vegetables |
|---|---|---|---|

## *Important Points To Remember from Chapter 9*

◉ We are born with an internal ability to sense our levels of hunger and fullness and respond appropriately. However, this ability is undermined by typically well-intended but inappropriate encouragement by

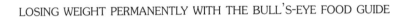

significant people in our lives to eat when we are not hungry. Mass media also encourage excessive consumption.

◉ Using the Bull's-Eye Food Guide swapping system and suggested daily menus in Menus and Recipes is an appropriate method to initiate weight loss. For long-term success, it is essential to develop a system to reconnect subtle internal signals of hunger and fullness to when and how much you eat.

◉ You should plan at least 1 day in advance to have high-quality, green inner circle foods available for your meals and snacks in the appropriate relative proportions. Monitor your level of hunger to determine when to eat, and your level of fullness to determine how much to eat or when to stop eating.

◉ With this more casual and physiologically connected method of determining when and how much to eat, use the guidelines on relative proportions of Grains & Starch Group swaps, Protein Group swaps, and Fat Group swaps to plan meals and snacks that are consistent with your selected eating style from Chapter 5.

# TOOLS, TOOLS,
# AND MORE TOOLS

### *What You Will Discover in Chapter 10*

⊚ There are many factors that influence your eating habits,
including your own biochemistry and physiology; interactions
among families, friends, and co-workers; and cultural trends in
society.

⊚ A new area of research on the palatability of foods reveals a
dynamic interaction among food components and your biochemical response to them. This dynamic relationship affects
your conditioned eating behaviors, as well as your ability to
sense hunger and fullness and respond appropriately.

⊚ To positively change your eating habits, you need to explore
your current habits and your relationship with food. This
process helps you identify opportunities to reshape them.

⊚ A variety of tools and techniques are recommended to reshape
your eating habits; these include mindful eating, goal ladders,
meditation, journaling, positive affirmations, and guided
imagery.

> ## What You Will Discover in Chapter 10
> ### (continued)
>
> ◉ Behavior changes occur in an expected sequence but do not progress in a simple straightforward fashion.
>
> ◉ It is important to develop a strategy of monitoring your weight in a nonemotional and objective way.

## The Changing Terrain

Travelers need many tools to negotiate their way through new and unfamiliar terrain. As you move along on your weight management journey, you will be challenged by new terrain as you negotiate changes in your relationship with food. There are many tools provided later in this chapter to help you explore and change your complex relationship with food. This relationship is only partially based on the need for calories and nutrients, as well as physiological hunger. Genetics also plays a role in this relationship—your body's chemistry and physiology partially dictate perceptions of hunger and appetite. For most people, these physiological aspects of their relationship with food are molded and shaped by their physical, social, and cultural environments. For example, food is often used as a way to express love. Parents, friends, and spouses often use food to show love, reward achievement, or as a focus of celebrations. Parents and child care providers often encourage children to eat past fullness, because doing so makes the adult feel like a successful care provider. This use of food is not new. However, the combination of food flavorings, such as sweeteners, salt, trans fats, and other chemicals, used in processed food has changed over recent years.

The dramatic increase in access to food also contributes to overeating. One sign of this is the increased number of vending machines in schools, work environments, and community agencies. Such access means that we rarely do anything (bowl, shop at the mall, or see a movie) without eating a meal or snack. Because the least healthy foods, such as chips, cookies, snack cakes, and candy, are cheapest and most readily and conveniently available, they are most often provided at meetings or clubs or in vending machines. In addition to increased availability of snack food items, there is an increased availability of convenience items for meals. This includes partially prepared items (rice or pasta mixes) and home replacement meals (rotisserie chicken and potato salad). Of course, there is also the wide variety of take-out foods, fast food restaurant fare, and car-friendly food for eating on the run. These foods are typically infused with sweeteners, sodium, and trans fats. Therefore, they perpetuate the desire for such strong processed tastes and make it difficult to appreciate the natural flavor of foods. They may also encourage eating past fullness. Their modest cost and convenience are additional factors that make them hard to resist. Therefore, although food has been used as a reward and a central part of celebrations for hundreds of years, the type, nutritional quality, and availability of foods have changed dramatically and to a greater extent than is generally understood by consumers. Consumers have not been provided with the tools to understand these rapid changes in the food supply.

Other factors that influence eating habits are associated with the complex issue of food palatability. From a food manufacturer's perspective, palatability equates to taste and is crucial to increase market share and profit. While food manufacturers are driven to provide palatable foods, researchers have shown that palatability is more than a matter of taste alone. There is a complex relationship between characteristics of food and biochemical responses within your body after eating food. These interactions are now the subject of active research, which is offering an expanded definition of the dynamic processes related to palatability. Palatability is now considered in two stages. The first stage is dominated by the characteristics of foods that are experienced while eating, such as flavor from added sweeteners, trans fats, sodium, and monosodium glutamate. The second stage deals with internal responses to chemical components of foods that are absorbed into your body after eating, including chemical messages sent from your gut to your brain, as well as biochemical responses by other body systems. This stage is influenced by each person's biochemistry and physiology. After your tongue, your gastrointestinal tract, or gut, is the next area of contact for the food you eat. Your gut readily communicates with your brain and other systems in your body, and food components have a direct impact on the production of many body chemicals, including neurotransmitters (chemicals produced by nerve cells in your brain).[1] For example, researchers have found evidence that enhanced activity in a specific area of the brain responsible for sensory processing of food may make overweight people more sensitive to palatability aspects of foods. In addition, some overweight people have a decreased ability to detect the presence of dopamine (a neurotransmitter normally produced in the brain) that increases feelings of satisfaction and pleasure in response to environmental stimuli, including food. This may lead some people to overeat in efforts to stimulate dopamine production and detection. Some researchers have noted that these interactions are similar to mechanisms of drug addictions.[2,3]

As the research in this area expands, more questions arise. Can combinations of sweeteners, trans fats, monosodium glutamate, and salt found in many foods increase palatability too much? Is there a potential for negative physiological effects in some people? These questions are especially timely because of the obesity epidemic and the dramatic increase in access to cheap, high-calorie foods with palatable combinations of sweeteners, trans fats, sodium, and monosodium glutamate. Essentially, there are complex interactions between individual factors (production and sensitivity to neurotransmitters, activity and responsiveness of specific areas of the brain to food, communication between the gut and brain, personality traits, and emotional states) and food characteristics (appearance, smell, texture, taste, and specific constituents). The interaction and feedback among these factors are likely to have a strong influence on initiation and termination of eating events, experiences of hunger and fullness, and development of learned patterns of eating. Your attention to these issues is necessary to increase awareness of your eating patterns and what appears to trigger overeating. With this information, you can develop strategies and coping mechanisms to change these patterns. Depending on various aspects of your chemical and physiological makeup, this may take more or less effort. For example, the hunger-fullness-scaling strategy presented in Chapter 9 may take longer to learn to use effectively for people who are more sensitive to food cues. However, it is the process of exploring, understanding, and changing your relationship with food and learned patterns of eating that will help you along your journey and lead to long-term success. Consider this process an opportunity to identify eating habits and patterns that you can change over time. The rest of this chapter will briefly review ideas about how people change behavior and then present a variety of strategies recommended to explore and change patterns of eating. Keep an open mind when reading about these strategies, and give each one a try. Then determine which you are willing to put into practice on a regular basis at this time. Reconsider using the other strategies periodically. In other words, this chapter should be read and reread many times as you work through these processes of reshaping your eating habits. These strategies also offer hope for true long-term success!

## Factors Influencing Your Eating Habits

Individuals' behaviors are shaped by factors at many levels: individual characteristics, relationships among individuals, institutions in which individuals operate, and the larger socio-cultural-political level.[4,5] Individual factors include biological makeup and learned behaviors. You have the most control at this level, but it is important to be aware of how factors at other levels influence your behavior. Over time you may choose to advocate change at multiple levels, such as within your home, your community, or at the level of public policy. By increasing your awareness and knowledge of factors at these levels, you can change your response to these factors, since you usually can't change factors at all of these levels quickly.

There are many ideas in behavioral research for you to consider regarding how people can successfully shape eating habits. Figure 10-1 reflects factors that influence how people form and shape their eating behaviors. Reviewing these ideas will help you identify opportunities and develop strategies to change undesirable eating behaviors and shape positive new ones. Factors that affect eating behavior are divided into three categories: individual factors, factors associated with family members and friends, and factors in our physical environment.

Biochemical and physiological factors, such as genetic predispositions, are very important but cannot be directly changed. However, you can change how these factors are expressed and the associated conditioned patterns of behaviors. Individual factors you can change include knowledge, such as detailed awareness of your current eating habits or how weight negatively affects your health. It would also include your knowledge of healthy foods, how to read food labels, and a your eating style. Healthy cooking techniques and hunger-fullness-scaling skills are also very important, as are skills to deal with stress and negative emotions. Meditation, guided imagery, and journaling are examples of such positive coping skills.

Perceptions and attitudes strongly influence behavior and acquisition of knowledge and skills. For example, your belief that you can positively change your eating habits and lose weight is critical for successfully navigating the long-term process of permanent weight loss. The way you perceive the relative balance of positive and negative consequences of changing your eating behaviors will determine the success of your behavior change. For example, if you believe that the benefits of eating healthier far outweigh potential inconveniences of learning to shop and cook differently, you are more likely to change your behaviors appropriately. Realistic short- and long-term expectations and patience are also important to develop. Chapter 11 reviews issues relevant to short- and long-term weight-loss goals and expectations. Positive perceptions and attitudes as just noted help build and sustain motivation to change eating habits. Once you have developed the knowledge, skills, and motivation, you need to secure the necessary resources. The most precious resource is time—it will take time for you to develop new cooking and food-shopping strategies,

**Figure 10-1.** Factors Affecting Your Eating Behaviors

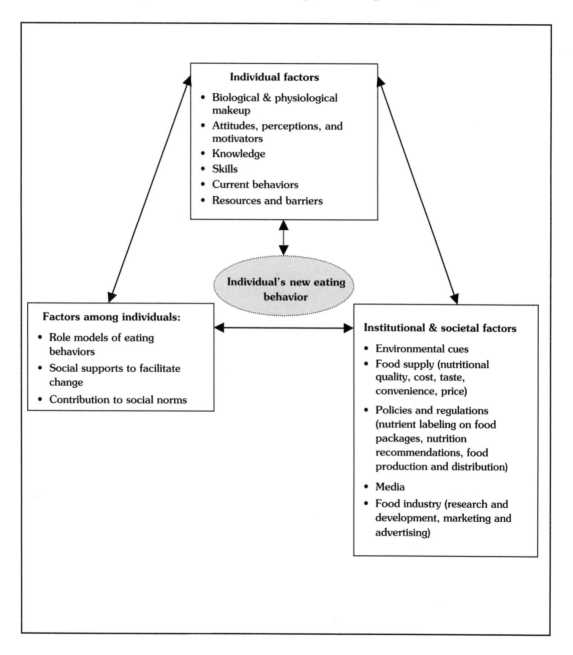

practice new coping skills, and change your relationship with food. You may need to reconsider how you allocate your time and the priorities you set for use of your time. Changes in your use of time may also affect other people in your family, so this has to be negotiated with significant others. The factors previously discussed influence the shaping of your new eating habits, and as just mentioned your behaviors and the behaviors of significant others interact and affect each other.

The eating behaviors of other people in your life are developed and molded by the same general factors discussed previously. As you are changing and improving your eating habits, significant people in your life may follow along or they may have already had healthy eating habits. If this is the case, they act as positive role models and supports for you. If this is not the case, and they are not willing or able to improve their eating habits, you need to use the strategies that follow to change your responses to their unsupportive attitudes and behaviors. This may slow your travel on your weight-loss journey, but need not prevent it or end it. To counterbalance those that are unsupportive, you may need to develop friendships with others who have similar goals to improve their eating habits and health. The behaviors of others are important, because it is through behaviors and actions that you interact with other people and influence each other's actions. Individuals interact and help shape the physical environment and policies within institutions, as well as social norms and the prevailing culture. Powerful factors at the level of culture and society include governmental policies guiding nutrition recommendations, nutrition labeling on food packages, and food advertising, as well as media messages. At first it may seem overwhelming to advocate for change at these levels. However, as you increase your knowledge and awareness of the nutritional quality of foods and change your behaviors you may want to affect gradual positive changes in your workplace, school district, and community. For example, you may want to work with a committee to select healthy food choices for vending machines in your workplace, or you may initiate a nutrition committee in your school district to draft nutrition policies for consideration by the board of education. Such changes will have a positive influence on your family, friends, and fellow community members, as well as reinforce your own healthy behaviors.

# New Navigation Tools

Now it is time to discover and practice new tools and strategies to influence some of the factors in Figure 10-1, and enable you to shape new healthy eating habits.

## Mindful Eating

One of the most important and basic strategies is mindful eating. Mindful eating is the practice of slowing the pace of daily living and using all your senses when eating to fully experience the food. Eating in this way helps you to successfully use the hunger-fullness scaling technique in Chapter 9, because it involves eating slowly and avoiding distractions. Here is an activity you can do to acquaint yourself with mindful eating. To do the activity, you will need one plump raisin. It is best to actually do the activity, but you can also get the general idea by just reading along.

- First take the raisin and place it in the center of your hand. Examine the raisin and notice the complexity of the color and texture. At first you may think the raisin is simply brown, but upon closer inspection you will notice that it has many shades of reddish-brown with a grayish-white sheen in the many creases and folds.

- Next, put the raisin in your mouth, but do not chew it. Instead, roll it around your tongue and feel the bumps and ridges. Do you notice a sweet taste? Is it sweeter on the front tip of you tongue? (Your taste buds for sweet are in the front of your tongue, and the taste buds for bitter are on the back of your tongue.) Notice the increase in saliva in your mouth.

- Now, bite the raisin just once. An intense sweet taste should flood over your tongue.

- Slowly chew the raisin 20 times before swallowing, and note the incredible amount of flavor derived from just one raisin.

⦿ Imagine the raisin traveling through your intestines and nutrients (or small components of the raisin) passing through your intestines to nourish your body.

During this exercise you involved your sense of taste, as well as your sense of touch and sight. With other types of foods, you can also involve your sense of smell and hearing (i.e., with crunchy foods).

This eating experience was probably in stark contrast to how you typically eat. Although it is unlikely that you will involve your senses to this degree every time you eat, you can strive to move in the direction of mindful eating. To do so, plan your meals to include a variety of colors, textures, smells, and flavors. When you eat, do not do other things such as watch television or do paperwork. Avoid thinking of stressful things. Instead concentrate on your food, putting your fork down between bites and chewing slowing and completely. You can also take time to consider the forces that brought the food to your table and express thankfulness. Eating in this way allows you to also be mindful of your internal signals of hunger and fullness, and to satisfy your hunger earlier. It also emphasizes that eating should be a pleasant experience that connects us to the world around us.

## Goal Ladders

A sample goal ladder worksheet is shown in Figure 10-2. A goal ladder is designed to build your confidence in crafting healthy eating behaviors and achieving a healthy weight. Although you wish to lose weight and improve your health, these concerns are not considered appropriate goals because they are not directly and completely within your control. A goal has to be specific, measurable, positively stated, and within your control. The goal ladder encourages you to establish short-term goals that are possible to achieve in a week. Each week you review your goal ladder and check off the goals you were able to achieve. If you were able to achieve the few goals set for the week, check them off and take the time to recognize and feel good about your achievements. Then establish new goals. If you were not able to achieve a goal, consider whether you think it is appropriate to try

**Figure 10-2.** Goal Ladder Worksheet

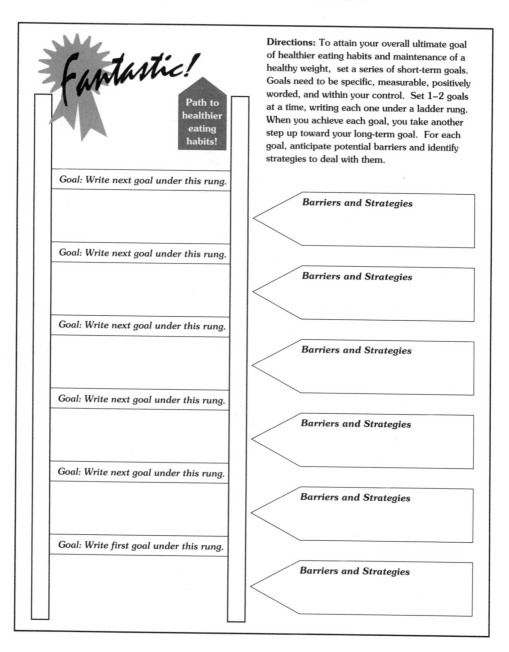

**Directions:** To attain your overall ultimate goal of healthier eating habits and maintenance of a healthy weight, set a series of short-term goals. Goals need to be specific, measurable, positively worded, and within your control. Set 1–2 goals at a time, writing each one under a ladder rung. When you achieve each goal, you take another step up toward your long-term goal. For each goal, anticipate potential barriers and identify strategies to deal with them.

Fantastic!

Path to healthier eating habits!

Goal: Write next goal under this rung.

Goal: Write next goal under this rung.

Goal: Write next goal under this rung.

Goal: Write next goal under this rung.

Goal: Write next goal under this rung.

Goal: Write first goal under this rung.

Barriers and Strategies

Barriers and Strategies

Barriers and Strategies

Barriers and Strategies

Barriers and Strategies

Barriers and Strategies

another week. You may need to reconsider whether a goal is actually achievable at this time. It may be better to put it on hold, revisit it another time, and set a different goal. Holding on to a goal for too long can lead to frustration and work against you. After a few weeks or months of setting and meeting goals, you will establish a sense that you can be successful in shaping healthy eating behaviors, one step at a time. It is important to take this stepwise approach as healthy eating involves changing so many behaviors that trying to change them all at once is difficult. When starting out, you may have adopted your selected eating style and the sample menus completely, because you were enthusiastic. However, many people find it difficult to continue to maintain all of these changes, and may revert back to some old habits. This is common and does not need to be the source of great concern if you start the suggested goal setting approach to *gradually* readopt the recommended eating style in steps on a more permanent basis.

Review the goal ladder worksheet in Figure 10-2. To start, set two small, specific, positively stated and measurable goals that are within your control. Here are some examples: (1) I will increase the number of vegetable swaps I eat each day from two to four; (2) I will decrease the cans of soda I drink each day from three to one; (3) I will increase the cups of water I drink a day from one to four; (4) I will eat breakfast at home according to my selected eating style and calorie level four times a week; or (5) I will switch from whole milk to 2% milk. Although each change may seem small, they will add up over time to equal calorie savings. In addition, you will be giving yourself the time necessary to practice changes in your lifestyle that will be required to attain such goals.

In addition to establishing goals, carefully consider what barriers might occur when trying to implement the goals and what you may do to prevent or overcome barriers. For example, when trying to increase your vegetable intake you may find you do not have enough time to clean and prepare fresh vegetables. Your strategy to overcome this anticipated barrier may be to plan leftovers when you do make fresh vegetables and to buy a variety of frozen vegetables to use when fresh is not possible. When trying to increase your water intake, availability during the day may be a barrier. Strategies to overcome this barrier may be to buy a few insulated water bottles to fill at home and bring with you.

This tool works best if you set aside the same time each week to review and set your goals. Like the other tools, it requires that you make time to increase your awareness of your eating habits and develop realistic and detailed plans to change.

## Meditation

Meditation is an excellent tool for dealing with stress and negative emotions. It is an incredibly healthy alternative to eating in response to stress or emotions. The key to meditation is focus—focusing on a word, a picture, or your breathing—in order to quiet and calm your busy mind. Sharply focusing your attention on such things allows you to be mindful of the moment and release thoughts of the past or future—to be free of stress and emotions. Meditation allows you to access the "relaxation response," which is characterized by a wakeful, relaxed state that is guided by the parasympathetic part of your autonomic nervous system. The other branch of this system, the sympathetic nervous system, is stimulated by emotional or physical stress and results in release of stress hormones, such as cortisol. Stress hormones increase heart rate, blood pressure, and the release of fats and sugar in the blood. In the days of cave people, this response helped them escape dangers such as a charging wooly mammoth. The increased blood flow and nutrients are necessary for muscular activity, for example, to run and escape. The stress people experience today, however, does not usually require a quick physical escape, and you rarely need to move in response to stress. Therefore, the results of the stress response are not helpful, and when not immediately followed by physical activity the resulting increase in blood pressure, heart rate, and fats in the blood are harmful. The relaxation response is associated with many positive physiological effects, such as decreased heart rate, breathing rate, blood pressure, and cortisol levels. The relaxation response can relieve stress and the associated risk for many chronic illnesses. It has been shown to decrease the severity of specific conditions associated with stress, such as tension headaches and high blood pressure.[6–9] Individuals with anxiety disorders, paranoia, or delusional thoughts should discuss the appropriateness of meditation with their health care provider before trying it.

When first learning to meditate it is important to create an appropriate setting. Each time you meditate re-create the same setting. Identify a quiet, private space to meditate in which you will not be distracted or interrupted. Select soothing instrumental music if you like. Wear loose, comfortable clothing. Your position is important. Sit in a chair or on the floor with your back straight and your weight comfortably balanced by gravity, rather than in a position that requires sustained muscular contractions. In other words, sit comfortably with your muscles relaxed. The goal is to start off alert, yet relaxed. Your point of focus can be a saying or your breathing. Breathe in and out through your nose. At first breathe in for 6 seconds, hold your breath for 4 seconds, and then slowly breathe out for 6 seconds. Breaths should be deep and fill your lungs, which will result in the rise of your stomach. This is called diaphragmatic breathing, which requires your diaphragm muscle to move down allowing for full inflation of your lungs. This is in contrast to common shallow breathing. With practice, you will be able to take longer to breath in and out, as you learn to take slower and deeper breaths. Your mind becomes focused on the rhythm of breathing and filled with a sense of calm and peace, and negative emotions such as stress and worry are released. Your state of mind is calm and nonreactive.

There are many resources available to learn and practice meditation: Your local library, health care facilities, or community centers may offer meditation classes. You can find audio- and videotapes on meditation and yoga, which is a type of movement meditation. You will also be able to find many resources by searching the Internet using the key words "meditation" or "meditative breathing." Here are a few tips. To begin meditation, close your eyes and breathe deeply and rhythmically, focusing on each inhalation and exhalation. Some people find it helpful to release tension by beginning their meditation with a body scan. Focus on each body part. Squeeze the associated muscles when you inhale, and then release the tension when you exhale, relaxing the body part. You can focus on your toes, feet, calves, thighs, pelvis, abdomen, shoulders, upper arms, forearms, hand, fingers, neck, jaws, and forehead, to name a few. Go through each body part in a detached, passive fashion without judging or evaluating the body part. With each body part relaxed, focus on the rhythm of your slow and deep breathing.

Although your goal is to clear your mind and simply focus on your breathing, you will find that your mind wanders. This is natural. As thoughts occur to you, acknowledge them and let them go. It may be helpful to imagine yourself sitting in a quiet, empty, peaceful room with two windows, one along the wall to the right and one along the wall to the left. As thoughts come to you, imagine a balloon coming in one window. Acknowledge the thought with a passive sense of detachment, put it in the balloon and let it float out the other window. In the beginning you may have a steady stream of balloons floating through your room. With practice, the thoughts will come less frequently, and you may only occasionally have a balloon floating through. Focus on the process not your performance. Unfortunately, many people give up on meditation, because they think they are not doing it correctly. Have confidence in yourself— everybody who is committed to the process can learn to meditate. Joining a meditation group or meditating with the assistance of an audio- or videotape may be helpful in the beginning.

When you are done meditating, you will be in a more relaxed state. Take your time to open your eyes and return to a normal state of awareness. Feeling the benefits of meditation may take weeks or months of practice—patience is key. You will be able to experience many of the benefits of meditation way before being able to completely clear your mind. Set aside a time to practice meditation, at least 10 minutes once or twice a day. After practicing for some time you will find that you can meditate in very busy places to deal with a stress or negative emotions when they occur, instead of using food. You can use modified meditative breathing techniques to elicit a relaxed state and to create a space or an opportunity in which to consider possible reactions to a situation or an emotion. Quite often, just focused, slow, deep rhythmic breathing, even in public with your eyes open, can elicit the relaxation response. It may also be helpful to assume a straight and balanced posture, and release muscular tension. Once you are relaxed and calm, you can check in on your hunger or fullness level and decide whether eating is appropriate. If you are hungry, you can also consider the quality of the food available, and decide whether to eat and how much you will eat or if you should choose to go someplace else to eat. Meditation followed by positive affirmations can be especially helpful to resume objective control of the situation and to avoid poor-quality food choices or eating beyond comfortable fullness. More about positive affirmations in the next section.

## Journaling and Positive Affirmations

The verbal or written expression of thoughts is a bridge between mind and body. The expression of thoughts is often suppressed—quiet self-talk not realized by the conscious self. In regards to weight, body image, food, and eating, this self-talk is often negative. It festers below the surface, driving negative emotions and non-hunger-related eating. It is an extremely powerful force. By actively changing the self-talk script and journaling about eating experiences, you can harness the power of expression to work for you—not against you!

Researchers have found that writing or talking about emotionally upsetting experiences can decrease symptoms of some chronic illnesses, enhance immune function, and result in fewer medical visits.[10,11] To establish a habit of journaling, set aside at least 20 minutes, 4 days a week to journal and reflect on your writings. You can journal by hand or by using a computer. Do not focus on spelling or grammar, just write continuously. If you experience a block, simply describe your eating-related activities in the past day or so, including details about your surroundings, the food and with whom you ate. Then describe any sensations you experienced or feelings you remember. Allow your emotions to run freely. Try to recapture the self-talk associated with these eating events in as much detail as possible. Most often self-talk associated with eating is emotionally charged and negative. Reflect on your self-talk. If it is negative, try putting a single line through the negative comments, and rewrite a positive script. For example, imagine that you selected a high-calorie dessert when eating out and felt so guilty that you ate it quickly before realizing the extent of your fullness. When journaling that night you describe the event and the meal, as well as the negative stream of thoughts that filled your head during and after eating dessert. Take some time to reflect on this negative self-talk and the factors that contributed to eating passed fullness. Next take a different color of pen and put a line through the negative thoughts. Write a new script, a stream of positive thoughts, above the negative writings. For example, your negative thoughts may have started after you ordered dessert. "I can't believe I just ordered that! What was I thinking! I am so stupid, I just blew the whole day. I might as well just give up, I'll never be able to change my eating habits and lose weight!" Upon reflecting on these thoughts, you realize that you set yourself up to fail when dessert was presented on the table. Next, you take a green pen and draw a line through the negative thoughts. On top write positive thoughts you would like to train yourself to say in similar situations—the automatic self-talk to replace the current script. "Everybody enjoys dessert-type foods at times, and I am no different. I can mindfully eat a dessert-type food while monitoring my level of fullness. Before I get too full, I will honor my body and my inner self and stop eating. Because I know it is okay for me to work these types of foods into my eating style I will have no guilt and simply save the rest for another time." When these words are expressed you set yourself up to succeed when dessert arrives. You implant in your mind a plan for success.

After writing the new script, read it out loud with conviction. Read your positive affirmations every time you journal (at least four times a week) and even daily if possible. Initially, you may not be completely successful in following through on your script, in this case eating only to comfortable fullness. This may be because old thoughts seep back into your mind. However, with practice over time you will become increasingly confident and successful in following through on your script and affirmation. Having success in this type of situation is a sign that you will have long-term success in establishing this type of casual and healthy relationship with food, and management of a healthy weight will follow.

If you have gone on a diet in the past, you may have written down all of the foods you ate each day. This is very different than journaling about your thoughts, feelings, experiences, and self-talk. However, for some people this is a familiar way to start journaling. This can be helpful, as long as the journaling does not stop with the list of foods but develops into the type of journaling described above. You'll be amazed at what you learn about yourself when you journal and what patterns are revealed. This type of self-exploration will help you design successful strategies and set appropriate goals to lead you to healthy eating habits. You will find many books and resources on journaling and positive self-talk or affirmations at your local library or on the Internet. A recommended CD set by Belleruth Naparstek that introduces meditation, positive affirmations, and guided imagery can be ordered at (800) 800-8661 or at the following Internet site: http://www.healthjourneys.com/product_detail.asp?id=116.

## Guided Imagery

There are many applications of guided imagery—for example, to prepare for surgery or to increase immune function—and research in this area is promising.[12–14] It is another tool you can use to shape your new eating behaviors. Like meditation, it is a technique to harness the power the mind can have over the body. It is also like meditation in that it is based on focusing your attention, but in this case you are also using your creativity and imagination to create an object of your focus—an image to influence your behavior on a day-to-day basis. To use this tool, you mentally create detailed images in which you successfully perform the new behaviors you are trying to achieve. You can also build into your guided images problems that may occur to deter you from following through with the intended behavior. Imagine how you will handle each problem in a way that allows you to follow through with the desired action. In essence, this is like practicing the behavior. It is recommended that you practice guided imagery one or two times a day for about 10 minutes. By the time you actually do have to perform the behavior, you will have the sense that you have already performed the desired behavior successfully, which provides a sense of confidence. Professional athletes recognize the power of this tool and successfully use guided imagery to perfect their performances.

The first step in guided imagery is selecting a time of day and a quiet place to practice. Then select a new eating-related behavior you would like to adopt. Begin with a meditation or relaxation breathing to create a relaxed, receptive frame of mind. Then create an image of the surroundings in which you will perform the behavior. For example, let us say that you eat dinner out with a friend twice a week, and you have not been able to appropriately manage your portion sizes. You would like to eat dinner out with a friend and eat an appropriate portion size rather than overeat and leave feeling stuffed. You are tempted to simply stop going out to eat until you get to your goal weight, but you decide to try guided imagery. First, schedule time to practice the guided imagery in the morning and evening. Imagine the restaurant you typically frequent, including the lobby area, smell of food cooking, lighting, flooring, arrangement of tables, and your usual table. Then imagine visualizing the guided imagery one last time while driving to the restaurant and feel the confidence washing over you. Imagine walking in with your friend, and the waitress taking you to the table. As you sit down, you feel the wooden chair beneath you, the feel of your sweater, the weight of the menu in your hands, your feet crossed at your ankles and resting on the tile floor. You hear the music playing and the noise of other diners chatting. Then you imagine ordering your entrée and speaking with your friend while you eat. You visualize yourself sipping water and successfully avoiding the bread at the table. When your food arrives, you imagine yourself eating slowly and mindfully, while continuing to speak and enjoy the music. You periodically check in with your level of hunger and fullness, and when you feel just comfortably full you put your knife and fork down on your plate. The waitress passes by and you ask her to wrap up your leftovers. You continue to chat with your friend, pay the bill, and then visualize yourself pushing back your chair and getting ready to leave. You walk across the dining area and feel the fresh air as you leave. Next you practice this guided imagery twice a day, sometime changing it a bit to reflect a barrier or deterrent to your successful performance. Rather than terminating the habit of going out to eat with this friend, you build your confidence that you can adopt a healthy eating style while enjoying this social event. As you practice more frequently, your performance will improve each time.

Guided imagery is an especially useful tool to shape behavior associated with social events that involve eating. Rather than isolate yourself and avoid these events you can create guided imageries to successfully handle a variety of events. As you master one set of guided images, you can begin crafting another set to improve a different eating habit. Periodically, review each of your guided imageries, as you build your repertoire. You should also consider keeping a journal of your images, because writing them down will further reinforce the imagery, as discussed in the journaling section. As you move throughout your day, you can summon up the appropriate images as needed. Similar to meditation, individuals with psychiatric or mental illnesses should check with their health care providers before practicing guided imagery. There may be classes on guided imagery in your community. There are many audio- and videotapes available at public libraries and on the Internet to help you learn this important skill.

## Food-Mood Dominos

The food-mood dominos worksheet, Figure 10-3, can help you explore your high-risk eating situations and pull the ideas and strategies presented in this chapter together into a single effective strategy. Thoughtfully completing the worksheet facilitates exploration of your relationship with food and allows you to tease apart habits that tie nonhunger eating or overeating with specific activities. First, consider your high-risk situations—situations in which you typically overeat—that occur on a regular basis. Two examples are eating when you get home from work before you start cooking or eating while watching television at night.

Consider the first example and the food-mood dominos worksheet. The worksheet depicts a series of dominos falling. The first domino represents the initial behavioral step that starts the series of dominos falling. The last fallen domino is the overeating activity. The behavior represented by this last domino is the most noticeable activity and the one most people try to change. However, it is much more difficult to keep this domino from falling after the momentum of all the other dominos accumulates and applies significant force. It is easier to prevent the first domino from falling, or pull out a domino early on in the series. The first step is to tease apart all of the little steps, that is the discrete dominos, that lead to the overeating event. Some of these steps may be powerful and negative self-talk scripts. Now, go back to the example and consider this potential series of steps: (1) you ate a very small lunch to try to cut back on calories; (2) you ignore hunger cues late in the afternoon; (3) you leave work and while driving home consider

**Figure 10-3.** Food-Mood Dominos Worksheet

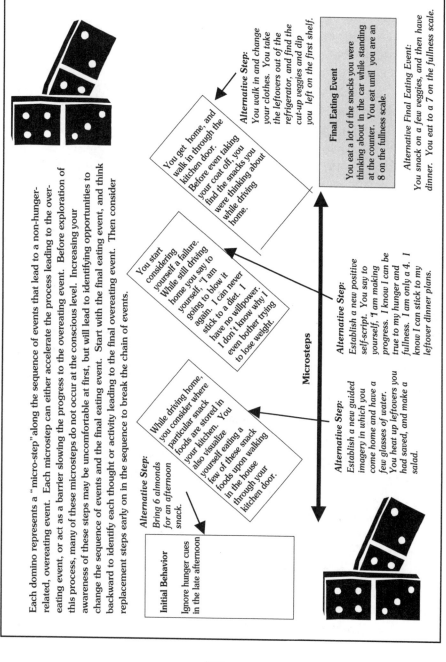

Each domino represents a "micro-step" along the sequence of events that lead to a non-hunger-related, overeating event. Each microstep can either accelerate the process leading to the overeating event, or act as a barrier slowing the progress to the overeating event. Before exploration of this process, many of these microsteps do not occur at the conscious level. Increasing your awareness of these steps may be uncomfortable at first, but will lead to identifying opportunities to change the sequence of events and the final eating event. Start with the final eating event, and think backward to identify each thought or activity leading to the final overeating event. Then consider replacement steps early on in the sequence to break the chain of events.

**Initial Behavior**
Ignore hunger cues in the late afternoon

*Alternative Step:*
*Bring 6 almonds for an afternoon snack.*

*Alternative Step:*
*Establish a new guided imagery in which you come home and have a few glasses of water. You heat up leftovers you had saved, and make a salad.*

While driving home, you consider where particular snack foods are stored in your kitchen. You also visualize yourself eating a few of these foods upon walking in the house through your kitchen door.

**Microsteps**

*Alternative Step:*
*Establish a new positive self-script. You say to yourself, "I am making progress. I know I can be true to my hunger and fullness. I am only a 4. I know I can stick to my leftover dinner plans.*

You start considering yourself a failure. While still driving home you say to yourself, "I am going to blow it again. I can never stick to a diet. I have no willpower. I don't know why I even bother trying to lose weight.

*Alternative Step:*
*You walk in and change your clothes. You take the leftovers out of the refrigerator, and find the cut-up veggies and dip you left on the first shelf.*

You get home, and walk in through the kitchen door. Before even taking your coat off, you find the snacks you were thinking about while driving home.

**Final Eating Event**
You eat a lot of the snacks you were thinking about in the car while standing at the counter. You eat until you are an 8 on the fullness scale.

*Alternative Final Eating Event:*
*You snack on a few veggies, and then have dinner. You eat to a 7 on the fullness scale.*

where particular snack foods are stored in your kitchen and which you will eat; (4) you think that this dieting attempt will be yet another failed attempt because you have no will power; (5) you arrive home and walk in through the kitchen door; (6) before even taking your coat off you find the snacks you were thinking about while driving; (7) you eat the snacks while standing at the counter until you are an 8 on the hunger-fullness scale. It is common to focus on eating the snack food at the counter and to think you can stop this behavior directly with sheer willpower. However, this approach is likely to fail. Consider instead using the tools presented in this chapter and Chapter 9 to prevent the dominos from ever falling. Try following these alternative steps: (1) develop the habit of planning your dinner meal at least one day before and having some of it partially preprepared or leftover so you don't feel overwhelmed with this chore when you get home; (2) be true to your hunger and fullness scale and bring adequate healthy foods for lunch and snack to avoid going too low on the hunger side of the scale; (3) create a positive and constructive guided imagery to visualize on the way home; (4) create a positive self-talk script that encourages you to be true to hunger and fullness and recognizes your successful efforts; (5) plan a different routine for when you come home that includes at least a few brief moments of meditative breathing; and (6) leave positive cues in your environment, such as sliced vegetables and healthy dip in the front of the refrigerator.

In summary, the food-mood worksheet helps you to tease apart complicated behavioral patterns that lead to overeating, especially non-hunger-related eating. Based on this information, you need to consider how to use the tools and strategies you have become familiar with to create a new sequence of healthy behaviors, a new healthy behavioral pattern. This process will take time. After you devise a new series of steps, create a timeline to work on each step. For example, you can schedule time to create and practice a guided imagery, and time to journal the current self-talk and rewrite a new positive script. After you successfully change a behavioral pattern, select the next high-risk situation and patterned behavioral response to tackle.

*As noted previously, the process of changing your relationship with food and creating new healthy eating habits is an exciting, insightful, and rewarding process. It does require a commitment of time and effort. However, the time and effort dedicated to this process will be well worth the gains in health and long-term management of a healthy weight.* Over time these new behaviors will become your new habits and require much less effort. The ultimate goal is to establish a casual relationship with food, in which you typically select healthy foods (although include some favorite dessert- or snack-type foods occasionally), eat when you are hungry, and stop when you are comfortably full.

## The Evolution of Changing Eating Habits

The tools described in the previous section can help you shape new and healthy eating habits. Long-term maintenance of these habits requires attention, monitoring, and management. These activities will become more automatic and less time-intensive as you proceed along your lifelong journey. The attention and management required will also depend on how strongly you are genetically predisposed to be overweight. Those with stronger predispositions will likely need to devote more time to this process. Over time you will learn the amount of attention necessary for you to successfully manage your weight, and you will learn to incorporate the appropriate management techniques into your daily living activities.

Changing your style of eating involves changing many discrete eating habits, such as the types and amounts of fat you eat, your style of cooking, your portion sizes, the beverages you drink, and so on. Each of these different habits may change at different times and at different rates. When developing new habits, researchers believe that you go through a series of ordered stages.[15] The first stage is precontemplation, during which time you are not aware that there is a need to change a specific behavior. The next stage, contemplation, is when you recognize the habit as a problem, but you are not yet ready to change it. The preparation stage is next; it represents the period when you gather information and develop a plan to change the behavior. The action stage is when you actually start changing and improving a specific habit. When in the maintenance stage you have demonstrated the ability to practice the new habit for about 6 months. Lastly, relapse is the stage in which you temporarily abandon your new habit and resume the older behavior. It is expected that you will shift back and forth along this continuum of stages, until you settle into a relatively stable maintenance period. For example, you may reach preparation and slide back to contemplation, before progressing back to preparation and then action. Lapses can be considered a short relapse, and are an expected part of the process. You may also find it difficult to make a good choice when eating out for lunch, but by dinnertime you are able to resume healthy choices. Or you may be in maintenance and have a big change in your lifestyle that prompts you to lapse back to older habits. In this case, you may need more time to cycle back through the stages of contemplation, preparation, action, and maintenance again. The longer you are in maintenance, the more resistant you become to lapses, and the lapses that do occur tend to be shorter and less frequent. It is important to fully expect that these lapses will occur, and to respond rationally and objectively to them. The trick is to find the balance between rational responses and excessive unproductive rationalizations. Rationalizations are just excuses with little acknowledged accountability and no plan for recovery. When you slip or lapse, it is important to stay positive, recognize the lapse, and consider what prompted it. Then you can develop a strategy and a time frame to get back on track. Rather than considering a relapse as a failure, consider it as an opportunity to develop stronger alternative strategies to resist non-hunger-related eating and stabilize healthy eating habits. Experiences with lapses also help you learn to anticipate high-risk situations, including the people, environments, or stressors that tend to prompt lapses.

When a lapse occurs, consider which tools would be most helpful considering your current situation. Keep all of your options open, including the tools discussed in this chapter, such as goal ladders and food-mood dominos, as well as resumption of the Bull's-Eye Food Guide swapping system and the daily menus in Menus and Recipes. Consider developing a time frame. Some situations may require stabilization of current eating habits—that is, avoiding further lapses, until you can resolve the other issues at hand and dedicate the time and effort necessary to re-create the healthier eating habits. During this time continue your positive self-talk and affirmations, because negative and self-deprecating thoughts are likely to lengthen or extend the scope of the lapse.

## Monitoring Weight

It is best to deal with the issue of monitoring your weight after practicing using the tools presented in this chapter. For many people, weighing themselves is a very negative event that leads to a series of negative self-thoughts, including a sense of failure and lapses in new healthy eating habits. Yet monitoring your weight is a part of the process of attaining and maintaining a healthy weight. It is important because monitoring your weight will help you understand how your weight naturally fluctuates, and to identify gradual trends in weight gain or loss. Therefore, you will be able to recognize a problem early on and develop a plan to cut back on calories. You will also be able to notice whether there is a gradual weight loss trend and whether you are on the right track. This may prevent you from prematurely changing more dietary habits that you are simply not ready to change at the moment, thereby preventing a future problem. Although some people are able to simply use how they feel in their clothes to monitor their weight, most people can gain a significant amount of weight before recognizing clothes getting tighter. On the other hand, they also many not notice if they are gradually losing weight, and therefore be missing out on positive reinforcement for their efforts. Therefore, it is a good idea to establish a habit of weighing yourself one morning a week with no clothes or the same light clothes.

If you have experienced negative consequences of weighing yourself in the past, you should prepare yourself to start this practice. You can use some of the tools discussed in the previous section. For example, you can create a guided imagery for yourself. Imagine the situation in which you would weight yourself in great detail, including the details of the room, the scale, and the clothes you would wear. Then imagine yourself putting the scale in position and stepping on the scale. Imagine how the scale will feel underfoot, imagine watching the needle or dial and determining the trend in your weight. Then visualize yourself responding appropriately—passively and objectively noting the number in a detached fashion, neither excessively jubilant nor excessively disappointed. Imagine yourself stating affirmations that acknowledge positive attributes about yourself and positive aspects of your efforts to date. Next visualize yourself, stepping off the scale and putting it away. Imagine yourself contently flowing out of the room, noting the weight on the scale as simply one factual piece of information, and moving on with your day as planned. The process of monitoring your weight leads us to Chapter 11, which presents relationships among patterns of weight loss, physical activity, and resting metabolic rate.

## Important Points To Remember from Chapter 10

- ◉ It is important to discover as much as possible about your current eating habits, including factors that prompt you to eat that are related to your own body's chemistry, interactions with others, cultural factors, and aspects of foods. This knowledge helps you tease apart habits that tie eating to nonhunger cues.

- ◉ Recognize that improving your eating habits requires changing a whole constellation of specific eating habits. At first you may want to change most, if not all, of your initial eating habits and follow the menus in Menus and Recipes perfectly. However, changing so many habits at once may prove difficult, and most people revert back to many old eating habits over time. Anticipate that this may happen, and establish a plan to reshape a few of these old habits at a time.

- ◉ There are many tools you can use to explore and change your eating habits, such as mindful eating, goal ladders, meditation, journaling, positive affirmations, and guided imagery. Many of these tools may be new to you. Keep an open mind and try each one to determine which combination of tools can help you with each eating behavior you target for change. The more of these strategies and skills you develop the easier it will be for you to attain and maintain a healthy weight. Your local library will have many additional resources to learn these tools (books, tapes, and videos). Other tools are available through the Internet by searching on the specified strategy. It is this process of exploration and practice that will take time and effort, but it is also this process that will lead to long-term success. Take your time and have fun with this process. You can use the eating plans in Chapters 6, 7, and 8 and the daily menus in Menus and Recipes to help you lose weight while you practice these skills.

11

# YOUR INTERNAL ENGINE AND FUEL-EFFICIENCY RATING

## *What You Will Discover in Chapter 11*

◉ Your body uses energy from the food you eat for maintaining bodily functions, digesting food, and physical activity. Your resting metabolic rate (RMR) is the amount of calories your body uses at rest to maintain bodily functions. When you reduce your calorie intake enough to lose weight, your body becomes more efficient and your RMR decreases. This makes continued weight loss difficult.

◉ You need to carefully plan your weight loss to prevent negative changes in RMR. A step-wise approach to weight loss minimizes negative changes in RMR and maximizes your chances for life-long maintenance of weight loss. With such an approach, you alternate periods of weight loss with *maintenance breaks* or periods of weight maintenance. In this chapter you will learn how to plan your step-wise weight-loss plan using a body mass index chart.

## What You Will Discover in Chapter 11
### (continued)

◉ During maintenance breaks, your RMR recovers and you practice the necessary lifestyle changes essential to lose weight and maintain weight loss.

◉ Carefully planning an exercise program will also help you lose weight and keep the weight off permanently. A combination of aerobic exercise and strength training increases fuel needs, making it necessary to use up fuel stored as fat. It also helps to minimize negative changes in RMR associated with losing weight by cutting calories alone. This chapter presents guidelines for developing such an exercise program.

## Issues of Fuel Efficiency

Fuel-efficiency issues are important to a traveler. For a traveler on a weight-management journey, the most important fuel-efficiency issue is resting metabolic rate (RMR). Fuel issues are related to the calories in the food you eat and the calories used by your body's cells to do chemical work (such as make a protein) or mechanical work (such as move a muscle). A smart and successful traveler learns how to manage his or her fuel efficiency to facilitate long-term weight management. Two strategies to facilitate this are presented in this chapter, after some necessary background information.

There are three factors that contribute to calorie use: RMR, eating and digestion, and physical activity. RMR is the amount of calories your body uses while resting to maintain your bodily functions, such as the pumping of your heart. RMR accounts for the majority of the calories your body uses in a day, about 50% to 80%. The more physically active you are, the lower this percentage, because physical activity would then account for a relatively greater percentage—between 10% and 40%. Your body size, especially your height, is the biggest determinant of your RMR. The taller you are, the higher your RMR—or the more calories you use up every minute of every day. As your weight increases, your RMR also increases. However, this increase is greater if the increased weight is from increased muscle mass. The increase is much less if the additional weight is from body fat. After the age of 35, increasing age is associated with a decrease in RMR. A large amount of this drop can be explained by decreasing hormone levels (estrogen in women and testosterone in men) as you age, which leads to decreasing muscle mass. Decreased daily physical activity as you get older also leads to loss of muscle mass, because there is less of a stimulus for maintenance of your muscles at their "younger" size. These losses can be largely prevented as discussed later in this chapter by increasing physical activity. In terms of weight management and balancing calories consumed with calories expended, less musculature means lower fuel needs.

Weight loss also affects your RMR, although the exact nature and extent of the relationship is still under debate by researchers. Scientists agree that when you cut calories to lose weight there is a decrease in your RMR. Therefore, there is a decrease in the number of calories you burn every minute of every day.[1-4] Some reduction in RMR would be expected since weight loss decreases your body size. However, the drop in RMR occurs very quickly after calorie intake is decreased—even before substantial weight loss. In addition, the extent of the drop is much greater than can be explained by the amount of weight loss. In other words, the drop in RMR is disproportionate to the drop in weight loss. So what explains this effect? Your body becomes a more efficient machine, using fuel or calories provided by the food you eat more carefully and completely. Prior to cutting the calories, your body's machinery was more apt to waste some calories and be less efficient in transferring the energy in food to work. This adaptation is partially controlled by your thyroid, but other factors play a role as well. For example, leptin, a chemical produced by your fat cells, and norepinephrin, a chemical secreted in response to stimulation from your central nervous system, are also important factors in RMR adaptation. A low fuel-efficiency rating facilitates weight loss and maintenance of weight loss. A high fuel-efficiency rating, such as when you are cutting back on calories enough to cause weight loss, slows weight loss.

The decrease in RMR while you continue to try to lose weight and decrease your calorie intake makes continued weight loss more difficult over time. In the past you may have experienced a *sticking point*, at which time you found it very difficult to lose more weight. This is common and typically very frustrating because this occurs before you are at your goal weight. At this point you may have just given up and started to resume your old eating habits that contributed to the weight gain. Alternatively, you may have tried decreasing your calorie intake even more in an effort to force the weight loss. After all, if you can't lose weight with the number of calories you are currently eating, you should decrease them further, right? No! Eating even fewer calories may initially work. However, after some time your metabolic rate is likely to decrease even further in response to the greater reduction in calorie intake—again making weight loss more difficult. In fact, the less you eat and the more weight you lose, the greater the reduction in your RMR and the greater your fuel-efficiency rating. Now the frustration really grows, because you know you are not overeating and yet the weight loss stalls. Strategies to prevent this problem are shared below, but first just one more point about metabolic rate.

The impact that changes in RMR have on maintenance of weight loss is another question, as of yet still controversial.[1-5] Some researchers have found that after weight loss and stabilization of weight, RMR recovers and is appropriate for the new weight. Other researchers have found that RMR remains lower than prior to attempting to lose weight, even after taking into account the amount of weight loss. For most people, the majority of the evidence points to a post-weight-loss recovery of RMR after a period of stabilizing weight. In other words, after losing weight and maintaining the new, lower weight for about 2 weeks, your resting metabolic rate will return to your normal level after it adjusts for your new, smaller body size. This is good news—your RMR does not seem to tie you to any level of overweightness.

Strategies to minimize negative effects on RMR are critical for both short-term and long-term success along your weight-management journey. You should carefully plan the amount and timing of your weight loss to avoid the negative effects that changes in RMR can have on managing your weight. Physical activity can play a key role in minimizing the drop in RMR during weight loss and in facilitating long-term maintenance of weight loss.

## Patterns of Weight Loss

Carefully planning your pattern of weight loss can limit negative effects of RMR on weight loss, especially preventing plateaus during which time weight loss slows down or stops despite a reduced calorie intake. Different patterns of weight loss were reflected in Chapter 1, Figure 1. In Figure 11-1 the recommended step-wise pattern of weight loss is shown, as well as an indication of RMR response. In this figure, the solid black line represents the recommended pattern of weight loss—alternating periods of

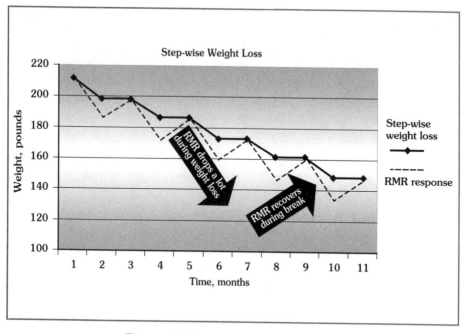

**Figure 11-1.** Step-Wise Weight Loss

weight loss and weight maintenance until a healthy weight is achieved. The dashed line reflects the RMR response, with a sharp decrease in RMR during the initiation of weight loss. During the maintenance break, weight is stable and RMR recovers. With this approach, you cut back on calories to initiate weight loss. This decrease in calories leads to an expected yet undesirable drop in RMR, which if ignored tends to lead to a weight plateau and resistance to further weight loss. This resistance can be avoided by building in periods of weight maintenance, referred to as *maintenance breaks*. Maintenance breaks are planned periods of weight maintenance. In other words, after losing about 15 to 20 pounds, you stop the weight loss on purpose. To create a maintenance break, you gradually increase the number of calories you eat over several days until your weight stabilizes. Calories are increased enough to stop weight loss, but not enough to gain weight. When calories are increased to this extent, your RMR can recover. In other words, your RMR will increase until it is appropriate for your new body size. This recovery has been shown to occur by 2 weeks of increasing calorie intake, and therefore maintenance breaks need to last for a minimum of 2 weeks. This normalization in RMR, as documented during weight stabilization, means that the amount of calories your body uses at rest is the same as before the weight loss after accounting for your new body size.[3,5] This recovery in RMR allows you to resume your selected eating style at the suggested calorie level and continue weight loss without the frustration of unplanned weight plateaus.

Sustaining weight loss is of critical importance. Thousands of research studies indicate that people can lose weight by following almost any diet. Similarly, you may have lost weight many times in the past by following a number of different diets, each time gaining the weight back. The difficulty in keeping the weight off is due to many related factors. First, most diets are unrealistic, absolutely eliminating too many foods and cutting calories too much. Second, during dieting RMR is decreased, which makes transitioning to a weight maintenance period tricky. Lastly, most diets require big changes in too many habits too quickly. This does not allow enough time to mentally and emotionally process the changes in habits and relations with others required to lose weight permanently. At some point, every dieter is likely to go off track and overeat. This increased calorie intake occurs at the point when RMR is very low due to a prolonged low calorie intake and weight loss. With an increased calorie intake, RMR will recover over time. However, if the initial increase in calorie intake is too great, rapid weight gain can occur (some of which is simply water weight) before this adjustment in RMR. Such weight gain leads to frustration and a sense of failure, leading to further increases in calorie intake and further weight gain. Therefore, it is much better to plan maintenance breaks and control these changes in your RMR so as to minimize the impact on your weight loss.

Maintenance breaks also provide time to practice the behavior changes you have made to date and to emotionally and mentally process these changes. The significance of this should not be overlooked, because difficulty in sustaining changes in habits often leads to gaining weight back. This is especially true if you took the initial step of immediately adopting the suggested eating plans and daily menus in Menus and Recipes. Such a complete adoption requires many changes in eating habits and lifestyle, as well as a commitment of time to learn new food shopping and cooking strategies. Maintenance breaks provide an opportunity to practice the tools presented in Chapter 10, such as mindful eating, meditation, positive self-talk, and guided imagery.

These breaks also provide time for you to consider how your relationships with other people have been influenced. For example, you may be cooking your meals separately if your spouse, partner, or children are not willing to change their eating habits. Although you may be able to do this for a while, it may be increasingly difficult to do so. Therefore, you need to consider compromises in planning family meals. If hamburgers are a family favorite, for example, make them with 90% lean ground beef. Pair up this family favorite with corn on the cob and salad instead of French fries. Or if you usually bread and fry chicken cutlets, try baking them instead. Serve them with family favorites like mashed potatoes (made with low-fat milk) and string beans. Allow family members to add butter to their potatoes if necessary, but don't add it to the pot. In other words, serve a family favorite with some new items. Cut up fruit at the end of each meal to make sure that those who don't like the new menu items have enough to eat. This will decrease resistance to the whole menu.

Your added time spent on cooking and exercising will take getting used to by your spouse, partner, or children. Your maintenance breaks also provide time for this process. Encourage others to join you in the kitchen. Make the environment pleasant and inviting by engaging family members in conversation. Try to encourage them to exercise with you as well—walking, running, or cycling together. Little children like games, such as tag, basketball, and soccer, and would willingly give up television viewing to be able to play and be active with you.

Next, take into consideration the influence friends have on your eating. Are there particular friends with whom you tend to overeat? Or, are there particular friends, co-workers, or relatives who encourage you to eat more once you start to lose weight? These other people may not even be aware of their influence on your eating habits. Take time during your maintenance break to examine these issues. Decide who you think you can depend on to support your efforts. You may need to let them know what type of support works best. For example, you spouse may think he or she is helping you by discouraging you from taking a second serving at dinner. However, such prompts may bother you and actually increase the likelihood that you will take the second portion. Perhaps, instead, you would rather that your spouse offer to walk with you after dinner. You need to communicate these types of details to your supporters. On the other hand, you may conclude that there are other people whose behavior you cannot change, and they will continue to tempt you to eat or skip exercise. In this case, you need to change your response to their comments or actions. Use guided imagery and positive affirmations as discussed in Chapter 10 to shape your new responses.

Lastly, during your maintenance breaks, you may need to get used to your new physical appearance and the attention it may or may not attract. Some people are comfortable with this increased attention, others are not. Others are disappointed by a lack of attention. Yet others are a bit uncomfortable or uneasy with changes in their physical appearance. Give some attention to exploring these issues. Journaling about such issues may facilitate added insight and self-awareness.

Maintenance breaks, therefore, serve two purposes. First, they allow time for recovery of RMR and, therefore, facilitate further weight loss and maintenance of weight lost in the future. Second, they allow time to process the necessary changes in lifestyle, appearance, and relationships, which are required to support behavior changes already made, as well as future behavior changes necessary for continued weight management. Maintenance breaks need to last at least 2 weeks to allow for the recovery of RMR. However, the time and effort needed to explore and process changes in lifestyle habits and relationships will take additional time and effort, perhaps as much as a few more weeks or even months. *It may be difficult to purposefully stop weight loss when you are in the process of successfully losing weight. However, maintenance breaks should be considered time well spent, because they increase the likelihood of sustaining the weight loss!*

### Directions for Maintenance Breaks

First, you need to determine when to take a maintenance break. Timing of maintenance breaks is based on changes in your weight and associated changes in your body mass index. Body mass index is a measure of your weight relative to your height. This measurement is closely related to your risk for diseases associated with obesity, such as insulin resistance syndrome, type 2 diabetes, and high blood pressure. As you decrease your body mass index, you decrease your risk for such diseases. Take a look at the body mass index chart in Appendix 1. Note that body mass index, or BMI, is indicated by the numbers along the top row. Height is indicated in the first column of the chart. Find your height, and underline the entire row associated with your height. The numbers in this row are weights. Find the weight closest to your current weight, and circle this number. Note the vertical column in which this weight belongs. Next follow that column all the way up to the row along the top that indicates the BMI resulting from your current height and weight. Circle this BMI. As an example, imagine that you are 5 feet, 6 inches (or a total of 66 inches) tall and 212 pounds. You would underline the entire row associated with 66 inches. Then find your weight. Your exact weight of 212 pounds is not shown on the chart. Your weight falls between 210 and 216 pounds, 210 pounds being closest. Circle the number 210. Now, follow the column associated with 210 pounds all the way up to the first row that is labeled BMI until you get to 34. Circle the number 34. Your current BMI would be 34. It is recommended that you take a maintenance break each time your BMI drops 2 units. In the example, this means that you would take a maintenance break when your BMI reaches 32. To determine what you would weigh at this new BMI, follow the column headed by 32 down until you get to the row you underlined that is associated with a height of 66 inches. In this example, you would stop at 198 pounds. Therefore, you first weight goal would be 198 pounds. You would start your first maintenance break at this weight. Following these same steps, your second maintenance break would be at 186 pounds, and your third at 173 pounds.

At each maintenance break you should also think about how your health has improved. Perhaps your blood sugar, cholesterol, or triglycerides have come down. Your blood pressure may have improved. You may be able to ask your health care provider about decreasing some of your medications. Many of these positive changes can happen with only about a 15- to 25-pound weight loss. Your final weight goal is hard to determine from the beginning of your weight-loss journey, because it will depend on how your health and feelings of fitness improve. Although it is often recommended that you lose weight until your BMI is equal to 25, this may not be possible or even necessary for you. Instead, you should continue to lose weight in increments of 2 BMI units until you feel fit, and you and your health care provider agree that you are at a healthy weight. Keep in mind that you may find that you lose 20 or 30 pounds, and at that point you are able to stop some of your medications and your health indicators are normal. You may decide to stop trying to lose weight and take a long maintenance break. During this time simply monitor your weight to ensure that you maintain your weight loss. Six months or a year later, you may decide you are ready to make some further changes in your diet and exercise habits, and decrease your weight an additional 2 BMI units. Consider your weight-management efforts a long-term project in which you are aiming for progress and improved health and fitness over time.

Determine your goal weight for your first maintenance break when you start changing your eating habits. When you get to this weight, take a moment to congratulate yourself on your efforts to get to this point. Although it may be tempting to continue the weight loss, convince yourself of the importance of taking the maintenance break by rereading the section above. The time you take to increase your metabolic rate and explore your changed habits will lead to long-term, permanent success. You will be practicing the art of maintaining your weight. This is truly an art and not an exact science, and it will require adjustments as you go through your maintenance break. You will need to weigh yourself daily or every other day during your maintenance break. Refer to the section in Chapter 10 on monitoring your weight in an objective, positive fashion. The first thing you need to determine is how much your weight normally fluctuates on a day-to-day basis. Most people's weights fluctuate about 3 pounds due to changes in water weight and timing of bowel movements. The larger you are, the more your weight may fluctuate. Therefore, initially, do not change your eating habits—you are simply on a fact-finding mission to determine how much your weight fluctuates. This is important, because adjustments in your eating plan will be based on trends in your daily weight. The goal is to maintain your weight; however, it is not realistic to expect your weight to stay exactly the same day to day. The goal is to keep your weight within a tight range, your current weight plus or minus the amount of weight your body normally fluctuates. In the above example, this would be 198 pounds plus or minus 3 pounds, or 195 to 201 pounds. If you were to continue the eating style that lead to the initial decrease in weight, your weight would continue to decrease until your RMR dropped to a problematic level. Therefore, when you get to 198 pounds and explore the extent of your natural weight fluctuations, you should gradually increase your calorie intake. On the first day of your maintenance break, increase your protein intake by 2 servings (from the green or yellow subgroups) and your fat intake by one serving (from the green subgroup). Monitor your weight for a few days to determine whether it has stabilized. If your weight continues to trend down, increase your whole-fruit intake by one swap. Continue to monitor your weight for a few days. If your weight increases remove a fruit and/or fat swap until it stabilizes over a few days. If weight continues to trend down, then increase your intake of grains and starches by one swap from the green inner circle. Again, monitor your weight. If you gain over a few days and exceed your range, than remove the grain swap. Lastly, if you still continue to lose weight and drop below your range, increase another grain swap from the green inner circle. During the beginning of your first mainte-nance break, you will need to monitor your weight and food intake carefully. Consider this a positive self-exploration process. As you gain more experi-ence with taking maintenance breaks, this process will become easier and require less practice. By the time you reach a healthy weight that you want to maintain permanently, you will have developed the strategies and skills necessary to maintain such a healthy weight. Because you have had a lot of practice in weight maintenance, and not just weight loss, you have increased the likelihood of maintaining your healthy weight for a lifetime.

## Physical Activity—A Unique Tool

Physical activity is a very effective tool to help you lose weight and then keep the weight off. Two types of exercise will be discussed: aerobic exercise and strength training. Each type of exercise is important, and each offers different benefits. The types of exercise and benefits will be discussed in the next two sections. In addition, practical tips for starting an exercise program are offered. It is highly recommended that you explore further practical tips at a gym in your neighborhood. Libraries also have a wide variety of books dedicated to exercise, as well as exercise videotapes or DVDs to help you get started. Lastly you can visit the American College of Sports Medicine's Web site, specifically the health and fitness information section for up-to-date articles on exercise (http://www.acsm.org). The site provides an online newsletter, as well as fact sheets on selecting home exercise equipment, gym/fitness facilities, or personal trainers. It is generally recommended that you obtain medical clearance from your health care provider before begin-ning an exercise program, especially if you are above the age of 35 years.

### Aerobic Exercise

Aerobic exercises include physical activities that involve your large muscle groups (legs and/or upper body, back, and abdominals) in rhythmic, contin-uous movement that results in a sustained elevation of your heart rate. Examples include walking, running, bicycling, elliptical trainers, and aerobic dance. Aerobic exercise increases your energy expenditure while you are performing the activity. Therefore, on the days you exercise aerobically you will use up more calories. If you are also cutting back on the number of calories you are eating, you will force your body to take fat out of storage to use as fuel for the exercising muscles. So when aerobic exercise is performed regularly and combined with a decreased calorie intake, body fat stores are decreased and you lose weight faster. Keep in mind that whole body fat stores are decreased, not just the fat stores near the exercising muscle. For example, even though you may be using your leg muscles when walking or running, fat may come from stores in your stomach, hips and legs—indeed from all over your body. Calories are, of course, expended during the aerobic activity session, and additional calories are also used an hour or so after your exercise session to repair cells and tissues and replace energy stores in the muscles involved in the exercise.

When you perform aerobic exercise on a regular basis, it also has very positive effects on your circulatory system and muscular-skeletal system. Aerobic exercise increases the effectiveness of your heart's pumping action so that more blood is pumped out with each beat. This allows your heart to beat fewer times per minute. Over days and years, this saves your heart a lot of work and preserves its work capacity. Regular exercise also leads to an increased number of small blood vessels feeding the muscles involved in the activity, thereby bringing more nutrients and oxygen to these muscles when needed. The cells making up these muscles also become more efficient at producing energy from fats and carbohydrates by actually increasing the amount of enzymes necessary to do so. In addition, baseline levels of some important chemicals in your blood change. For example, a decrease in the baseline levels of circulating epinephrine, one of the hormones associated with stress, leads to a decrease in baseline blood pressure. Regular aerobic exercise can be an effective way to lower high blood pressure.

All of the benefits described above also decrease your risk for many illnesses associated with being overweight or obese, such as insulin resistance, type 2 diabetes, hypertension, high cholesterol, and heart disease. Aerobic exercise also improves your quality of life—you are more easily able to walk long distances, climb stairs, carry your groceries, or play with your children or grandchildren.

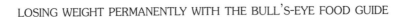

So how much do you need to do to get the benefits of aerobic exercise? There are a few different ways to answer this question. Most recent recommendations from the federal government suggest that you accumulate 30 minutes of physical activity most days (5 or 6) of the week. This can be achieved in many ways, such as three 10-minute walking sessions or two 15-minute sessions. This is a very reasonable recommendation for those just starting an exercise program, or for those who are not yet able to do 30 continuous minutes of aerobic exercise. Although several short exercise sessions throughout the day leads to many of the changes noted above, additional gains can be achieved by completing 20 to 30 *continuous* minutes of aerobic exercise at least 3 times a week. Lastly, if you can gradually increase your level of aerobic exercise to include 30 to 45 minutes, 5 to 6 times a week you will be able to maximize the resulting benefits for weight loss and maintenance of weight loss. Part of the reason for this is that it takes about 20 minutes for your body to be able to get fat out of storage and to the exercising muscles to be used for energy. Before this happens, the muscles involved in the exercise use carbohydrates stored right in the muscle. Therefore, exercise sessions lasting more than 20 minutes maximize the use of fat. If you just cannot exercise that long yet, keep in mind that your body will still dip into fat stores a bit after your exercise session to provide the energy necessary to replace the carbohydrate stores in the muscle.

Determining at what level of intensity to exercise is tricky, because exercising at too high an intensity can increase your risk of injury to your muscles and joints, as well as to your heart. You should discuss exercise intensity with your health care provider to determine the appropriate exercise intensity and any necessary limitations. Use your heart and breathing rate as a guide to measure the intensity of exercise. However, rather than use equations to determine your exercise heart rate, you can use a general rule of thumb—exercise at a pace at which "you can talk but not sing." If you are exercising so intensely that you could not have a brief conversation, you may be exercising too hard and increasing your risk for injury. If you are exercising at a pace that allows you to comfortably sing your favorite song, then you can probably increase the pace a bit. An exercise stress test ordered by your health care provider is the most accurate way to determine the safest and most efficient heart rate at which you should exercise. If it is not possible to have such a test, use the rule of thumb. Also be very aware of any pain you experience while exercising, as well as excessive shortness of breath or fatigue. These issues should be discussed with your health care provider.

Another important factor to maximize the efficiency of your exercise and minimize your risk for injury is to vary your aerobic activities. For example, walk or run on the treadmill two times a week, exercise on the elliptical machine two times a week, and cycle two times a week. Or you can alter walking with a variety of aerobic exercise tapes available. Your options will depend on whether you decide to join a fitness center or exercise at home. Refer to the American College of Sports Medicine's Web site for tips on selecting a gym or home exercise equipment (http://www.acsm.org). In addition, many communities sponsor walking or exercise groups. Your local YMCAs/YWCAs, adult education programs, or college continuing education programs also provide physical activity opportunities.

Thirty minutes of aerobic exercise is typically associated with an energy expenditure of 150 to 400 calories, depending on how intensely you can safely exercise. In addition, there will be some increase in calorie expenditure for an hour or so after exercise. This increase in energy demand will help create a need to dip into fat stores for energy to meet your daily calorie needs and therefore help use up fat stores. It also slows down the rate of fat moving into storage. However, keep in mind how easy it is to eat 150 to 400 calories, and resist justifying extra portions of food or beverages once you are exercising regularly. If you find you are hungrier after exercising, you may need to redistribute your planned food intake so as to plan for bigger servings for the meal or snack after you exercise.

Here is a summary of aerobic exercise recommendations. Your current level of fitness will determine your start point. It is important to progress slowly, so as to avoid injury and excessive pain, which would limit continued exercise.

◉ Prioritize your aerobic exercise sessions and schedule your sessions weekly.
  • Determine how many times a week you will exercise aerobically (three to six times a week).

- Determine how many times a day you will exercise aerobically and the length of each exercise session (three times a day for 10 minutes, two times a day for 15 minutes, one time a day for 30 to 45 minutes). The more fit you are, the longer your exercise sessions should last. If you cannot yet walk for 10 minutes at a time, start with walking 3 minutes three times a day and gradually add a minute to each exercise session until you can exercise for 10 minutes three times a day. In other words, you need to start with what you can physically do at this time, and gradually increase your fitness level. Increasing your fitness level is of critical importance and must be approached in a systematic and gradual fashion to avoid injuries and burnout.

- Determine what types of aerobic exercise you will do during each of your exercise sessions. Walking is the safest exercise and doesn't require special equipment. There are many in-home walking tapes that demonstrate appropriate walking form. This is very important to prevent injuries and maximize muscles incorporated during the walking sessions (such as arms and buttock muscles). You can walk in your home, around your neighborhood, on an outdoor track, or on a treadmill. Each can be effective. As your fitness level increases, consider varying the type of aerobic exercise by purchasing a gym membership, exercise videotapes, or home exercise equipment.

- Determine how intensely you will exercise aerobically. Discuss this with your health care provider, and ask if an exercise stress test is appropriate before you begin your exercise program.

## Strength Training

Strength is another component of physical fitness. Although strength training at all ages is an important aspect of fitness, it becomes increasingly important for weight management as you age. This is because of hormonal changes that occur as you age, specifically a decrease in estrogen and testosterone levels, which lead to a loss of muscle mass. This loss leads to a decrease in RMR, and therefore a decrease in calorie needs.

Because most people do not decrease their calorie intake as they age to accommodate for these decreased needs, they gain weight. Therefore, by the age of 35 or 40, strength training should be incorporated into a weight management program to increase muscle mass and the number of calories used each day.

Strength training is associated with many physiological benefits, and these benefits are different than those provided by aerobic training. Strength training leads to an increase in muscle mass and strength of the muscles involved in the training. It also leads to increased bone density of the bones to which the muscles involved in the exercise are attached. Most importantly for weight management, increased muscle mass leads to increased RMR and increased calorie expenditure every minute of every day. This increase counteracts age-related loss of muscle mass. When starting a strength-training program, you can increase muscle mass by 1 to 4 pounds in the first 4 to 6 months, and therefore increase energy expenditure by about 50 to 150 calories per day or more.[6,7] Therefore, at and above the age of 40 years, strength training is essential for weight management.

There are seven principles of strength training. If you have never strength-trained before, it will be necessary to be introduced to the process by a trained professional. Again, the American College of Sports Medicine provides tips on finding such a qualified person. An introduction to the principles of strength training follows.

⦿ Strength training requires that you overload a muscle during a training session, or, in other words, expose it to a greater weight than it typically is required to lift or move. During the strength training exercise, you work the muscle to fatigue. You should select a weight that you can properly lift through the exercise for 8 to 14 repetitions. The greater the weight you pick, the fewer the number of repetitions you would perform. If you pick a somewhat lighter weight, you would do more repetitions to get to the point of fatigue. Higher weights and lower repetitions tend to lead to greater muscle mass. Lighter weights and higher repetitions lead to a more gradual increase in muscle mass. A set is considered the number of repetitions you do with the amount of weight selected. In addition to the amount of weight and the number of repetitions, you need to consider how many sets of each exercise you will perform. Traditionally, it is recommended that you do three sets of each exercise, such as a bicep curl. The first set may include 14 repetitions with 20 pounds. The second set may include 12 repetitions with 20 pounds. By the third set you may be able to do only 8 repetitions. Three sets lead to maximum fatigue, and therefore maximum stimulus to increase muscle mass. However, completing three sets of each exercise takes a significant amount of time. You may not have this much time to dedicate to strength training. Therefore, keep in mind that you get about 80% of your gains from the first set. Therefore, if time is a limiting factor, simply do one or two sets. You will still see significant results. Over time, continued gains may require additional sets, but at that point it will most likely be sufficient to simply maintain the gains in muscle mass you have achieved, rather than continue to add more muscle mass. It is always a good idea to check with your health care provider when starting a new exercise program. This is especially necessary and highly recommended if you have any chronic conditions, such as heart disease, hypertension, or diabetes.

- It is necessary to train a muscle throughout its full range of motion for proper muscle development. For example, to train a bicep muscle you would start with you arm fully extended and hanging straight down by your side. You would lift the weight and curl your arm up until it was fully bent and your hand holding the weight was close to your shoulder. Then you would slowly return to the start position. Strength training machines may place your arm in a slightly different position during a particular exercise when compared to using free weights.

- It is necessary to move your muscle through its full range of motion at a controlled movement speed in both directions. You should be in full control of the speed and be able to stop at any point. This is important to maximize the effectiveness of the exercise and prevent injury.

- Proper strength training includes working muscles in pairs around the joint whose movement they control. For example, you should work both your biceps and triceps equally to fatigue.

◉ Strength training is highly specific, meaning that you only increase the strength and mass of the muscles involved in the exercise movement. Therefore, you need to do a variety of different strength-training exercises to increase whole-body muscle mass. It is generally recommended that you perform about 8 to 12 different exercises in order to work all of the major muscle groups.

◉ Because strength training provides a stimulus for the muscle to increase in size, you need to provide recovery time for this growth to occur. Therefore, you should not strength train the same muscle 2 days in a row. Plan to strength train every other day or three times a week—yet gains can be made with a 2-day-a-week program as well.

◉ As your muscles get bigger and stronger, you need to increase the weight used or the number of repetitions performed to continue to provide a stimulus for muscle growth. This is referred to as the progression principle. However, you will most likely be able to achieve sufficient gains in muscle mass the first 6 to 12 months of training, and at that point simply seek to maintain your gains in muscle mass.

In addition to these general principles, you should warm up your muscles before strength training to decrease your risk for injury.
Here is a summary of strength training recommendations:

◉ Similar to aerobic exercise, you need to prioritize your strength training sessions and schedule them weekly. If you are trying to increase muscle mass and strength, schedule three sessions per week. If you are simply trying to maintain increases in muscle mass, schedule two sessions per week. You will need to coordinate this with your aerobic exercise sessions.

◉ Before strength training, warm up you muscles by exercising aerobically first. For example, walk or run on the treadmill for 10 to 30 minutes.

◉ Select 8 to 12 muscles and corresponding exercises. If you have no experience with strength training, this will require the help of a personal trainer. Most reputable gyms will provide one orientation session to the strength-training machines and help you select the machines and appropriately adjust the settings. You can also investigate instructional resources at your local YMCAs/YWCAs, adult education programs, or colleges.

◉ Select the amount of weight, number of repetitions, and number of sets you will perform for each type of exercise. This will depend on how quickly you want to build muscle mass, how much muscle mass you want to gain, and how much time you can dedicate to the process. Pick a weight you can lift for 8 to 12 repetitions, and plan on one to three sets per exercise. When starting out, choose a relatively light weight to learn the motion and avoid injury.

Coordinating your aerobic and strength-training exercise sessions may require a bit more attention—especially if the amount of time you can dedicate to exercise is limited. Both types of exercise are equally important for weight management. Research indicates that combining aerobic exercise with strength training, while modestly decreasing calorie intake, leads to very important changes in body composition. For example, as you lose weight, more of the weight loss will be body fat as opposed to muscle mass. Researchers have found that subjects who combined aerobic and strength training exercise lost 97% of their weight as body fat, as opposed to only 78% being body fat when subjects only performed aerobic exercise and only 69% of weight loss being fat when subjects did not perform any structured exercise.[8] Therefore strength training protects muscle mass from being broken down, and, in fact, the amount of muscle can be increased by 1 to 4 pounds while body fat is being lost. This may look like slower progress with weight loss on the scale, but you will notice that your clothes feel looser and that you feel stronger. This increase in muscle mass while losing body fat is also associated with an increase in RMR from about 50 to 150 calories per day.[9,10] This increase in RMR offsets the typical decrease in RMR with weight loss achieved without exercise. Therefore, as your metabolism changes, your fuel needs increase, and dipping into fat stores for this fuel will lead to faster weight loss. Equally as important, you will increase your ability to maintain the weight loss and improve your health.

Therefore, to maximize the effects of exercise, consider how to include aerobic exercise and strength training into your weekly routines. Three times a week you will need to dedicate about 45 to 60 minutes for exercise. On these days you will warm up for 5 minutes, exercise aerobically for 20 to 30 minutes, and strength-train for 30 minutes (which is enough time to do one set of 10 different exercises). On another 2 to 3 days a week you will accumulate 30 to 45 minutes of aerobic exercise. It may take six months to one year to increase your fitness level enough to perform this amount of exercise, as well as to learn to prioritize exercise enough to accommodate this into your weekly schedule. This may require that you enlist the support of family members to pitch in and do household chores, or you may simply need to let some things go. This may also require giving up control over some family or household chores or issues. For example, others may not manage the laundry or mow the lawn the same way you do, and it may take you some time to get used to this. Your house may be a bit dustier and the yard may have a few more weeds, but if this is the cost of being healthier and more fit, it is worth it. The dust and weeds will be waiting for you after your exercise. In other words, if lifestyle choices are preventing you from dedicating a mere hour a day to exercise and realizing all of the health benefits that come along with it, you may need to consider your priorities and how you schedule your time. You may experience periods in your life in which unusual circumstances place a strain on your time commitments, but you should be able to look ahead to a time when such influences will dissipate.

## Important Points To Remember from Chapter 11

◉ Plan for step-wise weight loss, alternating periods of weight loss with periods of weight maintenance. Maintenance breaks should be planned after each 15- to 20-pound weight loss, which is about enough weight to decrease BMI two units. Use a BMI chart to plan your maintenance breaks and short-term weight goals in advance.

◉ Step-wise weight loss allows your RMR to recover along your weight-loss journey. This prevents a long-term increase in fuel efficiency, which leads to unplanned weight plateaus and makes continued weight loss difficult.

◉ An exercise program that includes both aerobic and strength-training exercises maximizes increases in muscle mass, as well as daily fuel needs. To meet these fuel needs, body fat stores are reduced. Increased muscle mass relative to decreased body fat stores also helps to protect RMR, minimizing reductions during weight loss and weight maintenance.

◉ Exercise aerobically at least 30 minutes most days of the week. Strength-train at least two times a week, completing 8 to 12 different exercises.

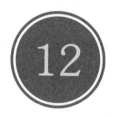

# TRAVELERS' DIARIES

**What You Will Discover in Chapter 12**

⊙  Establishing appropriate expectations for weight loss is very important for a successful weight-management journey.

⊙  It is important to define success in broad terms, including the establishment of healthier eating and exercise habits, improved indicators of health, and a greater level of self-confidence, as well as weight loss.

⊙  A step-wise approach to weight loss facilitates the gradual and permanent establishment of many healthy eating and exercise habits, as well as a positive self-identity.

⊙  Aerobic activity and strength training are key elements for permanent weight loss.

Travelers on a journey toward permanent weight loss can benefit from the wisdom of many successful travelers who have gone before them. Two success stories follow. Their stories will help you plan your personal journey, as well as to adjust your plan as you travel. The travelers' names and some details of their stories have been changed.

## Marie—Traveler One

Marie had been on the weight-loss and weight-gain roller coaster for most of her life before trying the Bull's-Eye Food Guide approach for permanent weight loss. She had tried most commercial weight-loss programs and books, losing 20 to 40 pounds in a few months each time. However, within a year or two of each weight loss effort she gained all of the weight back plus an extra 5 to 10 pounds. At the age of 52, these cumulative experiences have eroded her self-esteem and her confidence that she could manage her weight successfully over time. She now suffers from high blood pressure and high blood triglycerides, with blood sugar in the high normal range. She takes two medications to control her blood pressure. Her three children are grown, and she lives with her husband, who has never struggled with weight issues. He has a hard time understanding her difficulty in managing her weight. They share food shopping and cooking responsibilities, but she and her husband eat dinner out three to four times per week. She works part-time in a school. She brings her lunch to work, but stops at a deli for breakfast every morning. Two of her children live close by, and one daughter depends on her for after-school care for her two children aged 9 and 11. Marie drives the children to their after-school activities and supervises play time with their friends. At night Marie is exhausted. She watches television for about 2 hours, snacking often. She considers herself a sugar addict, stating that once she starts eating something sweet she can't stop. She is trying to cut back on her calorie intake and give up sugar altogether. Each day she wakes up promising herself that she will not eat anything sweetened, but gives up by afternoon or early evening. When she gives up and eats more than she knows she should, she gets angry with herself.

When Marie started the Bull's-Eye Food Guide program, she followed her 1500-calorie, lower-carb eating plan very carefully, avoiding all foods in the red outer circle. She followed the sample menus without deviating. She felt that she simply could not control her intake of outer circle foods and was better off avoiding them altogether. She was extremely pleased with her 16-pound weight loss in the first 10 weeks. She resisted the idea of a maintenance break, thinking that she did not want to stop her weight-losing momentum. All was going well, until she went to a wedding reception. At the reception she was faced with many different favorite food items that she had completely avoided for months. At first she told herself she would just have a small amount, but this was difficult. As she started to overeat a few items, negative thoughts about "failure" and "lack of willpower" came rushing back through her mind. She started to tell herself to just eat it all now, and that tomorrow she would start her strict plan again. As she ate, feelings of complete failure prevailed. Over the next few days she would start off trying to resume her strict plan, but by evening she was snacking like before. These extra calories soon resulted in slow, but gradual, weight gain.

Marie carefully reread Chapters 9, 10, and 11, and was able to step back long enough to explore the recent course of events. She did not want to repeat her past experiences and reconsidered adopting a more gradual approach. She made two initial decisions. The first was that she would try taking a walk after dinner and then listen to a meditation tape to clear her mind and distract her from her usual television time and associated uncontrolled snacking. She also decided to plan to have a dessert-type snack with her grandchildren in the afternoon. This was a big step, because she usually ate these types of foods alone after her husband had gone to bed. By planning the snack into her eating plan and eating it with others, she could more completely experience the food and eat slowly enough to be mindful of her level of hunger and fullness. She also practiced not feeling guilty over eating these foods because they were planned into her daily calorie intake.

Over the next few months she talked to her daughter about cutting back on the number of days she took care of the children after school. She increasingly realized that she needed to build in time to grocery shop and plan meals for the week so she could cut back on the number of times she ate breakfast and dinner out. Marie began watching her grandchildren only 2 days a week. On the other 3 weekdays and on Saturdays, she started a walking program. She had a long discussion with her husband about their different propensities regarding weight and her need for them to change some of their shared habits. They discussed limiting eating out to one time per week, and planning and cooking meals together. Soon her husband was joining her on many of her walking excursions.

With this newly nurtured family support, Marie was also able to develop a more positive self-esteem and habitual self-talk scripts. She began to truly believe that she could be successful and would visualize herself making appropriate choices in situations that used to be difficult for her. These images became reality over time. Through these efforts Marie was able to resume her weight loss, albeit it at a slower pace. She planned her first maintenance break, and this time when the time came she welcomed the opportunity to practice maintenance and new lifestyle habits she had developed. She decided to make her first maintenance break a full month, and then she planned her next series of lifestyle changes to get to her second maintenance break. After her second maintenance break, she visited her doctor and found that her blood sugar and triglycerides dropped well into the normal range. Her blood pressure also dropped, and her health care provider agreed to taper down her dose of one of her blood pressure medications to determine whether it was still necessary to control her blood pressure. She was well on her way to a successful weight-management journey and permanent weight loss.

## Bill—Traveler Two

Bill was very athletic in high school and college, playing on many different teams and intramural leagues. He also did a lot of strength training. He was always considered a "big kid." After college Bill got a sales job and within another 2 years was married. Over the next 10 years, Bill gained about 50 pounds due to frequent eating out with clients, a long work day, and a dramatic drop in physical activity. There were also problems in Bill's marriage, and within another 2 years he was divorced. Bill found life as a divorcee very difficult, and he was exceptionally angry over how the situation developed. Bill found himself using food to deal with his anger and loneliness. He was now eating breakfast, lunch, and dinner out, as well as snacking while watching television late into the night. The weight piled on at an alarming rate. At 33 years of age he was 6 feet 2 inches, was 325 pounds, and had health concerns—high (LDL) cholesterol and borderline high blood pressure. Bill felt uncomfortable moving around and became short of breath easily. Fortunately, his weight was evenly distributed, and he did not have a family history for diabetes or heart disease. His health care provider encouraged him to try losing weight before starting medication. He was given 3 months to lose about 30 pounds before returning to have his cholesterol and blood pressure checked.

The diagnosis of high cholesterol and blood pressure forced Bill to confront his current health and physical condition. He was, of course, disappointed with the choices he had made and how his health and fitness level had deteriorated. However, he decided this was not how he wanted to continue his life. Bill discovered the Bull's-Eye Food Guide program through a friend and decided to change his diet before tackling exercise. First, he had to modify his work schedule. He discovered he could be much more efficient at work, and that he had really been spending more time than necessary with clients in order to avoid being home alone. He spent more time grocery shopping, reading food labels, and reading the background information in Chapters 3 and 4. He then decided on his appropriate meal plan—2400-calorie, moderate-carb. He decided he could limit eating out to four meals a week without compromising business relationships. He prepared simple meals at home that were consistent with his plan and ordered carefully at restaurants. After about 2 weeks he started walking 10 minutes, three times a day. His most difficult time was still when he was home alone at night. Therefore, he decided to join a local gym and start some light strength training. When he came home from the gym he planned a light snack and then read before going asleep. With the exercise, healthy eating habits, and greater amounts of sleep, Bill was feeling more energetic and content. This translated into more effective business negotiations and a greater sense of self-confidence. He began to adopt a successful perceived identity, which helped sustain his healthy eating and physical activity habits. He began visualizing himself in various high-risk situations making the healthy choice, and he developed a keen sense of awareness of his hunger and fullness levels. By markedly increasing the amount of salads and vegetables he ate, Bill felt full more quickly and was able to decrease his portion sizes at meals. He also made sure he had 8 to 12 cups of water a day.

By the time Bill returned to his health care provider 3 months later, he had lost 28 pounds. He discovered that although his cholesterol had not completely normalized, it was very close to normal. His blood pressure was now well within the normal range. Bill decided to take a 3-week maintenance break to practice all of the habits he had changed. He even worked in some favorite snack items, while maintaining his weight. He realized he still had a long way to go, but felt confident that he was on his way to a healthy weight that he would be able to maintain.

## Parting Thoughts

In addition to considering the path taken by individual travelers, researchers have identified common characteristics of travelers who successfully lose weight and keep it off. Here are some points of wisdom from this research for you to consider and determine how best to incorporate into own your travel plans.

First, set realistic expectations. Many people determine their expectations for the amount and timing of their weight loss based on media messages that bombard them every day: "lose 10 pounds in a week" or "lose 25 pounds without dieting or exercise." It takes a bit of effort to resist the influence of the media and advertisements and to set realist weight management expectations that include a series of short-term weight goals over time, as discussed in Chapter 11. This is a critical first step, as research shows that most people's expectations are unrealistic and that they typically hope to lose 22% to 34% of their starting weight. This is in contrast to the 5% to 10% necessary for improvements in health and the 10% weight loss resulting from most short-term (12 to 20 weeks) weight-loss treatments.

When expectations are set too high, subsequent disappointment leads to frustration, resumption of old habits, and weight gain.[1,2] The Bull's-Eye Food Guide approach helps you prevent such disappointment and plan a step-wise approach to weight loss and management over an extended period of time. This long-term approach may be difficult to accept at first, because it is so at odds with most other programs and media hype. The suggested maintenance breaks help you to adapt to the lifestyle changes made to date, acknowledge your current level of success, and get ready for the next series of behavior changes that will move you along your journey to your next short-term weight goal.

Acknowledging other indicators of success, besides just weight loss, helps focus you on the big health picture. The following positive effects can be seen after only a 10% weight loss (for example, after losing 20 pounds if your starting weight is 200 pounds): decreased blood pressure, decreased blood sugar, improved insulin sensitivity, decreased cholesterol levels, decreased triglyceride levels, decreased fatigue or increased feeling of energy, and improved fitness and ability to complete necessary daily activities more easily. Many people report having more energy to do things they enjoy, such as hiking, biking, or playing actively with children or grandchildren. They can more fully live their lives!

A second point of wisdom is to recognize that successful long-term weight management requires changing many, many behaviors and that this complex process takes time. At the beginning of most weight-loss efforts, most people adopt a completely new way of eating prescribed by the diet program and underestimate the magnitude of these changes. In anticipation of starting a diet, many dieters eat a lot the day before, which only magnifies these differences. In the beginning, your enthusiasm and hope facilitate these dramatic changes, but they are difficult to sustain. Although it is important to consider many aspects of your eating and exercise habits and to work on changing many behaviors, this process should be approached in a step-wise fashion over time in coordination with your step-wise weight loss.[2,3] Therefore, the preferred strategy is to establish a few behavior changes that will get you to your first short-term weight goal. For example, your first set of behavior changes might include the following: cutting back on eating dinner out to once a week, starting to walk 20 minutes three times a week, and avoiding sweetened sodas and iced teas. Adopting these habits may seem easy at first, but time constraints, social pressures, and well-established taste preferences make maintaining these new habits difficult. After reaching your first goal weight, take a planned maintenance break. Refer to Chapter 11 for detailed information on planning your maintenance break. During your maintenance break you take the time to practice these new habits, establish new taste preferences, and help your family and friends adjust and support your new habits. When this is accomplished, you determine your next set of habits to change—perhaps reducing your number of snacks, bringing your lunch to work from home, and adding a 30-minute strength-training routine two times a week. These changes bring you to your next short-term weight goal and your second maintenance break. This process continues, as you work on improving your eating habits and move towards your recommended meal plan and as you improve your physical activity and exercise habits. This process maximizes your chance for long-term maintenance of new habits and, therefore, weight loss.

Those who decide to start this program by adopting their entire eating plan all at once should anticipate some slips back to old eating habits. If this occurs, use the step-wise approach described above to reinforce clusters of habits. Avoid extended periods of frustration, guilt, or disappointment, and consider slips as part of the learning process—a diversion from your weight-management journey.

Another point of wisdom is regarding your method of changing your eating behaviors. You may choose a strict control approach—a black-white or on-off approach—or a flexible approach.[2,4] The strict approach is often adopted because in the short-term it requires less thought and seems easier. You don't have to deal with moderating amounts of high-calorie foods eaten or how to compensate for the calories later in the day—you simply avoid them. You are "on" or in the "white." In the long-term, however, it becomes increasingly difficult to avoid these high-calorie foods completely. Eventually you find yourself in a situation in which they are available, and you are unable to resist. Once the self-imposed rule to not eat these foods is broken, a complete lack of inhibition follows with the consumption of large amounts of the food. You are "off" or in the "black." Negative feelings and guilt usually fuel the overconsumption and spirals into subsequent overeating episodes. This spiraling process is difficult to stop and often leads to weight gain. A flexible approach has been shown to be associated with better weight control.[2,5,6] A system of flexible control may require more initial effort to determine how to include moderate amounts of favorite, high-calorie foods when desired. This requires the development of a sense of self-confidence, knowledge in manipulating swaps of different food groups, and mindful eating skills to fully experience the pleasure of eating and successfully monitor hunger and fullness while eating. Positive self-talk also helps to reaffirm to yourself the appropriateness of eating favorite foods. The development of such skills takes time and practice. In addition, development of these skills may be complicated by attempts to subconsciously and inappropriately rationalize excessive amounts or frequency of eating high-calorie foods. This is especially true if you are not mindfully eating these foods, but using the consumption of such foods as a strategy to deal with negative emotions or boredom. You need to develop a sense of self-awareness regarding the reasons you are eating and the amounts or frequency you are eating such foods. In other words, you need to establish a balance between incorporating favorite, high-calorie foods without rationalizing inappropriately excessive amounts of these foods. This takes thought, self-awareness, and practice, and it is necessary for long-term weight management. Refer to Chapters 9 and 10 for tools that help you develop the necessary skills.

Another factor reported by those who have successfully maintained weight loss is the change in perceived identity. They no longer see themselves as the "fat one." They also encourage others to change their perceptions so that they are no longer known to be the one to finish off the pizza or take the cake home. Such a change in self-identity is a long-term process that researchers have found requires a series of steps.[7] The first step would be a self-evaluation of your weight, which includes consideration of health issues and fitness level, and a comparison of this evaluation with your goals and values. Such a comparison reveals a conflict, which you become increasing uncomfortable with and eventually decide to resolve. Unfortunately, this decision is often delayed for many reasons, including the resistance to change or social reinforcements of negative eating behaviors. Eventually, many people are able to convince themselves of the benefits of change, and this decision leads to the first attempt to change. This is when you are ready to try to change your eating habits. If this first attempt leads to some level of success, and you can access sufficient social supports or self-determination, it can initiate the change in your perceived identity. Using the skills of guided imagery and tools such as the goal ladder and the food-mood dominos worksheet will help you craft this new perceived identity and build support from family and friends. This growing new perceived identity increases the importance of healthy changes in eating behaviors, because you perceive more of a vested interest in maintaining your new identity. This further supports full adoption of these new healthy eating behaviors as habits. The growing new perceived identity and healthy eating and exercise habits become mutually reinforcing, leading to successful long-term weight management.

Some researchers have studied individuals who have lost 30 pounds or more and kept the weight off for at least 1 year. The average weight loss was 66 pounds for an average of 5½ years .[8] These individuals report frequent self-monitoring, including monitoring weight and food intake, and a high level of physical activity. Seventy-five percent of the roughly 3,000 individuals followed by these researchers report weighing themselves once a week or more. This allows participants to identify weight gain trends very early on, when such weight gain is minor and fairly easily corrected. Monitoring food intake increases awareness of calorie intake and can help you identify negative patterns that need to be changed. Ninety-one percent of individuals studied report an increase in physical activity. Fifty-two percent reported exercising enough to burn 1000 calories per week. How much exercise this equates to is dependent on how intensely you exercise. If you are exercising at a light-to-moderate intensity, this would equate to about 30 minutes of walking 6 or 7 days a week. An additional 20% of individuals studied exercise enough to expend 2000 calories per day, or up to an hour of walking most days. Twenty-four percent of men and 20% of women report strength training. Suffice it to say, maintaining an exercise program is very important to lose weight, as well as to maintain the weight loss and improve your health. Refer back to Chapter 11 for more details on developing your exercise program.

The Bull's-Eye Food Guide approach establishes a strategy for substantial weight loss and improvements in health and well-being over time.

To get the maximum benefits from the program, you need to put substantial time and energy into these efforts initially. Over time, habits will become firmly established, and your confidence in your ability to manage your weight will improve. You will soon be well along on your journey to healthy weight loss—weight that you lose permanently.

## Important Points To Remember from Chapter 12

◉ Step-wise weight loss leads to improvements in health indicators, which are typically observed in the first or second weight-maintenance break. It also allows for the establishment and/or reinforcement of healthy eating and exercise habits in clusters. Such an approach allows adequate time to adjust to such habits.

◉ Establish a flexible approach to changing your eating and exercise habits. Avoid strict rules about the types of foods you can eat and the number of times you exercise. However, be on alert for inappropriate rationalizing of poor choices that can spiral into a long-term lapse back to unhealthy habits. Developing this sense of flexibility without inappropriate rationalizing takes practice.

◉ As you begin to lose weight and change your habits, reconsider how you identify yourself. Take time to purposively adopt a healthier, more self-confident perceived identity.

◉ Significantly increase your chances for a successful long-term weight management journey by adopting an exercise plan that includes both aerobic exercise and strength training.

# FRUIT GROUP SWAPS*

| Inner Circle | Amount=1 Swap |
|---|---|
| Apple | 1 medium |
| Applesauce | ½ cup |
| Apricots, medium, raw | 4 apricots |
| Apricots, canned | 1 cup |
| Banana | ½, 4-inches |
| Berries, black or blue | ¾ cup |
| Cantaloupe | ½ or 1 cup |
| Cherries | 12 cherries |
| Figs, raw, 2-inch across | 2 figs |
| Fruit salad, fresh | ¾ cup |
| Grapefruit | ½ grapefruit |
| Grapes | 10 grapes |
| Guava | ¾ cup |
| Honeydew melon | ⅛ or 1 cup |
| Kiwi | 1 kiwi |
| Mandarin orange | ¾ cup |
| Mango | ½ mango |
| Muscadines | 17 muscadines |
| Nectarine | 1 nectarine |
| Orange | 1 medium |
| Papaya | 1 cup cubed |
| Peach | 1 medium peach |
| Pear | 1 small pear |
| Persimmon | 2 medium |
| Pineapple, raw | ¾ cup |
| Plum | 2 plums |
| Pomegranate | ½ pomegranate |
| Raspberries, raw | 1 cup |
| Strawberries, raw whole | 1¼ cup |
| Tangerine | 2 tangerines |
| Watermelon | 1¼ cup cubed |
| Zapote | ¼ piece |

*Dried Fruits*

| | |
|---|---|
| Apples, dried | 4 rings |
| Apricots, dried | 8 halves |
| Dates, dried | 2½ medium dates |
| Figs, dried | 1½ figs |
| Prunes, dried | 3 prunes |
| Raisins | 2 Tbsp |
| Zapote | ¼ fruit |

| Middle Circle | Amount = 1 Swap |
|---|---|
| Fruit cocktail or fruit, canned in water | ½ cup |
| Fruit cocktail or fruit, canned in juice | ½ cup |
| Fruit cocktail or fruit, canned in light syrup | ⅓ cup |
| Juice, apple, grapefruit, orange, or pineapple | ½ cup |
| Juice, cranberry, grape, or prune | ⅓ cup |
| Peaches, canned unsweetened | ½ cup or 2 halves |
| Pears, canned, unsweetened | ½ cup or 2 halves |

| Outer Circle | Amount = 1 Swap |
|---|---|
| Figs, candied | 2 Tbsp |
| Fruit, canned, heavy syrup | ⅓ cup |
| Fruit, dried, sweetened | Variable; some also have added fat |
| Fruit drink or fruit punch | ½ cup |
| Fruit, dried, candied | ½ ounce |

* For an introduction on how to use the Swap Lists, refer to Chapter 4.

# VEGETABLE GROUP SWAPS

| Inner Circle | Amount=1 Swap | Middle Circle | Amount = 1 Swap | Outer Circle | Amount = 1 Swap |
|---|---|---|---|---|---|
| Artichoke | ½ medium | Marinara sauce | ½ cup | Deep fried vegetables | Variable number of added fats; if breaded, add starches |
| Asparagus | ½ cup | Tomato sauce | ⅓ cup | | |
| Beans (green, wax, Italian) | ½ cup | Vegetable juice | ½ cup | | |
| Beets | ½ cup | | | | |
| Broccoli | ½ cup | | | | |
| Brussel sprouts | ½ cup | | | | |
| Cabbage, cooked | 1 cup | | | | |
| Carrots | ½ cup | | | | |
| Cauliflower | 1 cup | | | | |
| Celery, Chinese | ½ cup | | | | |
| Chayote | ½ cup | | | | |
| Eggplant | 1 cup | | | | |
| Greens (collard, mustard, turnip), steamed | 1 cup | | | | |
| Jicama | ½ cup | | | | |
| Kale, cooked | ½ cup | | | | |
| Kohlrabi | ½ cup | | | | |
| Leeks | ½ cup | | | | |
| Mung bean sprouts, seed attach | 1 cup | | | | |
| Mushrooms, cooked | ½ cup | | | | |
| Okra | ½ cup | | | | |
| Onions, raw or cooked | ½ cup | | | | |
| Pea pods | ½ cup | | | | |
| Peppers, sweet | 1 cup | | | | |
| Rutabaga | ½ cup | | | | |
| Salsa, fresh | ½ cup | | | | |
| Sauerkraut (high in sodium) | ½ cup | | | | |
| Spinach, cooked | ½ cup | | | | |
| Summer squash | ½ cup | | | | |
| Tomato | 1 large or 1 cup | | | | |
| Tomato, crushed | ½ cup | | | | |
| Turnips | 1 cup | | | | |
| Water chestnuts | ½ cup | | | | |
| Zucchini, cooked | 1 cup | | | | |

## MILK & YOGURT GROUP SWAPS

| Inner Circle | Amount=1 Swap |
| --- | --- |
| Dry nonfat milk | ⅓ cup |
| Skim milk | 1 cup |
| Skim milk, evaporated | ½ cup |
| Soymilk, low-fat, low-sugar (less than 2.5 grams of fat and less than 12 grams of sugar per cup, or about 100 calories) | 1 cup |
| Yogurt cheese (homemade with plain, nonfat, unsweetened yogurt) | 8 Tbsp |
| Yogurt, nonfat, unsweetened | 1 cup |

| Middle Circle | Amount = 1 Swap |
| --- | --- |
| Buttermilk, low-fat | 1 cup |
| Milk, 1% | 1 cup |
| Soymilk, (less than 3 grams of fat and 18 grams of sugar) | 1 cup |
| Yogurt, plain, low-fat | 1 cup |
| Yogurt, nonfat, sweetened with aspartame | 1 cup |

| Outer Circle | Amount = 1 Swap |
| --- | --- |
| *Fatty Milk Products* | |
| Milk 2% | 1 cup<br>Counts As: 1 milk & 1 fat |
| Soymilk, whole fat | 1 cup<br>Counts As:1 milk & 1 fat |
| *Very Fatty Milk Products* | |
| Whole milk | 1 cup<br>Counts As: 1 milk & 1½ fats |
| Whole milk, evaporated | ½ cup<br>Counts As:1 milk & 1½ fats |
| Yogurt, whole fat | 1 cup<br>Counts As: 1 milk & 1½ fats |
| *Sugary Milk Products* | |
| Low-fat fruit yogurt, sweetened | 1 cup<br>Counts As: 1 milk & 1 fruit & 1 starch |
| Soymilk, low-fat or fat-free, sweetened (more than 20 grams of sugar) | 1 cup<br>Counts As: 1 milk & 1 starch |

# FAT GROUP SWAPS

| Inner Circle | Amount=1 Swap |
|---|---|
| Avocado | ⅛ medium |
| Natural peanut butter | 2 tsp |
| Nuts, almonds | 6 whole nuts |
| Nuts, cashews | 6 whole nuts |
| Nuts, chestnuts | 2 whole nuts |
| Nuts, hazelnuts/filberts | 1 Tbsp |
| Nuts, macadamias | 1 Tbsp |
| Nuts, peanuts, dry roasted | 10 |
| Nuts, pecans | 2 whole nuts |
| Nuts, pistachios, dry roasted | 1 Tbsp |
| Nuts, walnuts | 1½ whole |
| Nuts, pine nuts | 1 Tbsp |
| Nuts, other | 1 Tbsp |
| Oil, olive, canola or peanut | 1 tsp |
| Oil, flaxseed or walnut oil | 1 tsp |
| Olives, black | 8 |
| Olives, green stuffed | 10 small |
| Pesto sauce | 2 tsp |
| Seeds, flax | 1½ Tbsp |
| Seeds, pumpkin | 1 Tbsp |
| Seeds, sunflower | 1 Tbsp |
| Seeds, sesame | 1 Tbsp |
| Seeds, sesame paste | 2 tsp |

| Middle Circle | Amount = 1 Swap |
|---|---|
| Margarine-like spread, trans free | 1 tsp |
| Salad dressing, vinaigrette | 2 tsp |
| Salad dressing, diet, vinaigrette | 2 Tbsp |
| Vegetable oils, most varieties (corn, safflower, sunflower) | 1 tsp |

| Outer Circle | Amount = 1 Swap |
|---|---|
| Bacon | 1 slice |
| Butter | 1 tsp |
| Chitterlings | 1 ounce |
| Coconut milk | 1 Tbsp |
| Coconut, shredded | 2 Tbsp |
| Coffee whitener, liquid | 3 Tbsp |
| Coffee whitener, powder | 4 tsp |
| Cream, heavy, whipping | 1 Tbsp |
| Cream, half & half | 2 Tbsp |
| Cream cheese | 1 Tbsp |
| Cream cheese, light | 1½ Tbsp |
| Fat back | ¼ ounce |
| Gravy, homemade | ¼ cup |
| Lard | 1 tsp |
| Margarine or mayonnaise | 1 tsp |
| Margarine or mayonnaise, diet | 1 Tbsp |
| Salad dressing, creamy | 2 tsp |
| Salad dressing, diet, creamy | 1 Tbsp |
| Salt pork | ¼ ounce |
| Sauce, alfredo | 1 Tbsp |
| Sauce, bearnaise | 2 tsp |
| Sauce, hollandaise | 2 tsp |
| Sauce, tartar | 2 tsp |
| Sauce, white | 2 Tbsp |
| Sour cream | 2 Tbsp |
| Sour cream, light | 3 Tbsp |

## GRAIN & STARCH GROUP SWAPS—INNER CIRCLE

| Inner Circle | *Amount=1 Swap* |
|---|---|
| Beans, split peas, lentils, cooked | ⅓ cup |
| Beans, lima | ⅓ cup |
| Bread, whole wheat | 1 slice |
| Bread, whole wheat, light, 40 calories per slice | 2 slices |
| Bread, whole wheat, pita | ½, 6 inches |
| Cereals, bran | ½ cup |
| Cereals, whole grain, unsweetened | ¾ cup |
| Cereals, Grapenuts | 3 Tbsp |
| Cereals, cooked, (such as oatmeal) | ½ cup |
| Cereals, shredded wheat | ½ cup |
| Corn on the cob | 1, 8 inches |
| Corn or sweet peas | ½ cup |
| Cornmeal, dry | 2½ Tbsp |
| Crackers, whole wheat, low-fat | 4 to 6 |
| Grains, bulgur, cooked | ½ cup |
| Grains, couscous, whole | ⅓ cup |
| Grains, kasha, cooked | ½ cup |
| Grains, other, cooked | ½ cup |
| Grains, millet, cooked | ¼ cup |
| Hominy | ¾ cup |
| Melba toast, whole grain | 4 |
| Muffin, low fat, whole grain | 1 small (½-cup size) |
| Pancake, whole wheat, low-fat | 2, 4 inch |
| Pasta, whole wheat, cooked | ½ cup |
| Parsnip | ½ cup |
| Plantain | ½ cup |
| Popcorn, no fat | 3 cups |
| Potato, baked or boiled | 1 small (3 ounce) or ½ cup cubed |
| Potato, mashed, no fat | ½ cup |
| Potato, sweet or yam | ½ cup (3 ounce) |

| Inner Circle (cont'd) | *Amount=1 Swap* |
|---|---|
| Pumpkin | 1 cup |
| Rice, brown, cooked | ⅓ cup |
| Roll, whole wheat, plain | 1 small |
| Squash, spaghetti | 1½ cups |
| Squash, winter (acorn, butternut) | ¾ cup |
| Succotash | ½ cup |
| Tortilla, whole grain, no-fat, soft | 1, 6 inches |
| Waffle, low-fat, whole grain | 1, 4 inches |
| Water chestnuts, Chinese | ½ cup |
| Wheat germ | 3 Tbsp |

# GRAIN & STARCH GROUP SWAPS—MIDDLE CIRCLE

| Middle Circle | *Amount = 1 Swap* |
|---|---|
| Bagel, frozen, 1–2 ounces | (½ bagel) |
| Bagel, fresh, 4 ounces | (¼ bagel) |
| Bread, English muffin | ½ muffin |
| Bread, white | 1 slice |
| Bread, white, light (40 calories per slice) | 2 slices |
| Bread, white, pita | ½, 6 inches |
| Bread, raisin, unfrosted | 1 slice |
| Bread, sticks | 2, 4 inches |
| Bun, hamburger or frankfurter | ½ bun |
| Cereal, unsweetened, refined grain | ¾ cup |
| Cereal, puffed cereals | 1½ cups |
| Cereal, grits | ½ cup |
| Couscous, refined | ⅓ cup |
| Crackers, oyster | 24 crackers |
| Crackers, saltine-type | 6 |
| Matzoh | ¾ ounce |
| Melba toast, white flour | 4 pieces |
| Muffin, low-fat | 1 small muffin |
| Noodles, cellophane or mung bean | ½ cup |
| Pasta, cooked | ½ cup |
| Pancake, low-fat | 2, 4 inches |
| Pretzels | ¾ ounce |
| Rice, white, cooked | ⅓ cup |
| Rice cakes (40 calories each) | 2 cakes |
| Roll, plain, small, 1 ounce | 1 roll |
| Tortilla, no fat, soft | 1, 6 inches |

# GRAIN & STARCH & GROUP SWAPS—OUTER CIRCLE

| Outer Circle | Amount=1 Swap | Counts As: |
|---|---|---|
| *Sugary Foods:* | | |
| Angel food cake | ½₂ cake | 2 starches |
| Animal crackers | 8 | 1 starch |
| Barbecue sauce | 2 Tbsp | 1 starch |
| Cereal, sweetened | ½ cup | 1 starch |
| Cookies, low-fat | 3, small | 1 starch |
| Cranberry sauce | 3 Tbsp | 1 starch |
| Frozen fruit yogurt | ⅓ cup | 1 starch |
| Graham crackers | 3 squares | 1 starch |
| Hard candy | 1 ounce | ½ starch |
| Iced tea, sweetened | 16 ounces | 2 starches |
| Jelly | 1½ Tbsp. | 1 starch |
| Pudding, sugar-free | ¼ cup | 1 starch |
| Sherbert | ½ cup | 1 starch |
| Soda | 12 ounces | 2 starches |
| Sugar | 5 tsp. | 1 starch |
| Syrup | 1½ Tbsp. | 1 starch |
| | | |
| *Sugary-Fatty Foods:* | | |
| Banana bread | 1 slice | 1 starch & 1 fat & 1 fruit |
| Cake (no icing) | ½₂ cake | 2 starches & 2 fats |
| Chocolate, plain (about 6 kisses) | 1 ounce | 1 starch & 1½ fats |
| Cookies | 2 small | 1 starch & 1 fat |
| Cookies, vanilla wafers | 6 small | 1 starch & 1 fat |
| Ice cream | ½ cup | 1 starch & 2 fats |
| Ice milk | ½ cup | 1 starch & 1 fat |
| M&Ms, 1.6 ounces | 1 pkg. | 2 starches & 2½ fats |
| Snickers bar, 2 ounces | 1 bar | 2 starches & 2½ fats |
| | | |
| *Starchy-Fatty Foods* | | |
| Biscuit or churro | 1, 2 inches | 1 starch & 1 fat |
| Corn bread square | 2 inches | 1 starch & 1 fat |
| Croissant | 1 croissant | 1 starch & 1 fat |
| Croutons | 1 cup | 1 starch & 1 fat |
| French fries, deep fried | Small order | 2 starches & 2 fats |
| French fries, frozen, baked | 3 ounces | 1 starch & ½ fat |
| Granola | ¼ cup | 1 starch & 1 fat |
| Hash browns | 3 ounces | 1 starch & 1 fat |
| Muffin, small, 1 ounce | 1 muffin | 2 starches & 1 fat |
| Pancake, waffle | 1, medium | 1 starch & 1 fat |
| Popped corn, no extras | 3 cups | 1 starch & 1 fat |
| Potato chips | 12 chips | 1 starch & 1 fat |
| Snack chips | 1 ounce | 1 starch & 1 fat |
| Stuffing, bread | ¼ cup | 1 starch & 1 fat |
| Taco shell, 6 inches across | 1 shell | 1 starch & 1 fat |
| Tortilla, fat added | 1, 6 inches | 1 starch & 1 fat |

# PROTEIN GROUP SWAPS—INNER CIRCLE

| Inner Circle | Amount=1 Swap |
|---|---|
| *Eggs* | |
| Egg whites | 3 whites |
| Egg substitutes, less than 55 calories per ¼ cup | ½ cup |
| *Fish* | |
| Herring (uncreamed or smoked) | 1 ounce |
| Medium-fatty to fatty fish (bluefish, mackerel, salmon, tuna steak) | 1 ounce |
| Shellfish (fresh, frozen, or canned in water—shrimp, clams, crab, lobster, scallops) | 2 ounces |
| Squid | 2 ounces |
| Tuna fish, canned in water | ¼ cup or 2 ounces |
| White fish (such as flounder) | 2 ounces |
| *Vegetable Protein Foods* | |
| Soy cheese, low-fat | 1 oz |
| Soy protein powder | 1 scoop |
| Tofu (regular, soft, firm) | 3 ounces or ¼ block |
| Textured soy protein | ¾ ounce |

| Inner Circle (cont'd) | Amount = 1 Swap | Counts As |
|---|---|---|
| *Vegetable-Starchy Protein Foods* | | |
| Beans (kidney) | ⅔ cup | 1 protein & 1 starch |
| Lentils | ⅔ cup | 1 protein & 1 starch |
| Lima beans | ⅔ cup | 1 protein & 1 starch |
| Soybeans | ½ cup | 1 protein & 1 starch |
| Split peas | ⅔ cup | 1 protein & 1 starch |
| Tempeh | 4 ounces | 3 proteins & 1 starch |
| Veggie burgers with less than 10 grams of carbohydrates and more than 15 grams of protein | | 2 proteins & ½ starch |
| Veggie burgers with more than 15 grams of carbohydrate and less than 8 grams of protein | | 1 protein & 1 starch |
| *Vegetable-Fatty Protein Foods* | | |
| Natural peanut butter | 4 tsp | 1 protein & 1 fat |

# PROTEIN GROUP SWAPS—MIDDLE CIRCLE

| Middle Circle | Amount = 1 Swap |
|---|---|
| *Meat* | |
| Beef (90% lean ground sirloin, eye round, flank, or tenderloin steak) | 1 ounce |
| Lamb (loin and sirloin) | 1 ounce |
| Luncheon meats, 95%–98% lean | 1 ounce |
| Opossum | 1 ounce |
| Ox tail | 1 ounce |
| Pork (tenderloin, center loin) | 1 ounce |
| Tripe | 1 ounce |
| Veal (lean chops and roasts) | 2 ounces |
| Wild game (rabbit, venison) | 1 ounce |
| | 1 ounce |
| *Poultry* | |
| Chicken, white meat, no skin | 1 ounce |
| Cornish hen, no skin | 1 ounce |
| Turkey, white meat, no skin | 1 ounce |
| Egg | 1 egg |
| *Cheese* | |
| Cheeses, low-fat (less than 3 or 4 grams of fat per oz) | 1 ounce |
| Cheeses, fat-free | 2 ounces |
| Cottage cheese, low-fat | ¼ cup |
| Grated Parmesan | 2 Tbsp |

# PROTEIN GROUP SWAPS—OUTER CIRCLE

| Outer Circle | Amount=1 Swap | Counts As: |
|---|---|---|
| *Fatty Proteins* | | |
| Ham hock | 1 ounce | 1 protein & ½ fat |
| Lamb, loin | 1 ounce | 1 protein & ½ fat |
| | | |
| *Very Fatty Proteins* | | |
| Beef, most cuts | 1 ounce | 1 protein & 1 fat |
| Cheese, lower in fat, | | |
| 5-8 grams of fat | 1 ounce | 1 protein & 1 fat |
| Chicken with skin | 1 ounce | 1 protein & 1 fat |
| Duck or goose | 1 ounce | 1 protein & 1 fat |
| Fish, fried | 1 ounce | 1 protein & 1 fat |
| Lamb, most cuts | 1 ounce | 1 protein & 1 fat |
| Peanut butter, reg. | 1 Tbsp | 1 protein & 1 fat |
| Pig tail | 1 ounce | 1 protein & 1 fat |
| Pork, most cuts | 1 ounce | 1 protein & 1 fat |
| Tuna, canned in oil | ¼ cup | 1 protein & 1 fat |
| Turkey with skin | 1 ounce | 1 protein & 1 fat |
| Turkey, ground | 1 ounce | 1 protein & 1 fat |
| | | |
| *Extremely Fatty Proteins* | | |
| Beef, ribs | 1 ounce | 1 protein & 2 fats |
| Bratwurst | 1 ounce | 1 protein & 2 fats |
| Canadian bacon | 1 ounce | 1 protein (high sodium) |
| Cheese, whole fat | 1 ounce | 1 protein & 2 fats |
| Chorizo | 1 ounce | 1 protein & 2 fats |
| Knockwurst | 1 ounce | 1 protein & 2 fats |
| Frankfurter | 1 ounce | 1 protein & 2 fats |
| Luncheon meats | | |
| (bologna, salami, | | |
| liverwurst) | 1 ounce | 1 protein & 2 fats |
| Pork, spareribs | 1 ounce | 1 protein & 2 fats |
| Sausage, any type | 1 ounce | 1 protein & 2 fats |

## FREE FOODS

Bouillon, low-fat, low-sodium
Cabbage, Chinese cabbage
Candy, hard, sugar-free (not recommended)
Carbonated drinks, sugar-free (not recommended)
Carbonated water (seltzer)
Celery
Coffee or tea
Cucumber
Endive
Escarole
Gingerroot, raw
Green onions (scallions)
Herbs and spices
Horseradish
Hot peppers
Jam or jelly, sugar-free (not recommended)
Lettuce
Mushrooms
Mustard
Nonstick cooking spray
Nopales, raw
Pickles, dill, unsweetened (high in sodium)
Radishes
Romaine lettuce
Spinach
Sugar-free gelatin (not recommended)
Sugar substitutes (not recommended)
Taco sauce
Vinegar
Zucchini

## ALMOST FREE FOODS

Nonfat mayonnaise (limit 1 Tbsp)
Nonfat margarine (limit 1 Tbsp)
Nonfat cream cheese (limit 1 Tbsp)
Nonfat sour cream (limit 1 Tbsp)
Cocoa powder, unsweetened (limit 1 Tbsp)
Pancake syrup, sugar-free (limit 2 Tbsp)
Rhubarb, unsweetened (limit 1 Tbsp)
Whipped topping (limit 2 Tbsp)
Salad dressing, fat-free (limit 2 Tbsp)

## COMBINATION FOODS *

| | Amount=1 Swap | Counts As: |
|---|---|---|
| Baked beans | 1 cup | 1 starch & 2 fats |
| Bean soup | 1 cup | 1 starch, 1 protein, & 1 vegetable |
| California roll | 9 pieces | 3 starches, ½ protein, & ½ vegetable |
| Casseroles | 1 cup | 2 starches, 2 proteins, & 2 fats |
| Cheeseburger on bun | 1 large | 3 starches, 8 proteins, & 6 fats |
| Chicken parmesan with spaghetti | 2½ cups | 5 starches, 8 proteins, 2 vegetables, & 8 fats |
| Chili, beans with meat | 1 cup | 2 starches, 2 proteins, & 2 fats |
| Chunky soup | 1 cup | 1 starch, 1 protein, 1 vegetable, & 1 fat |
| Cream soup | 1 cup | 1 starch & 1 fat |
| Fajita, lean beef with 2 tortillas, salsa, no other condiments | | 2 starches, 4 proteins, & 2 vegetables |
| French onion soup | 1 bowl | 2 starches, 2 proteins, 2 vegetables, & 4 fats |
| Hummus | ⅓ cup | 1 starch & 1 fat |
| Macaroni & cheese | 1 cup | 2 starches, 1 protein, & 3 fats |
| Pizza | 1 slice | 2 starches, 2 proteins, & 2 fats |
| Ravioli & tomato sauce | 8 ounces | 2 starches, 1 protein, & 1 vegetable |
| Stir fry, chicken | 2 to 2½ cups | 2 starches, 2 proteins, & 3 vegetables |

* The nutrition content of combination foods varies based on specific recipes and quality of ingredients.

# DESSERT FOODS

| | Amount=1 Swap | Counts As: |
|---|---|---|
| Apple cobbler | 1 serving | 1 starch & 1 fat |
| Apple pie | 1 slice | 2 starches & 2 fats |
| Boston cream pie | 1 slice | 2 starches & 1 fat |
| Brownies | 1, 2 inch sq | 1 starch & 1 fat |
| Cheesecake | 1 slice | 1½ starches & 3 fats |
| Chocolate milkshake | 1, medium | 2½ starches, 1 milk, & 1 fat |
| Chocolate mousse pie | 1 serving | 1½ starches & 1 fat |
| Chocolate pudding | 1 cup | 2 starches, 1 milk, & 1 fat |
| Chocolate cake w/ icing | 1 slice | 3 starches & 3 fats |
| Cupcake, with icing | 1 item | 2 starches & 1 fat |
| Danish | 1 item | 2½ starches & 2 fats |
| Doughnut, plain | 1 item | 1½ starches & 2 fats |
| Doughnut, glazed | 1 item | 2 starches & 2 fats |
| Eclair with icing | 1 item | 2 starches & 2 fats |
| Ice cream sundae with hot fudge | 1 item | 2½ starches & 2 fats |
| Lemon meringue pie | 1 slice | 2½ starches & 2 fats |
| Pecan pie | 1 slice | 4 starches & 4 fats |
| Pound cake | 1 slice | 1½ starches & 1½ fats |
| Pumpkin pie | 1 slice | 2 starches & 2½ fats |
| Rice pudding with raisins | 1 cup | 3 starches, 1 milk, & 1 fat |

# ALCOHOLIC BEVERAGES

| | Amount=1 Swap | Counts As: |
|---|---|---|
| Beer, light | 12 ounces | 2 fats |
| Beer, regular | 12 ounces | 1 starch & 2 fats |
| Brandy, dry | 1 ounce | 1½ fats |
| Liquor (gin, rum, scotch, vodka, whiskey) | | |
| 80 proof | 1½ ounces | 2 fats |
| 100 proof | 1½ ounces | 3 fats |
| Sherry | 2 ounces | 1½ fats |
| Sherry, sweet | 2 ounces | ½ starch & 1½ fats |
| Wine, dry, unsweetened | 3½ ounces | 1½ fats |

## EXCHANGES FOR THE COOK

| *Food* | *Volume, Dry* | *Weight* | *# Swaps and Food Group* |
|---|---|---|---|
| *Vegetables* | | | |
| Tomato paste | 1 cup | 9 ounces | 8½ vegetables |
| | 1 can | 6 ounces | 5½ vegetables |
| *Grain, Starch, & Sugar* | | | |
| Beans, kidney, dry | 1 cup | 6½ ounces | 7 starches & 2 proteins |
| | ¼ cup | | 1 starch & 1 protein |
| Bread crumbs | 1 cup | 3½ ounces | 5 starches |
| Cornmeal, dry | | | |
| whole | 1 cup | 4 ounces | 5½ starches |
| degermed | 1 cup | 5 ounces | 6 starches |
| Cornstarch | 1 cup | 4½ ounces | 6 starches |
| | 1 Tbsp | ⅓ ounces | ⅓ starch |
| Flour, unsifted | 1 cup | 5 ounces | 6½ starches |
| | 3 tbsp | | 1 starch |
| Flour, whole wheat | 1 cup | 4 ounces | 5 starches |
| Honey | 1 cup | 12 ounces | 13 starches |
| | 1 Tbsp | 1 ounce | 1 starch |
| Molasses, blackstrap | 1 cup | 11½ ounces | 11 starchew |
| | 1 Tbsp | 1 ounce | ¾ starch |
| Pasta, uncooked | ¼ cup | | 1 starch |
| | | 1 ounce | 1⅓ starches |
| | (One ounce of raw pasta equals ⅔ cup cooked. Volume measures equal to 1 ounce. dry is dependent on the shape of the pasta.) | | |
| Oatmeal, dry | 1 cup | 3 ounces | 4 starches |
| | 3 Tbsp | | 1 starch |
| Rice | 1 cup | 3 ounces | 4½ starches |
| | 2 Tbsp | | 1 starch (⅓ cup cooked) |
| Sugar | 1 cup | 7 ounces | 9½ starches |
| | 1 Tbsp | ½ ounce | ¾ starch |
| Sugar, brown | 1 cup | 8 ounces | 10¼ starches |

# INTRODUCTION TO THE
# MENUS AND RECIPES

The menus and recipes in this section provide detailed road maps for you to reach your destination—a healthy, maintainable weight. To get started on your journey, you first need to select a calorie level and eating style as described in Chapter 5. Then locate the corresponding menus in this section—lower-carb menus and recipes are in section A; moderate-carb menus and recipes are in section B; and high-carb menus and recipes are in section C. In each section, one week's worth of daily menus are provided by calorie level—1200 calories/day; 1500 calories/day; 1800 calories/day; 2100 calories/day and 2400 calories/day. For many meals simple food items are combined. In addition, there are many recipes for you to try. After each serving of a food item or recipe, the equivalent number and types of swaps are provided in parentheses according to the following code—V = Vegetable Group, Fr = Fruit Group, S = Grain & Starch Group, P = Protein Group, M = Milk & Yogurt Group, Fa = Fat Group. After all menus for a particular eating style are presented, the recipes used in the menus are provided.

As you begin to follow the menus, read the rest of the book to fully understand the Bull's-Eye Food Guide system. Familiarize yourself with the Bull's-Eye Food Guide corresponding to your selected eating style in the front of the book, read Chapter 2, and review the swap lists that start on page 263. Then read Chapter 4, as the information provided in this chapter will help you gain an in-depth understanding of how the menus are put together and, even more importantly, how to modify them to suit your taste preferences. In general, if you do not like a particular menu item or do not have it available, use the swap lists to make a change. For example, you may not like a particular menu item, such as ⅓ cup of hummus, shown as being equivalent to 1 Grain & Starch Group swap and 1 Fat Group swap. Therefore, you would go to the swap list for these two food groups and pick replacement food items. You might select 4 to 6 whole wheat crackers to provide the 1 Grain & Starch Group swap and 6 almonds to provide the 1 Fat Group swap. This system provides you with infinite flexibility to create new menus.

The daily menus are based on the information provided for each eating style—Chapter 6 for the lower-carb eating style, Chapter 7 for the moderate-carb eating style and Chapter 8 for the high-carb eating style. Specifically, the second table in each of these chapters provides the organizational structure for the daily menus. As shown in these tables and explained in these chapters the swaps are combined to get the desired distribution of calories among carbohydrates, proteins, and fats. You can move swaps around between meals and snacks on occasion, as you will note in the menus provided. However, if you do this too often or to too great an extent, the intended distribution will be altered substantially. In addition, you can distribute the food items listed as snacks to times during the day when you are experiencing hunger. If you decide to move swaps around, simply monitor your weight and hunger to determine if the changes are having the desired effect—weight loss without excessive hunger.

It is best to plan your daily menus at least 1 day in advance, but a week in advance is ideal. Such planning allows you to have the appropriate foods available when you need them. Over time, you will find that the lead time for planning decreases. As you commit the swaps for each meal and snack to memory, you will be able to pull healthy meals together quickly. You will also learn to incorporate free foods, herbs and spices to flavor food according to your food preferences. If you prefer to put foods together yourself, you do not have to follow the recipes provided. The first day in each week's menu does not incorporate recipes, and provides you with a simple structure to follow without recipes.

The week's menus incorporate smaller amounts of many different types of foods—such as 1 swap of 2 or 3 different vegetables or grains/starches —rather than larger amounts of fewer types of foods—such as 2 or 3 swaps of one type of vegetable or grain/starch. This allows for a wide variety of flavors and textures, as well as nutrients and phytochemicals. You can modify the menus to increase or decrease variety according to your taste preferences and time available for food preparation.

Beverages are not included in the menus. The recommended beverages are water, seltzer, flavored seltzer (without sweeteners/calories as well as artificial sweeteners), and iced herbal teas. If you have not been told by your health care provider to limit caffeine, you can also add coffee or tea. Keep in mind that you may need to save part of a Milk Group swap to add to your coffee or tea throughout the day. Flavored/sweetened creamers are not recommended and are often high in hydrogenated fats and sweeteners. If you need to add more than 1 to 2 teaspoons of sugar a day to your coffee or tea you will also need to save a full or part of a Grain & Starch Group swap for this purpose (1 Grain & Starch swap = 5 teaspoons of sugar).

In terms of specific foods, there are a few things to remember. You can always add Vegetable Group swaps to meals and snacks to help control hunger. Amounts of foods presented in menus refer to cooked foods, such as cooked pasta or cooked rice. Amounts given in recipes refer to raw amounts, unless specified. Salt is typically used in recipes. If you are reducing your intake of processed foods (for example most canned, packaged, and frozen items) as suggested, the relatively small amounts of salt added when cooking would not be problematic. If, however, you have been told by your health care provider to avoid or limit sodium use pepper, herbs, and spices instead of salt. If you have allergies or intolerances use the swap lists to replace foods to which you are intolerant or allergic. For example, use soy milk and soy milk products (soy cheese or soy yogurt) instead of cow's milk and cow's milk products (cheese or yogurt) if you are lactose intolerant or if you have a milk allergy. Rice milk and rice milk-based cheeses are also available. Select soy- and rice-based products that are fortified with calcium, as well as riboflavin and vitamins A and D. If you decide not to use soy or rice milk products you can substitute the 2 daily Milk and Yogurt swaps as follows: 1) if you are following the lower-carb or moderate-carb eating styles replace with 2 Protein Group swaps and 1 Grain & Starch Group swap; 2) if you are following the high-carb eating style replace with 2 Grain & Starch Group swaps and 1 Protein Group swap. Nuts and natural peanut butter are often used due to the high quality fats, protein, fiber, and/or nutrients they provide. If you have a peanut allergy or do not like nuts or natural peanut butter use the swap lists to find alternatives. Lastly, if you have celiac disease or a wheat allergy, you will benefit from avoiding processed foods and using the swap lists to find alternatives to wheat-based breads, pastas, and cereals. For example, substitute rice, potatoes, beans, or winter squashes, as well as rice, or tapioca-based breads, pastas, or crackers and corn-based cereals.

Lastly, when selecting fish keep in mind advisories to avoid some types of fish that are high in mercury. Women who are pregnant, women who might become pregnant, breastfeeding women, and young children should not eat shark, swordfish, king mackerel, tilefish, or albacore tuna. These individuals should eat up to (but not greater than) 12 ounces of fish and shellfish that are lower in mercury such as shrimp, canned light tuna (but not albacore tuna), salmon, pollock, or catfish a week.

Enjoy the menus and recipes as you read through the book to gain an in-depth understanding of the Bull's-Eye Food Guide weight management system. The unique strategies and tools presented will empower you to navigate your way to successful and permanent weight loss.

# LOWER-CARB
# DAILY

## MENUS

### 1200 Calories per Day
#### DAY 1

*Breakfast*
- 2 slices of light whole-wheat bread (1 S) with 4 teaspoons of natural peanut butter (1 P, 1 Fa)
- ½ cup 1% milk or soymilk (½ M)

*Lunch*
- Salad: lettuce, ¼ cup sliced carrots, ¼ cup diced red peppers, ¼ cup tomato slices, and ½ cup broccoli (2 V); ⅓ cup garbanzo beans (1 S); 1-ounce chicken breast (1 P), cooked and cubed; 2 teaspoons olive oil (2 Fa); balsamic vinegar, salt (optional), and pepper to taste (freebies)
- 1 cup honeydew melon (1 Fr), cubed, topped with ½ cup plain low-fat yogurt (½ M)

*Tip: You can mix in 1 tablespoon vanilla yogurt until you get accustomed to plain low-fat yogurt.*

*Dinner*
On nights that you do not want to follow a recipe, use the swap lists and this suggested guideline to create a simple dinner menu.
- 1 cup of vegetables (2 V) sautéed with 2 teaspoons olive oil (2 Fa) and garlic (freebie)

- 1 small baked potato (3-ounce); OR ½ cup whole-wheat pasta tossed with sautéed vegetables; OR ⅓ cup brown rice topped with sautéed vegetables (1 S)
- 3 ounces of baked or grilled white-meat chicken or turkey (no skin); OR 3 ounces of lean grilled beef or pork; OR 3 ounces of grilled or baked salmon or other fatty fish; OR 6 ounces of baked or grilled flounder, other white fish, or shellfish (3 P)

*Snack*
- Simple Smoothie: ½ banana (1 Fr) blended with 1 cup 1% milk or soymilk (1 M) and ice (freebie)
- 6 almonds (1 Fa)

# DAY 2

*Breakfast*
- Breakfast Protein Smoothie: 1 scoop soy protein powder (1 P) blended with 2 teaspoons of natural peanut butter (1 Fa), ½ cup 1% milk or soymilk (½ M), and ice (freebie)
- ¾ cup whole-grain cereal squares OR 4–6 whole-grain crackers (1 S)

*Tip: Look for cereals with less than 5–7 grams of sugar. Avoid cereals and crackers with trans- or partially hydrogenated fats or oils.*

*Lunch*
- Turkey Sandwich: 2 slices whole-wheat light bread (1 S) with 1 ounce thinly sliced turkey breast (1 P), ⅛ avocado (1 Fa), sliced, and mustard (freebie)
- ½ cup baby carrots and 1 cup red pepper slices (2 V)
- ½ cup plain low-fat yogurt (½ M) topped with 2 tablespoons raisins (1 Fr) and 10 peanuts (1 Fa)

*Dinner*
- Steak and Roasted Vegetables over Field Greens—see recipe section; use 12 ounces of steak for 4 servings (1 serving = 3 P, 2 V, 2 Fa)
- 1 small (3-inch) whole-wheat pita bread (1 S)

*Snack*
- 1 apple (1 Fr), sliced and dipped in 2 teaspoons natural peanut butter (1 Fa)
- 1 cup 1% milk or plain soymilk (1 M)

# DAY 3

*Breakfast*
- 2 slices whole-wheat light bread (1 S) with 1 teaspoon butter (1 Fa)
- ¼ cup low-fat cottage cheese (1 P)
- ½ cup 1% milk or plain soymilk (1/2 M)

*Lunch*
- Egg Salad Sandwich:
  — 1 small whole-wheat pita bread (3 inches; 1 S), sliced open
  — 1 hard-boiled egg (1 P) crumbled and mixed with 1 teaspoon
    mayonnaise (1 Fa); add ½ teaspoon Dijon mustard and minced
    red onion to taste (freebies)
  — ⅛ avocado (1 Fa) sliced and placed in pita with egg salad
- 1 cup string beans (2 V), cooked and chilled (marinated overnight with
  balsamic vinegar and whole cloves of garlic)
- 10 grapes (1 Fr)
- ½ cup 1% milk or plain soymilk (½ M)

*Dinner*
- Scallop, Spinach, and Tomato Sauté—see recipe section; use 1½
  pounds of scallops for 4 servings (1 serving = 3 P, 2 V, 2 Fa)
- ⅓ cup cooked brown rice (1 S)

*Snack*
- 4 dried apricot halves (1 Fr) tossed with 6 almonds (1 Fa)
- 1 cup 1% milk, plain soymilk, or plain low-fat yogurt (1 M)

# DAY 4

*Breakfast*
- 1 small whole-wheat pita bread (3-inch; 1 S) spread with 2 tablespoons
  Homemade Yogurt Cheese (¼ M)—see recipe section
- 1 ounce smoked salmon (1 P) on pita bread, topped with 1 teaspoon
  capers (freebie)

*Note: ¼ Milk Group swap saved for snack and 1 Fat Group swap saved for snack.*

*Lunch*
- Lentil Salad—see recipe section (1 P, 1 S, 1 V, 2 Fa)
- ½ cup baby carrots (1 V)
- ½ cup cantaloupe (½ Fr—save the other half for dinner recipe), cubed
- ½ cup 1% milk or soymilk (½ M)

*Dinner*
- Apple Pork—see recipe section; use 4, 3-ounce center loin or tender-loin pork medallions for 4 servings (3 P, ½ Fr, 1 Fa)
- 1 cup boiled beets (2 V), peeled and sliced
- ½ cup baked sweet potato (1 S)
- 10 pistachios (1 Fa)

*Snack*
- ½ banana (1 Fr) with 2 teaspoons natural peanut butter to spread on banana (1 Fa)
- 6 almonds (1 Fa—extra fat borrowed from breakfast)
- 10 ounces of 1% milk or soymilk (1 M—extra ¼ swap saved from breakfast)

# DAY 5

*Breakfast*
- Omelet: 3 egg whites (1 P) with sautéed onions, red pepper, and tomato (extra vegetables are freebies) in 1 teaspoon olive oil (1 Fa)
- 1 whole-grain tortilla (6-inch, no added fat; 1 S) to wrap omelet
- ½ cup 1% milk or plain soymilk (½ M)

*Lunch*
- Stuffed Baked Potato: 1 small baked or microwaved potato (3-ounce; 1 S) topped with 1 cup fresh or frozen broccoli (2 V), steamed or microwaved and placed on top of potato; and 1 ounce cheddar cheese (1 P, 2 Fa), shredded and melted over the top of the potato and broccoli
- 12 cherries (1 Fr)
- ½ cup 1% milk or plain soymilk (½ M)

*Dinner*

- Spicy Peanut Chicken—see recipe section; use 12 ounces of chicken breast for 4 servings (3 P, 1 V, 2 Fa)
- ½ cup steamed or microwaved cauliflower (1 V)
- ⅓ cup whole-wheat couscous (1 S)

*Snack*

- Simple Smoothie: ¾ cup berries (1 Fr) blended with 1 cup 1% milk or plain soymilk (1 M) and ice
- 6 cashews (1 Fa)

*Note: You can use fresh or frozen berry mixtures with no added sweeteners. In other words, the ingredient list should just list berries—no sugar, high-fructose corn syrup, corn syrup, honey, or other added sweetener.*

# DAY 6

*Breakfast*

- 1 soft-boiled egg (1 P) with 2 slices whole-wheat light bread (1 S) and 1 teaspoon butter (1 Fa)
- 1/2 cup 1% milk or plain soymilk (1/2 M)

*Lunch*

- Simple Pasta Salad: ½ cup whole-wheat pasta (1 S), cooked and chilled, tossed with 1 teaspoon olive oil (1 Fa), 1 large diced tomato (1 V), ¼ cup tuna fish (light and packed in water, 1 P), drained, and mixed with 1 teaspoon mayonnaise (1 Fa) and 1/2 teaspoon mustard (freebie)
- ½ cup baby carrots
- 1 orange (1 Fr)
- ½ cup 1% milk or plain soymilk (1 M)

*Dinner*

- Turkey with Corn Salsa—see recipe section; use 12 ounces of turkey breast for 4 servings (3 P, 1 S, 1 V, 2 Fa)
- ½ cup steamed string beans (1 V)

*Snack*

Once in a while, you can combine the calories from your some of your snack swaps to have a typical dessert food. In this case, you have 1 Fruit Group swap, 1 Fat Group swap, and 1 Milk & Yogurt Group swap (60 calories + 45 calories + 90 calories), or 195 calories, to spend on a dessert. Use food labels to determine the amount of a particular food you can have that provides 195 calories. For example, you can have ½ to ¾ cup of ice cream (depending on the flavor and brand) OR have 3–4 cookies.

# DAY 7

*Breakfast*
- ¾ cup whole-grain cereal (1 S) with ½ cup plain low-fat yogurt (½ M)
- 6 almonds (1 Fa)

*Notes: Save 1 Protein Group swap for lunch. You can mix 1 tablespoon of vanilla yogurt into the plain yogurt until you get accustomed to the plain low-fat yogurt.*

*Lunch*
- 1 veggie burger (2 P, ½ S—1 Protein Group swap borrowed from breakfast) on 1 slice of whole-wheat light bread (½ S) and topped with spinach leaves, red onion slices, and ½ tomato (1 V), sliced, and ¼ avocado (2 Fa), sliced
- 1 cup sliced red pepper (1 V)
- ½ cup honeydew melon (½ Fr—½ saved for dinner recipe)
- ½ cup 1% milk or plain soymilk (½ M)

*Dinner*
- 6 ounces of flounder fillet (3 P), baked, and brushed lightly with olive oil and topped with onion slices, 1 teaspoon capers, and juice of 1 lemon wedge (freebies)
- 1 cup steamed asparagus (2 V)
- Wild Rice with Pecans and Cranberries—see recipe section (1 S, 2 Fa, ½ Fr—borrowed from lunch)

*Snack*
- Peanut Butter Smoothie: ½ banana (1 Fr) blended with 1 cup 1% milk or plain soymilk (1 M), 2 teaspoons natural peanut butter (1 Fa), and ice (freebie)

# 1500 Calories per Day

## DAY 1

*Breakfast*
- 2 slices of light whole-wheat bread (1 S) with 4 teaspoons of natural peanut butter (1 P, 1 Fa)
- ½ cup 1% milk or soymilk (½ M)

*Lunch*
- Salad: lettuce, ¼ cup sliced carrots, ¼ cup diced red peppers, ¼ cup tomato slices, and ½ cup broccoli (2 V); ⅓ cup garbanzo beans (1 S); 2-ounce chicken breast (2 P), cooked and cubed; 2 teaspoons olive oil (2 Fa); balsamic vinegar, salt (optional), and pepper to taste (freebies)
- 1 cup honeydew melon (1 Fr), cubed, topped with ½ cup plain low-fat yogurt (1/2 M)

*Tip: You can mix in 1 tablespoon vanilla yogurt until you get accustomed to plain low-fat yogurt.*

*Dinner*
On nights that you do not want to follow a recipe, use the swap lists and this suggested guideline to create a simple dinner menu.
- 2 cups of vegetables (4 V) sautéed with 2 teaspoons olive oil (2 Fa) and garlic (freebie)
- 1 medium baked potato (6-ounce); OR 1 cup whole-wheat pasta tossed with sautéed vegetables; OR ⅔ cup brown rice topped with sautéed vegetables (2 S)
- 4 ounces of baked or grilled white-meat chicken or turkey (no skin); OR 4 ounces of lean grilled beef or pork; OR 4 ounces of grilled or baked salmon or other fatty fish; OR 8 ounces of baked or grilled flounder, other white fish, or shellfish (4 P)

*Snack*
- Smoothie: ½ banana (1 Fr) blended with 1 scoop soy protein powder (1 P), 1 cup 1% milk or soymilk (1 M), and ice (freebie)
- 6 almonds (1 Fa)

# DAY 2

*Breakfast*
- Breakfast Protein Smoothie: 1 scoop soy protein powder (1 P) blended with 2 teaspoons of natural peanut butter (1 Fa), ½ cup 1% milk or soymilk (½ M), and ice (freebie)
- ¾ cup whole-grain cereal squares OR 4–6 whole-grain crackers (1 S)

*Tip: Look for cereals with less than 5–7 grams of sugar. Avoid cereals and crackers with trans- or partially hydrogenated fats or oils.*

*Lunch*
- Turkey Sandwich: 2 slices whole-wheat light bread (1 S) with 2 ounces thinly sliced turkey breast (2 P), ⅛ avocado (1 Fa), sliced, and mustard (freebie)
- ½ cup baby carrots and 1 cup red pepper slices (2 V)
- ½ cup plain low-fat yogurt (½ M) topped with 2 tablespoons raisins (1 Fr) and 10 peanuts (1 Fa)

*Dinner*
- Steak and Roasted Vegetables over Field Greens—see recipe section; use 1 pound of steak for 4 servings (1 serving = 4 P, 2 V, 2 Fa)
- 1 cup string beans (2 V)
- 1 large (6-inch) whole-wheat pita bread (2 S)

*Snack*
- 1 apple (1 Fr), sliced and dipped in 4 teaspoons natural peanut butter (1 P, 1 Fa)
- 1 cup 1% milk or plain soymilk (1 M)

# DAY 3

*Breakfast*
- 2 slices whole-wheat light bread (1 S) with 1 teaspoon butter (1 Fa)
- ¼ cup low-fat cottage cheese (1 P)
- ½ cup 1% milk or plain soymilk (½ M)

*Lunch*
- Egg Salad Sandwich:
  — 1 small whole-wheat pita bread (3-inch; 1 S), sliced open
  — 2 hard-boiled eggs (2 P) crumbled and mixed with 1 teaspoon mayonnaise (1 Fa); add ½ teaspoon Dijon mustard and minced red onion to taste (freebies)
  — ⅛ avocado (1 Fa) sliced and placed in pita with egg salad
- 1 cup string beans (2 V), cooked and chilled (marinated overnight with balsamic vinegar and whole cloves of garlic)
- 10 grapes (1 Fr)
- ½ cup 1% milk or plain soymilk (½ M)

*Dinner*
- Scallop, Spinach, and Tomato Sauté—see recipe section; use 2 pounds of scallops for 4 servings (1 serving = 4 P, 2 V, 2 Fa)
- 1 cup steamed or microwaved carrots (2 V)
- ⅔ cup cooked brown rice (2 S)

*Snack*
- ¼ cup cottage cheese (1 P) topped with 1¼ cup strawberries (1 Fr), sliced
- 6 almonds (1 Fa)
- 1 cup 1% milk or plain soymilk (1 M)

## DAY 4

*Breakfast*
- 1 small whole-wheat pita bread (3-inch; 1 S) spread with 2 tablespoons Homemade Yogurt Cheese (¼ M)—see recipe section
- 2 ounces smoked salmon on pita bread (2 P—1 Protein Group swap borrowed from lunch) topped with 1 teaspoon capers (freebie)

*Note: ¼ Milk Group swap saved for snack; 1 Fat Group swap saved for lunch.*

*Lunch*
- Lentil Salad—see recipe section (1 P, 1 S, 1 V, 2 Fa)
- ½ cup baby carrots (1 V)
- ½ cup cantaloupe (½ Fr—save the other half for dinner recipe), cubed

- ½ cup 1% milk or soymilk (½ M)

Dinner
- Apple Pork—see recipe section; use 4, 4-ounce center loin or tender-loin pork medallions for 4 servings (4 P, ½ Fr, 1 Fa)
- 1 cup boiled beets (2 V), peeled and sliced, and 1 cup steamed or microwaved cauliflower (2 V)
- 1 cup baked sweet potato (2 S)
- 10 pistachios (1 Fa)

Snack
- ½ banana (1 Fr) with 4 teaspoons natural peanut butter to spread on banana (1 P, 1 Fa)
- 10 ounces of 1% milk or soymilk (1 M—plus extra ¼ swap borrowed from breakfast)

# DAY 5

Breakfast
- Omelet: 3 egg whites (1 P) with sautéed onions, red pepper, and toma-to (extra vegetables are freebies) in 1 teaspoon olive oil (1 Fa)
- 1 whole-grain tortilla (6-inch, no added fat; 1 S) to wrap omelet
- ½ cup 1% milk or plain soymilk (½ M)

Lunch
- Stuffed Baked Potato: 1 small baked or microwaved potato (3-ounce; 1 S) topped with 1 cup fresh or frozen broccoli (2 V), steamed or microwaved and placed on top of potato; 1 ounce lean ham (1 P), diced; and 1 ounce cheddar cheese (1 P, 2 Fa), shredded and melted over the top of the potato and broccoli
- 12 cherries (1 Fr)
- ½ cup 1% milk or plain soymilk (½ M)

Dinner
- Spicy Peanut Chicken—see recipe section; use 1 pound of chicken breast for 4 servings (4 P, 1 V, 2 Fa)
- 1½ cups steamed or microwaved cauliflower (3 V)

- ⅔ cup whole-wheat couscous (2 S)

*Snack*
- Protein Smoothie: 3/4 cup berries (1 Fr) blended with 1 scoop soy protein powder (1 P), 1 cup 1% milk or plain soymilk (1 M), and ice (freebie)
- 6 cashews (1 Fa)

*Note: You can use fresh or frozen berry mixtures with no added sweeteners. In other words, the ingredient list should just list berries—no sugar, high-fructose corn syrup, corn syrup, honey, or other added sweetener.*

# DAY 6

*Breakfast*
- 1 soft-boiled egg (1 P) with 2 slices whole-wheat light bread (1 S) and 1 teaspoon butter (1 Fa)
- ½ cup 1% milk or plain soymilk (½ M)

*Lunch*
- Simple Pasta Salad: ½ cup whole-wheat pasta (1 S), cooked and chilled, tossed with 1 teaspoon olive oil (1 Fa), 1 large diced tomato (1 V), ½ cup tuna fish (light and packed in water, 2 P), drained, and mixed with 1 teaspoon mayonnaise (1 Fa) and ½ teaspoon mustard (freebie)
- ½ cup baby carrots (1 V)
- 1 orange (1 Fr)
- ½ cup 1% milk or plain soymilk (1 M)

*Dinner*
- Turkey with Corn Salsa—see recipe section; use 1 pound of turkey breast for 4 servings (4 P, 1 S, 1 V, 2 Fa)
- 2, 4-inch bread sticks (1 S)
- 1½ cups steamed string beans (3 V)

*Note: Look for whole-wheat bread sticks without hydrogenated oils.*

*Snack*
Once in a while, you can combine the calories from some of your snack swaps to have a typical dessert food. In this case, you have 1 Fruit Group

swap, 1 Protein Group swap, 1 Fat Group swap, and 1 Milk & Yogurt Group swap (60 calories + 55 calories + 45 calories + 90 calories), or 250 calories, to spend on a dessert. Use food labels to determine the amount of a particular food you can have that provides 250 calories. For example, you can have about 1 cup of ice cream (depending on the flavor and brand) OR have 3–4 cookies and 1 cup of 1% milk.

# DAY 7

*Breakfast*
- ¾ cup whole-grain cereal (1 S) with ½ cup plain low-fat yogurt (½ M)
- 6 almonds (1 Fa)

Notes: *Save 1 Protein Group swap for lunch. You can mix 1 tablespoon of vanilla yogurt into the plain yogurt until you get accustomed to the plain low-fat yogurt.*

*Lunch*
- 1 veggie burger (2 P, ½ S) with 1 ounce soy cheese melted over top (1 P—1 Protein Group swap borrowed from breakfast) on 1 slice of whole-wheat light bread (½ S) and topped with spinach leaves, red onion slices, and ½ tomato (1 V), sliced, and ¼ avocado (2 Fa), sliced
- 1 cup sliced red pepper (1 V)
- ½ cup honeydew melon (½ Fr—½ saved for dinner recipe)
- ½ cup 1% milk or plain soymilk (½ M)

*Dinner*
- 8 ounces of flounder fillet (4 P), baked and brushed lightly with olive oil and topped with onion slices, 1 teaspoon capers, and juice of 1 lemon wedge (freebies)
- 2 cups steamed asparagus (4 V)
- Wild Rice with Pecans and Cranberries—see recipe section (1 S, ½ Fr—borrowed from lunch, 2 Fa)

Note: *Save 1 Grain & Starch Group swap for snack.*

*Snack*
- Peanut Butter Smoothie: ½ banana (1 Fr) blended with 1 cup 1% milk or plain soymilk (1 M), 4 teaspoons natural peanut butter (1 P, 1 Fa), and ice (freebie)

- 4–6 whole-wheat crackers (1 S)

# 1800 Calories per Day

## DAY 1

*Breakfast*
- 2 slices of light whole-wheat bread (1 S) with 4 teaspoons of natural peanut butter (1 P, 1 Fa)
- ½ cup 1% milk or soymilk (½ M)

*Lunch*
- Salad: lettuce, ¼ cup sliced carrots, ¼ cup diced red peppers, ¼ cup tomato slices, and ½ cup broccoli (2 V); ⅔ cup garbanzo beans (2 S); 3-ounce chicken breast (3 P), cooked and cubed; 2 teaspoons olive oil (2 Fa); balsamic vinegar, salt (optional), and pepper to taste (freebies)
- 1 cup honeydew melon (1 Fr), cubed, topped with ½ cup plain low-fat yogurt (½ M)

*Tip: You can mix in 1 tablespoon vanilla yogurt until you get accustomed to plain low-fat yogurt.*

*Dinner*
On nights that you do not want to follow a recipe, use the swap lists and this suggested guideline to create a simple dinner menu.
- 2 cups of vegetables (4 V) sautéed with 3 teaspoons olive oil (3 Fa) and garlic (freebie)
- 1 large baked potato (9-ounce); OR 1½ cups whole-wheat pasta tossed with sautéed vegetables; OR 1 cup brown rice topped with sautéed vegetables (3 S)
- 4 ounces of baked or grilled white-meat chicken or turkey (no skin); OR 4 ounces of lean grilled beef or pork; OR 4 ounces of grilled or baked salmon or other fatty fish; OR 8 ounces of baked or grilled flounder, other white fish, or shellfish (4 P)

*Snack*
- Smoothie: ½ banana (1 Fr) blended with 1 scoop soy protein powder (1 P), 1 cup 1% milk or soymilk (1 M), and ice (freebie)
- 12 almonds (2 Fa)

# DAY 2

*Breakfast*
- Breakfast Protein Smoothie: 1 scoop soy protein powder (1 P) blended with 2 teaspoons of natural peanut butter (1 Fa), ½ cup 1% milk or soymilk (½ M), and ice (freebie)
- ¾ cup whole-grain cereal squares OR 4–6 whole-grain crackers (1 S)

*Tip: Look for cereals with less than 5–7 grams of sugar. Avoid cereals and crackers with trans- or partially hydrogenated fats or oils.*

*Lunch*
- Turkey Sandwich: 2 slices whole-wheat bread (2 S) with 3 ounces thinly sliced turkey breast (3 P), ⅛ avocado (1 Fa), sliced, and mustard (freebie)
- ½ cup baby carrots and 1 cup red pepper slices (2 V)
- ½ cup plain low-fat yogurt (½ M) topped with 2 tablespoons raisins (1 Fr) and 10 peanuts (1 Fa)

*Dinner*
- Steak and Roasted Vegetables over Field Greens—see recipe section; use 1 pound of steak for 4 servings (1 serving = 4 P, 2 V, 2 Fa); top with 8 black olives (1 Fa).
- 1 cup string beans (2 V)
- 1½ large (6-inch) whole-wheat pita bread (3 S)

*Snack*
- 1 apple (1 Fr), sliced and dipped in 4 teaspoons natural peanut butter (1 P, 1 Fa)
- 1 cup 1% milk or plain soymilk (1 M)
- 10 peanuts (1 Fa)

# DAY 3

*Breakfast*
- 2 slices whole-wheat light bread (1 S) with 1 teaspoon butter (1 Fa)
- ½ cup low-fat cottage cheese (2 P—1 Protein Group swap borrowed from lunch)

- ½ cup 1% milk or plain soymilk (½ M)

*Lunch*
- Egg Salad Sandwich:
    — 1 large whole-wheat pita bread (6-inch; 2 S), sliced open
    — 2 hard-boiled eggs (2 P) crumbled and mixed with 1 teaspoon mayonnaise (1 Fa); add ½ teaspoon Dijon mustard and minced red onion to taste (freebies)
    — ⅛ avocado (1 Fa), sliced and placed in pita with egg salad
- 1 cup string beans (2 V), cooked and chilled (marinated overnight with balsamic vinegar and whole cloves of garlic)
- 10 grapes (1 Fr)
- 1/2 cup 1% milk or plain soymilk (½ M)

*Note: 1 Protein Group swap saved for breakfast.*

*Dinner*
- Scallop, Spinach, and Tomato Sauté—see recipe section; use 2 pounds of scallops for 4 servings (1 serving = 4 P, 2 V, 2 Fa)
- 1 cup steamed or microwaved carrots (2 V)
- 1 cup cooked brown rice (3 S)
- 6 cashews (1 Fa)

*Snack*
- ¼ cup cottage cheese (1 P) topped with 1¼ cup strawberries (1 Fr), sliced
- 12 almonds (2 Fa)
- 1 cup 1% milk or plain soymilk (1 M)

# DAY 4

*Breakfast*
- 1 small whole-wheat pita bread (3-inch; 1 S) spread with 2 tablespoons Homemade Yogurt Cheese (¼ M)—see recipe section
- 2 ounces smoked salmon on pita bread (2 P—1 Protein Group swap borrowed from lunch), topped with 10 green olives (1 Fa), chopped

*Note: ¼ Milk Group swap saved for snack.*

*Lunch*
- Lentil Salad—see recipe section (1 P, 1 S, 1 V, 2 Fa)
- ½ cup baby carrots (1 V)
- 4–6 whole-wheat crackers (1 S) with 1 ounce low-fat cheese (1 P), cut into small cubes
- ½ cup cantaloupe (½ Fr—save the other half for dinner recipe), cubed
- ½ cup 1% milk or soymilk (½ M)

Note: *1 Protein Group swap borrowed from breakfast.*

*Dinner*
- Apple Pork—see recipe section; use 4, 4-ounce center loin or tenderloin pork medallions for 4 servings (4 P, 1 Fa, ½ Fr—borrowed from lunch)
- 1 cup boiled beets (2 V), peeled and sliced, and 1 cup steamed or microwaved cauliflower (2 V)
- 1½ cups baked sweet potato (3 S)
- 20 pistachios (2 Fa)

*Snack*
- ½ banana (1 Fr) with 4 teaspoons natural peanut butter to spread on banana (1 P, 1 Fa)
- 6 almonds (1 Fa)
- 10 ounces of 1% milk or soymilk (1 M—plus extra ¼ swap saved from breakfast)

# DAY 5

*Breakfast*
- Omelet: 3 egg whites (1 P) with sautéed onions, red pepper, and tomato (extra vegetables are freebies) in 1 teaspoon olive oil (1 Fa)
- 1 whole-grain tortilla (6-inch, no added fat; 1 S) to wrap omelet
- ½ cup 1% milk or plain soymilk (½ M)

*Lunch*
- Stuffed Baked Potato: 1 medium baked or microwaved potato (6-ounce; 2 S) topped with 1 cup fresh or frozen broccoli (2 V), steamed or microwaved and placed on top of potato; 2 ounces lean ham (2 P), diced; and 1 ounce cheddar cheese, shredded and melted over top of potato and broccoli (1 P, 2 Fa)

- 12 cherries (1 Fr)
- ½ cup 1% milk or plain soymilk (½ M)

*Dinner*
- Spicy Peanut Chicken—see recipe section; use 1 pound of chicken breast for 4 servings (4 P, 1 V, 2 Fa)
- 1½ cup steamed or microwaved cauliflower (3 V)
- 1 cup whole-wheat couscous (3 S)
- 10 peanuts (1 Fa)

*Snack*
- Protein Smoothie: ¾ cup berries (1 Fr) blended with 1 scoop soy protein powder (1 P), 1 cup 1% milk or plain soymilk (1 M), and ice (freebie)
- 12 cashews (2 Fa)

*Note: You can use fresh or frozen berry mixtures with no added sweeteners. In other words, the ingredient list should just list berries—no sugar, high-fructose corn syrup, corn syrup, honey, or other added sweetener.*


# DAY 6

*Breakfast*
- 1 soft-boiled egg (1 P) with 2 slices whole-wheat light bread (1 S) and 1 teaspoon butter (1 Fa)
- ½ cup 1% milk or plain soymilk (½ M)

*Lunch*
- Simple Pasta Salad: 1 cup whole-wheat pasta (2 S), cooked and chilled, tossed with 1 teaspoon olive oil (1 Fa), 1 large diced tomato (1 V), ¾ cup tuna fish (light and packed in water, 3 P), drained, and mixed with 1 teaspoon mayonnaise (1 Fa), and ½ teaspoon mustard (freebie)
- ½ cup baby carrots (1 V)
- 1 orange (1 Fr)
- ½ cup 1% milk or plain soymilk (½ M)

*Dinner*
- Turkey with Corn Salsa—see recipe section; use 1 pound of turkey breast for 4 servings (4 P, 1 S, 1 V, 2 Fa)
- 4, 4-inch bread sticks (2 S)
- 1½ cup steamed string beans (3 V)
- 2 walnuts (1 Fa)

Note: *Look for whole-wheat bread sticks without hydrogenated oils.*

*Snack*
Once in a while, you can combine the calories from some of your snack swaps to have a typical dessert food. In this case, you have 1 Fruit Group swap, 1 Protein Group swap, and 2 Fat Group swaps (60 calories + 55 calories + 90 calories), or 205 calories, to spend on a dessert that you have with your Milk Group swap. Use food labels to determine the amount of a particular food you can have that provides 205 calories. For example, you can make an ice cream shake with 1 cup of 1% milk or plain soymilk blended with about ¾ cup ice cream (depending on the flavor and brand) OR have 3–4 cookies and 1 cup of 1% milk.

# DAY 7

*Breakfast*
- ¾ cup whole-grain cereal (1 S) with ½ cup plain low-fat yogurt (½ M)
- 6 almonds (1 Fa)

Notes: *Save 1 Protein Group swap for lunch. You can mix 1 tablespoon of vanilla yogurt into the plain yogurt until you get accustomed to the plain low-fat yogurt.*

*Lunch*
- 1 veggie burger (2 P, ½ S) with 2 ounces soy cheese melted overtop (2 P—1 Protein Group swap borrowed from lunch) on 2 slices of whole-wheat light bread (1 S) and topped with spinach leaves, red onion slices, and ½ tomato (1 V), sliced, and ¼ avocado (2 Fa), sliced
- 1 cup sliced red pepper (1 V)
- ½ cup honeydew melon (½ Fr—½ saved for dinner recipe) topped with ½ cup plain low-fat yogurt (½ M) and 1½ tablespoons Grape-Nuts cereal (½ S)

*Dinner*
- 8 ounces of flounder fillet (4 P), baked and brushed lightly with olive oil and topped with onion slices, 1 teaspoon capers, and juice of 1 lemon wedge (freebies)
- 2 cups steamed asparagus (4 V)
- Wild Rice with Pecans and Cranberries—see recipe section (1 S, 2 Fa, ½ Fr borrowed from lunch)
- ½ cup corn (1 S)
- 2 pecans (1 Fa)

*Note: Save 1 Grain & Starch Group swap for snack.*

*Snack*
- Peanut Butter Smoothie: ½ banana (1 Fr) blended with 1 cup 1% milk or plain soymilk (1 M), 4 teaspoons natural peanut butter (1 P, 1 Fa), and ice (freebie)
- 2 slices whole-wheat light bread (1 S—borrowed from dinner) with 2 teaspoons natural peanut butter (1 Fa)

# 2100 Calories per Day

## DAY 1

*Breakfast*
- 2 slices of whole-wheat light bread (1 S) with 8 teaspoons of natural peanut butter (2 P, 2 Fa)
- ½ cup 1% milk or soymilk (½ M)

*Lunch*
- Salad: lettuce, ¼ cup sliced carrots, ¼ cup diced red peppers, ¼ cup tomato slices, and ½ cup broccoli (2 V); ⅔ cup garbanzo beans (2 S); 4-ounce chicken breast (4 P), cooked and cubed; 2 teaspoons olive oil (2 Fa); balsamic vinegar, salt (optional), and pepper to taste (freebies)
- 1 cup honeydew melon (1 Fr), cubed, topped with ½ cup plain low-fat yogurt (½ M)

*Tip: You can mix in 1 tablespoon vanilla yogurt until you get accustomed to plain yogurt.*

*Dinner*

On nights that you do not want to follow a recipe, use the swap lists and this suggested guideline to create a simple dinner menu.

- 2 cups of vegetables (4 V) sautéed with 3 teaspoons olive oil (3 Fa) and garlic (freebie)
- 1 large baked potato (9-ounce); OR 1½ cups whole-wheat pasta tossed with sautéed vegetables; OR 1 cup brown rice topped with sautéed vegetables (3 S)
- 4 ounces of baked or grilled white-meat chicken or turkey (no skin); OR 4 ounces of lean grilled beef or pork; OR 4 ounces of grilled or baked salmon or other fatty fish; OR 8 ounces of baked or grilled flounder, other white fish, or shellfish (4 P)

*Snack*

- Smoothie: ½ banana (1 Fr) blended with 1 scoop soy protein powder (1 P), 1 cup 1% milk or soymilk (1 M), and ice (freebie)
- Crunchy Trail Mix: ¾ cup whole-grain cereal squares (1 S), 2 tablespoons raisins (1 Fr), and 12 almonds (2 Fa)

# DAY 2

*Breakfast*

- Breakfast Protein Smoothie: 2 scoops soy protein powder (2 P) blended with 2 teaspoons of natural peanut butter (1 Fa), ½ cup 1% milk or soymilk (½ M), and ice (freebie)
- ¾ cup whole-grain cereal squares OR 4–6 whole-grain crackers (1 S)
- 6 almonds (1 Fa)

*Tip: Look for cereals with less than 5–7 grams of sugar. Avoid cereals and crackers with trans- or partially hydrogenated fats or oils.*

*Lunch*

- Turkey Sandwich: 2 slices whole-wheat bread (2 S) with 4 ounces thinly sliced turkey breast (4 P), ⅛ avocado (1 Fa), sliced, and mustard (freebie)
- ½ cup baby carrots and 1 cup sliced red pepper (2 V)
- ½ cup plain low-fat yogurt (½ M) topped with 2 tablespoons raisins (1 Fr), and 10 peanuts (1 Fa)

*Dinner*
- Steak and Roasted Vegetables over Field Greens—see recipe section; use 1 pound of steak for 4 servings (1 serving = 4 P, 2 V, 2 Fa); top with 8 black olives (1 Fa)
- 1 cup string beans (2 V)
- 1½ large (6-inch) whole-wheat pita bread (3 S)

*Snack*
- 1 apple (1 Fr), sliced and dipped in 4 teaspoons natural peanut butter (1 P, 1 Fa)
- 1 cup 1% milk or plain soymilk or 1 cup plain low-fat yogurt (1 M)
- Crunchy Trail Mix: 4 dried apricot halves (1 Fr), ¾ cup whole-grain cereal squares (1 S), 10 peanuts (1 Fa)

Note: *Try the yogurt topped with the Crunchy Trail Mix.*

# DAY 3

*Breakfast*
- 2 slices whole-wheat light bread (1 S) with 1 teaspoon butter (1 Fa)
- 1 cup low-fat cottage cheese (4 P—2 Protein Group swaps borrowed from lunch)
- ½ cup 1% milk or plain soymilk (½ M)

Note: *Save 1 Fat Group swap for lunch.*

*Lunch*
- Egg Salad Sandwich:
  — 1 large whole-wheat pita bread (6-inch; 2 S), sliced open
  — 2 hard-boiled eggs (2 P) crumbled and mixed with 1 teaspoon mayonnaise (1 Fa); add ½ teaspoon Dijon mustard and minced red onion to taste (freebies)
  — ¼ avocado, sliced and placed in pita with egg salad (2 Fa—1 Fat Group swap borrowed from breakfast)
- 1 cup string beans (2 V), cooked and chilled (marinated overnight with balsamic vinegar and whole cloves of garlic)
- 10 grapes (1 Fr)
- ½ cup 1% milk or plain soymilk (½ M)

Note: *2 Protein Group swaps saved for breakfast.*

*Dinner*
- Scallop, Spinach, and Tomato Sauté—see recipe section; use 2 pounds of scallops for 4 servings (1 serving = 4 P, 2 V, 2 Fa)
- 1 cup steamed or microwaved carrots (2 V)
- 1 cup cooked brown rice (3 S)
- 6 cashews (1 Fa)

*Snack*
- ¼ cup cottage cheese (1 P) topped with 1¼ cups strawberries (1 Fr), sliced
- 4–6 whole-wheat crackers (1 S)
- 12 almonds (2 Fa) eaten with 1 peach (1 Fr)
- 1 cup 1% milk or plain soymilk (1 M)

# DAY 4

*Breakfast*
- 1 small whole-wheat pita bread (3-inch; 1 S) spread with 2 tablespoons Homemade Yogurt Cheese (¼ M)—see recipe section
- 2 ounces smoked salmon on pita bread (2 P), topped with 10 green olives (1 Fa), chopped

Note: *¼ Milk Group swap saved for snack; 1 Fat Group swap saved for lunch.*

*Lunch*
- Lentil Salad—see recipe section (1 P, 1 S, 1 V, 2 Fa)
- ½ cup baby carrots (1 V)
- 4–6 whole-wheat crackers (1 S) with 3 ounces low-fat cheese (3 P), cut into small cubes
- ½ cup cantaloupe (½ Fr—save the other half for dinner recipe), cubed
- 2 walnuts (1 Fa—borrowed from breakfast)
- ½ cup 1% milk or plain soymilk (½ M)

Note: *Try crumbling the walnuts and sprinkling on top of the Lentil Salad.*

*Dinner*
- Apple Pork—see recipe section; use 4, 4-ounce center loin or tender-loin pork medallions for 4 servings (4 P, 1 Fa, ½ Fr—borrowed from lunch)

- 1 cup boiled beets (2 V), peeled and sliced, and 1 cup steamed or microwaved cauliflower (2 V)
- 1½ cups baked sweet potato (3 S)
- 20 pistachios (2 Fa)

*Note: 1 Fat Group swap saved for snack.*

*Snack*
- ½ banana (1 Fr) with 4 teaspoons natural peanut butter (1 P, 1 Fa) to spread on banana
- ½ cup 1% milk or plain soymilk (½ M)
- ¾ cup whole-grain cereal (1 S), ¾ cup blueberries (1 Fr), and 6 ounces milk (½ M—plus extra 1/4 Milk Group swap saved from breakfast)
- 6 almonds (1 Fa)

# DAY 5

*Breakfast*
- Omelet: 3 egg whites and 1 whole egg (2 P) with sautéed onions, red pepper, and tomato (extra vegetables are freebies) in 2 teaspoons olive oil (2 Fa)
- 1 whole-grain tortilla (6-inch, no fat added; 1 S) to wrap omelet
- ½ cup 1% milk or plain soymilk (½ M)

*Lunch*
- Stuffed Baked Potato: 1 medium baked or microwaved potato (6-ounce; 2 S) topped with 1 cup fresh or frozen broccoli (2 V), steamed or microwaved and placed on top of potato; 3 ounces lean ham (3 P), diced; and 1 ounce cheddar cheese (1 P, 2 Fa), shredded and melted over top of potato and broccoli
- 12 cherries (1 Fr)
- ½ cup 1% milk or plain soymilk (½ M)

*Dinner*
- Spicy Peanut Chicken—see recipe section; use 1 pound of chicken breast for 4 servings (4 P, 1 V, 2 Fa)
- 1½ cups steamed or microwaved cauliflower (3 V)
- 1 cup whole-wheat couscous (3 S)
- 10 peanuts (1 Fa)

Snack
- Protein Smoothie: ¾ cup berries (1 Fr) blended with 1 scoop soy protein powder (1 P), 1 cup 1% milk or plain soymilk (1 M), and ice (freebie)
- 4–6 whole wheat crackers (1 S)
- 12 cashews (2 Fa) eaten with 1 orange (1 Fr)

Note: *You can use fresh or frozen berry mixtures with no added sweeteners. In other words, the ingredient list should just list berries—no sugar, high-fructose corn syrup, corn syrup, honey, or other added sweetener.*

# DAY 6

Breakfast
- 2 soft-boiled eggs (2 P) with 2 slices whole-wheat light bread (1 S) and 2 teaspoons butter (2 Fa)
- ½ cup 1% milk or plain soymilk (½ M)

Lunch
- Simple Pasta Salad: 1 cup whole-wheat pasta (2 S), cooked and chilled, tossed with 1 teaspoon olive oil (1 Fa), 1 large diced tomato (1 V), ¾ cup tuna fish (light and packed in water, 3 P), drained, and mixed with 1 teaspoon mayonnaise (1 Fa) and ½ teaspoon mustard (freebie)
- ½ cup baby carrots (1 V)
- 1 orange (1 Fr)
- ½ cup 1% milk or plain soymilk (½ M)

Note: *Save 1 Protein Group swap for snack.*

Dinner
- Turkey with Corn Salsa—see recipe section; use 1 pound of turkey breast for 4 servings (4 P, 1 S, 1 V, 2 Fa)
- 4, 4-inch bread sticks (2 S)
- 1½ cups steamed string beans (3 V)
- 2 walnuts (1 Fa)

Note: *Look for whole-wheat bread sticks without hydrogenated oils.*

Snack
Once in a while, you can combine the calories from some of your snack swaps to have a typical dessert food. In this case, you have 1 Fruit Group

swap, 2 Protein Group swaps (1 Protein Group swap borrowed from lunch), and 2 Fat Group swaps (60 calories + 110 calories + 90 calories), or 260 calories, to spend on a dessert that you have with your Milk Group swap. Use food labels to determine the amount of a particular food you can have that provides 260 calories. For example, you can make an ice cream shake with 1 cup of 1% milk or plain soymilk blended with about 1 cup ice cream (depending on the flavor and brand) OR 3–4 cookies and 1 cup of 1% milk.

# DAY 7

*Breakfast*
- ¾ cup whole-grain cereal (1 S) with ½ cup plain low-fat yogurt (½ M)
- 12 almonds (2 Fa)

*Notes: Save 2 Protein Group swaps for snack. You can mix 1 tablespoon of vanilla yogurt into the plain yogurt until you get accustomed to the plain low-fat yogurt.*

*Lunch*
- 1 veggie burger (2 P, ½ S) with 2 ounces soy cheese melted over top (2 P) on 2 slices of whole-wheat light bread (1 S) and topped with spinach leaves, red onion slices, and ½ tomato (1 V), sliced, and ¼ avocado (2 Fa), sliced
- 1 sliced red pepper (1 V)
- ½ cup honeydew melon (½ Fr—½ saved for dinner recipe) topped with ½ cup plain low-fat yogurt (½ M) and 1½ tablespoons Grape-Nuts cereal (½ S)

*Dinner*
- 10 ounces of flounder fillet (4 P—plus 1 Protein Group swap borrowed from breakfast), baked and brushed lightly with olive oil and topped with onion slices, 1 teaspoon capers, and juice of 1 lemon wedge (freebies)
- 2 cups steamed asparagus (4 V)
- Wild Rice with Pecans and Cranberries—see recipe section (1 S, ½ Fr borrowed from lunch, 2 Fa)
- ½ cup corn (1 S)
- 2 pecans (1 Fa)

*Note: Save 1 Grain & Starch Group swap for snack.*

*Snack*
- Peanut Butter Smoothie: ½ banana (1 Fr) blended with 1 cup 1% milk or plain soymilk (1 M), 2 teaspoons natural peanut butter (1 Fa), and ice (freebie)
- 2 slices whole-wheat bread (2 S—1 Grain & Starch Group swap saved from dinner) with 3 ounces turkey (3 P—2 Protein Group swaps borrowed from breakfast) and ⅛ avocado (1 Fa), sliced; 10 grapes (1 Fr)

# 2400 Calories per Day

## DAY 1

*Breakfast*
- 2 slices of whole-wheat bread (2 S) with 8 teaspoons of natural peanut butter (2 P, 2 Fa)
- ½ cup 1% milk or soymilk (½ M)

*Lunch*
- Salad: lettuce, ½ cup sliced carrots, ½ cup diced red peppers, ½ cup tomato slices, and ½ cup broccoli (3 V); ⅔ cup garbanzo beans (2 S); 4-ounce chicken breast (4 P), cooked and cubed; 2 teaspoons olive oil (2 Fa); balsamic vinegar, salt (optional), and pepper to taste (freebies)
- 1 cup honeydew melon (1 Fr), cubed, topped with ½ cup plain low-fat yogurt (½ M)

*Tip: You can mix in 1 tablespoon vanilla yogurt until you get accustomed to plain low-fat yogurt.*

*Dinner*
On nights that you do not want to follow a recipe, use the swap lists and this suggested guideline to create a simple dinner menu.
- 2½ cups of vegetables (5 V) sautéed with 3 teaspoons olive oil (3 Fa) and garlic (freebie)
- 1 large baked potato (9-ounce); OR 1½ cups whole-wheat pasta tossed with sautéed vegetables; OR 1 cup brown rice topped with sautéed vegetables (3 S)
- 6 ounces of baked or grilled white-meat chicken or turkey (no skin); OR 6 ounces of lean grilled beef or pork; OR 6 ounces of grilled or baked

salmon or other fatty fish; OR 12 ounces of baked or grilled flounder, other white fish, or shellfish (6 P)
- 1 apple (1 Fr)

*Snack*
- Smoothie: ½ banana (1 Fr) blended with 1 scoop soy protein powder (1 P), 1 cup 1% milk or soymilk (1 M), and ice (freebie)
- Crunchy Trail Mix: ¾ cup whole-grain cereal squares (1 S), 2 tablespoons raisins (1 Fr), and 12 almonds (2 Fa)

## DAY 2

*Breakfast*
- Breakfast Protein Smoothie: 2 scoops soy protein powder (2 P) blended with 2 teaspoons of natural peanut butter (1 Fa), ½ cup 1% milk or soymilk (½ M), and ice (freebie)
- 1½ cup whole-grain cereal squares OR 8–12 whole-grain crackers (2 S)
- 6 almonds (1 Fa)

*Tip: Look for cereals with less than 5–7 grams of sugar. Avoid cereals and crackers with trans- or partially hydrogenated fats or oils.*

*Lunch*
- Turkey Sandwich: 2 slices whole-wheat bread (2 S) with 4 ounces thinly sliced turkey breast (4 P), ⅛ avocado (1 Fa), sliced, and mustard (freebie)
- 1 cup baby carrots and 1 cup red pepper slices (3 V)
- ½ cup plain low-fat yogurt (½ M) topped with 2 tablespoons raisins (1 Fr) and 10 peanuts (1 Fa)

*Dinner*
- Steak and Roasted Vegetables over Field Greens—see recipe section; use 1½ pounds of steak for 4 servings (1 serving = 6 P, 2 V, 2 Fa); top with 8 black olives (1 Fa) and 1 cup grape tomatoes (1 V), halved
- 1½ large (6-inch) whole-wheat pita bread (3 S)
- 1 pear (1 Fr)

*Note: 2 Vegetable Group swaps saved for snack.*

*Snack*
- 1 apple (1 Fr), sliced and dipped in 4 teaspoons natural peanut butter (1 P, 1 Fa)
- 1 cup 1% milk or plain soymilk (1 M)
- 1 cup mixed fresh or steamed vegetable sticks (such as carrots, celery, asparagus, and string beans; 2 V—borrowed from dinner) with hummus dip (1 S, 1 Fa); 2 plums (1 Fr)

# DAY 3

*Breakfast*
- 2 slices whole-wheat bread (2 S) with 1 teaspoon butter (1 Fa)
- 1 cup low-fat cottage cheese (4 P—2 Protein Group swaps borrowed from lunch)
- ½ cup 1% milk or plain soymilk (½ M)

*Note: Save 1 Fat Group swap for lunch.*

*Lunch*
- Egg Salad Sandwich:
  — 1 large whole-wheat pita bread (6-inch; 2 S), sliced open
  — 2 hard-boiled eggs (2 P) crumbled and mixed with 1 teaspoon mayonnaise (1 Fa); add ½ teaspoon Dijon mustard and minced red onion to taste (freebies)
  — ¼ avocado (2 Fa—1 Fat Group swap borrowed from breakfast), sliced and placed in pita with egg salad
- 1½ cups string beans (3 V), cooked and chilled (marinated overnight with balsamic vinegar and whole cloves of garlic)
- 10 grapes (1 Fr)
- ½ cup 1% milk or plain soymilk (½ M)

*Note: 2 Protein Group swaps saved for breakfast.*

*Dinner*
- Scallop, Spinach, and Tomato Sauté—see recipe section; use 3 pounds of scallops for 4 servings (1 serving = 6 P, 2 V, 2 Fa)
- 1½ cups steamed or microwaved carrots (3 V)
- 1 cup cooked brown rice (3 S)
- 1 orange (1 Fr)
- 6 cashews (1 Fa)

*Snack*
- ¼ cup cottage cheese (1 P) topped with 1¼ cup strawberries (1 Fr), sliced
- 4–6 whole-wheat crackers (1 S)
- 12 almonds (2 Fa) eaten with 1 peach (1 Fr)
- 1 cup 1% milk or plain soymilk (1 M)

# DAY 4

*Breakfast*
- 1 large whole-wheat pita bread (6-inch; 2 S) spread with 2 tablespoons Homemade Yogurt Cheese (¼ M)—see recipe section
- 2 ounces smoked salmon on pita bread (2 P), topped with 10 green olives (1 Fa), chopped

Note: ¼ Milk Group swap saved for snack; 1 Fat Group swap saved for lunch.

*Lunch*
- Lentil Salad—see recipe section (1 P, 1 S, 1 V, 2 Fa)
- 1 cup baby carrots (2 V)
- 4–6 whole-wheat crackers (1 S) with 3 ounces low-fat cheese (3 P), cut into small cubes
- ½ mango (1 Fr), cubed
- 2 walnuts (1 Fa—borrowed from breakfast)
- ½ cup 1% milk or plain soymilk (½ M)

Note: *Try crumbling the walnuts and sprinkling on top of the Lentil Salad.*

*Dinner*
- Apple Pork—see recipe section; use 4, 6-ounce center loin or tenderloin pork medallions for 4 servings (6 P, ½ Fr, 1 Fa)
- 1 cup boiled beets (2 V), peeled and sliced, and 1½ cup steamed or microwaved cauliflower (3 V)
- 1½ cups baked sweet potato (3 S)
- ½ cup cantaloupe (½ Fr)
- 20 pistachios (2 Fa)

*Snack*
- ½ banana (1 Fr) with 4 teaspoons natural peanut butter to spread on banana (1 P, 1 Fa)

- ½ cup 1% milk or plain soymilk (½ M)
- ¾ cup whole-grain cereal, ¾ cup blueberries, and 6 ounces milk (½ M—plus extra ¼ Milk Group swap saved from breakfast)
- 6 almonds (1 Fa )

# DAY 5

*Breakfast*
- Omelet: 3 egg whites and 1 whole egg (2 P) with sautéed onions, red pepper, and tomato (extra vegetables are freebies) in 2 teaspoons olive oil (2 Fa)
- 2 whole-grain tortillas (6-inch, no added fat; 2 S) to wrap omelet
- ½ cup 1% milk or plain soymilk (½ M)

*Lunch*
- Stuffed Baked Potato: 1 medium baked or microwaved potato (6-ounce; 2 S) topped with 1½ cups fresh or frozen broccoli (3 V), steamed or microwaved and placed on top of potato; 3 ounces lean ham (3 P), diced; and 1 ounce cheddar cheese (1 P, 2 Fa), shredded and melted over top of potato and broccoli
- 12 cherries (1 Fr)
- ½ cup 1% milk or plain soymilk (½ M)

*Dinner*
- Spicy Peanut Chicken—see recipe section; use 1½ pounds of chicken breast for 4 servings (6 P, 1 V, 2 Fa)
- 2 cups steamed or microwaved cauliflower (4 V)
- 1 cup whole-wheat couscous (3 S)
- ¾ cup fresh fruit salad (1 Fr)
- 10 peanuts (1 Fa)

*Snack*
- Protein Smoothie: ¾ cup berries (1 Fr) blended with 1 scoop soy protein powder (1 P), 1 cup 1% milk or plain soymilk (1 M), and ice (freebie) with 4–6 whole-wheat crackers (1 S)
- 12 cashews (2 Fa) eaten with 1 orange (1 Fr)

*Note: You can use fresh or frozen berry mixtures with no added sweeteners. In other words, the ingredient list should just list berries—no sugar, high-fructose corn syrup, corn syrup, honey, or other added sweetener.*

# DAY 6

*Breakfast*
- 2 soft-boiled eggs (2 P) with 2 slices whole-wheat bread (2 S) and 2 teaspoons butter (2 Fa)
- ½ cup 1% milk or plain soymilk (½ M)

*Lunch*
- Simple Pasta Salad: 1 cup whole-wheat pasta (2 S), cooked and chilled, tossed with 1 teaspoon olive oil (1 Fa), 1 large diced tomato (1 V), 1 cup diced zucchini (1 V), ¾ cup tuna fish (light and packed in water, 3 P), drained, and mixed with 1 teaspoon mayonnaise (1 Fa) and ½ teaspoon mustard (freebie)
- ½ cup baby carrots (1 V)
- 1 orange (1 Fr)
- ½ cup 1% milk or plain soymilk (½ M)

*Note: Save 1 Protein Group swap for snack.*

*Dinner*
- Turkey with Corn Salsa—see recipe section; use 1½ pounds of turkey breast for 4 servings (6 P, 1 S, 1 V, 2 Fa)
- 4, 4-inch bread sticks (2 S)
- 2 cups steamed string beans (4 V)
- 1 cup cubed papaya (1 Fr)
- 2 walnuts (1 Fa)

*Note: Look for whole-wheat bread sticks without hydrogenated oils.*

*Snack*
Once in a while, you can combine the calories from some of your snack swaps to have a typical dessert food. In this case, you have 1 Fruit Group swap, 2 Protein Group swaps (1 Protein Group swap borrowed from lunch), and 2 Fat Group swaps (60 calories + 110 calories + 90 calories), or 260 calories, to spend on a dessert that you have with your Milk Group swap. Use food labels to determine the amount of a particular food you can have that provides 260 calories. For example, you can make an ice cream shake with 1 cup of 1% milk or plain soymilk blended with about 1 cup ice cream (depending on the flavor and brand) OR have 3–4 cookies and 1 cup of 1% milk.

# Day 7

*Breakfast*
- 1½ cups whole-grain cereal (2 S) with ½ cup plain low-fat yogurt (½ M)
- 12 almonds (2 Fa)

Notes: *Save 2 Protein Group swaps for snack. You can mix 1 tablespoon of vanilla yogurt into the plain yogurt until you get accustomed to the plain low-fat yogurt.*

*Lunch*
- 1 veggie burger (2 P, ½ S) with 2 ounces soy cheese melted over top (2 P) on 2 slices of whole-wheat light bread (1 S) and topped with spinach leaves, red onion slices, and ½ tomato (1 V), sliced, and ¼ avocado (2 Fa), sliced
- 1 sliced red pepper (1 V) and 1 cup sliced zucchini (1 V)
- 1 cup honeydew melon (1 Fr) topped with ½ cup plain low-fat yogurt (½ M) and 1½ tablespoons Grape-Nuts cereal (½ S)

*Dinner*
- 12 ounces of flounder fillet (6 P), baked and brushed lightly with olive oil and topped with onion slices, 1 teaspoon capers, and juice of 1 lemon wedge (freebies)
- 2½ cups steamed asparagus (5 V)
- Wild Rice with Pecans and Cranberries—see recipe section (1 S, 2 Fa, ½ Fr borrowed from lunch)
- ½ cup corn (1 S)
- 1 plum (1/2 Fr)
- 2 pecans (1 Fa)

Note: *Save 1 Grain & Starch Group swap for snack.*

*Snack*
- Peanut Butter Smoothie: ½ banana (1 Fr) blended with 1 cup 1% milk or plain soymilk (1 M), 2 teaspoons natural peanut butter (1 Fa), and ice (freebie)
- 2 slices whole-wheat bread (2 S—1 Grain & Starch Group swap saved from dinner) with 3 ounces turkey (3 P—2 Protein Group swaps saved from breakfast) and ⅛ avocado (1 Fa), sliced; 10 grapes (1 Fr)

# RECIPES

### Apple Pork (serves 4)

*Ingredients*

- Center loin or tenderloin pork medallions (amount used depends on calorie level, refer to menu)
- ½ teaspoon black pepper
- 1 teaspoon pumpkin pie spice
- ½ teaspoon ground coriander
- 2 teaspoons canola oil, cold pressed or mechanically extracted
- 1 medium onion, chopped
- 1 large apple, cored and coarsely chopped
- ¼ cup apple juice diluted with 1/4 cup water

*Directions*

Combine black pepper and pumpkin pie spice and rub on both sides of medallions. Heat oil in a large nonstick skillet over medium-high heat and brown both sides of medallions. Set aside. Add onions and apple to pan and sauté until tender. Add diluted apple juice to pan, and simmer. Add pork medallions to pan, cover, and simmer for 5 minutes or until pork thoroughly cooked.

### Homemade Yogurt Cheese

*Ingredients*

- 1 cup plain, fat-free yogurt

*Directions*

Line a strainer with a coffee filter, and place the strainer over a bowl. Scoop 1 cup of plain, fat-free yogurt into the coffee filter and cover with plastic wrap or aluminum foil. Refrigerate the yogurt for 24 hours, then drain the liquid that collects in the bowl. Continue to refrigerate the yogurt for another 12–24 hours, until the yogurt has thickened. Remove the thickened yogurt and place it in a resealable container. You can flavor the yogurt according to your taste preferences. For example, you can add minced scallions and olives to the yogurt or add vanilla extract and cinnamon.

## Lentil Salad (serves 4)

*Ingredients for Lentils*
- ¾ cup dried lentils
- 3 cups of water
- 1 small onion, cut into wedges
- 2 cloves garlic, cut in halves
- 1 bay leaf

*Salad Ingredients*
- ¼ cup black olives, pitted and chopped
- ¾ cup celery, chopped
- ¾ cup red bell pepper, chopped
- 2 tablespoons parsley, chopped
- ¼ cup fresh lemon juice
- 2 tablespoons olive oil
- 2 cloves garlic, crushed
- ½ teaspoons dried thyme leaves
- Salt and pepper to taste (optional)

*Directions:*
Wash the lentils well. Place lentils, water, onion wedges, garlic halves, and bay leaf in pot, and bring to a boil. Reduce heat and simmer until the lentils are just tender—about 20 minutes. Drain, discarding onion, garlic, and bay leaf. Refrigerate the lentils in cold water. While lentils are chilling, combine all salad ingredients, mixing well. When lentils are chilled, toss them together with the other salad ingredients.

## Scallop, Spinach, and Tomato Sauté (serves 4)

*Ingredients*
- 8 teaspoons olive oil
- 4 cloves garlic, crushed
- Scallops, rinsed (amount used depends on calorie level, refer to menu)
- 1 tablespoons fresh basil, chopped (or 2 teaspoons dried basil)
- 3 large tomatoes, diced
- 12 ounces baby spinach, washed, stems removed
- Salt and pepper to taste (optional)

*Directions:*

In a large nonstick skillet gently heat olive oil and garlic over low heat for 1 minute or until garlic is lightly browned. Stir in scallops, cover, and cook for 1 minute. Stir in basil, tomatoes, and rinsed spinach. Add salt and pepper to taste (optional). Cook and cover for 4 to 5 minutes more, stirring occasionally until the scallops whiten. Spoons the scallops and sauce over brown rice.

## **Spicy Peanut Chicken** (serves 4)

*Ingredients*

- 1 teaspoon ground cumin
- 1 teaspoon cinnamon
- Chicken breast, no skin (amount used depends on calorie level, refer to menu)
- 4 teaspoon olive oil
- 1 small onion, sliced
- 2 cloves garlic, crushed
- 2 teaspoon jalapeno pepper, minced
- 4 plum tomatoes, diced
- 4 tablespoons tomato puree
- 4 teaspoons natural peanut butter

*Directions*

Mix the cumin and cinnamon, and rub the mixture on both sides of the chicken breast. Heat oil in a large skillet and sauté onion, garlic, jalapeno pepper, and chicken. When both sides of the chicken breast are seared, add plum tomatoes and cook for 3–5 minutes. Add tomato puree and natural peanut butter and stir until all ingredients are well-incorporated. Cover the pan and simmer 5 minutes or until the chicken is thoroughly cooked. Serve over a bed of couscous and with steamed carrots.

## **Steak and Roasted Vegetables over Field Greens** (serves 4)

*Ingredients*

- Eye round beef steak (amount used depends on calorie level, refer to menu)
- 1 medium zucchini, 1-inch diagonal slices

- 1 medium eggplant, peeled, 1-inch slices
- 1 medium onion, 1-inch wedges
- 1 portabella mushroom, 1-inch slices
- Salt and pepper to taste (optional)
- Field greens, 16-ounce bag

*Marinade Ingredients*
- 2 tablespoons balsamic vinegar
- 4 teaspoons olive oil
- 2 large cloves garlic, crushed
- 1 teaspoon dried rosemary leaves, crushed
- ¼ teaspoon pepper

*Salad Dressing Ingredients*
- ½ cup balsamic vinegar
- 2 teaspoons honey
- 1 teaspoon mustard
- 4 teaspoons cold water
- 6 teaspoons olive oil
- ½ teaspoon basil
- ¼ teaspoon thyme
- Salt and pepper to taste

*Directions*
Heat oven to 425°F. Wipe the baking sheet with olive oil. Place the vegetables on the sheet. Combine marinade ingredients and drizzle the mixture over the vegetables. Roast the vegetables in a heated oven for 30 minutes, or until tender. Halfway through baking, turn the vegetables. While the vegetables are cooking, heat a large nonstick skillet over medium heat. Place the eye round steak in skillet and cook for 15 minutes or until the steak is cooked through. (Alternatively, grill or barbeque the steak.) Cut the steak into thin slices. While the steak and vegetables are cooking, make the salad dressing. Dissolve honey in vinegar by microwaving for 25 seconds. Whisk them together, and continue whisking vigorously while adding other ingredients. Equally divide the field greens onto 4 plates. Equally divide the steak and vegetables on top of the field greens. Drizzle 2 tablespoons of dressing over each serving of steak, vegetables, and greens.

### Turkey and Corn Salsa (serves 4)

*Ingredients*
- Turkey breast, no skin (amount used depends on calorie level, refer to menu)
- 2 tablespoons fresh lime juice
- 2 teaspoons olive oil
- ½ teaspoon ground cumin
- ½ teaspoon dried oregano
- Salt and pepper to taste (optional)

*Salsa*
- ½ teaspoon minced hot green chili pepper (optional)
- 1 pound tomatoes, seeds removed and diced
- 2 cups corn kernels, fresh or thawed frozen
- 3 scallions, chopped
- 2 tablespoons chopped cilantro
- 2 tablespoons lime juice
- 2 teaspoons olive oil
- ½ avocado, diced
- Salt and pepper to taste

In a shallow dish, arrange the turkey breasts. Combine lime juice, olive oil, cumin, oregano, salt (optional), and pepper and drizzle or brush the mixture over the turkey breasts. Cover and marinate at least 1 hour or overnight, if possible. Meanwhile, make the salsa by gently combining all ingredients. Set the salsa aside. Grill the turkey breast, turning it occasionally until thoroughly cooked. Serve with the salsa.

### Wild Rice with Pecans and Cranberries (serves 4)

*Ingredients*
- ⅔ cup wild rice
- 4 cups water
- ¼ cup pecan halves, lightly toasted
- 1 yellow pepper, seeded and diced
- ¼ cup dried cranberries
- ¼ cup minced parsley
- 4 scallions, sliced thinly

*Dressing*
- 3 teaspoons raspberry vinegar
- 3 teaspoons balsamic vinegar
- 4 teaspoons olive oil
- ½ cup vegetable broth or bouillon (low sodium)
- Pepper to taste

*Directions*
Place the rice and water in a saucepan and bring to a boil. Cover the rice and reduce the heat to simmer and cook approximately 45 minutes, or until the rice is tender. Drain the rice. While the rice is cooking, combine toasted pecans, yellow pepper, cranberries, parsley, and scallions in a container large enough to hold the rice and dressing. In a smaller bowl, combine all the ingredients for dressing and whisk them together. Pour over pecan and cranberry mixture and mix well. Add the rice and continue to mix until all the ingredients are evenly distributed.

# MODERATE-CARB
# DAILY

## MENUS

### 1200 Calories per Day

#### DAY 1

*Breakfast*
- 2 slices whole-wheat light bread (1 S) with 4 teaspoons of natural peanut butter (1 P, 1 Fa) and ½ banana sliced on top (1 Fr)
- 1 cup 1% milk or plain soymilk (1 M)

*Lunch*
- Salad: lettuce (freebie), ¼ cup sliced carrots, ¼ cup diced red pepper, ¼ tomato, sliced, ½ cup broccoli (2 V); ⅓ cup garbanzo beans (1 S); 1-ounce chicken breast (1 P), cooked and cubed; 1 teaspoon olive oil (1 Fa); and balsamic vinegar, salt, and pepper to taste (freebies)

*Dinner*
On nights that you do not want to follow a recipe, use the swap lists and this suggested guideline to create a simple dinner menu.
- 2 ounces of baked or grilled white-meat chicken or turkey; OR 2 ounces of salmon or fatty fish; OR 4 ounces of baked or grilled flounder, other white fish, or shellfish; OR 2 ounces lean meat (2 P)
- 2 cups vegetables sautéed (4 V) with 1 teaspoon olive oil (1 Fa) and garlic (freebie)

- 1 medium baked potato (6-ounce); OR 1 cup whole-wheat pasta tossed with sautéed vegetables; OR ⅔ cup brown rice topped with sautéed vegetables (2 S)

*Snack*
- Simple Smoothie: 1¼ cup sliced strawberries (1 Fr) blended with 1 cup 1% milk (1 M) and ice (freebie)
- 6 almonds (1 Fa)

## DAY 2

*Breakfast*
- Breakfast Protein Smoothie: ½ banana (1 Fr) blended with 1 scoop soy protein powder (1 P), 1 cup 1% milk or plain soymilk (1 M), 2 teaspoons natural peanut butter (1 Fa), and ice (freebie)
- ¾ cup whole-grain cereal squares OR 4–6 whole-wheat crackers (1 S)

*Lunch*
- 2 slices whole-wheat light bread (1 S) with 1 ounce thinly sliced turkey breast (1 P), lettuce (freebie), and ⅛ avocado (1 Fa), sliced
- ½ cup baby carrots (1 V) and 1 cup red pepper slices (1 V)

*Dinner*
- Beef Stir-Fry—see recipe section; use ½ pound of eye round steak for 4 servings (2 P, 4 V, ½ S, 1 Fa) over ½ cup brown rice (1½ S)

*Snack*
- 1 apple (1 Fr), sliced, and 6 cashews (1 Fa)
- 1 cup 1% milk or plain soymilk (1 M)

## DAY 3

*Breakfast*
- ¼ cup cottage cheese (1 P) topped with 3/4 cup blueberries (1 Fr)
- 4–6 whole-wheat crackers (1 S)
- 2 walnuts (1 Fa)
- 1 cup 1% milk or plain soymilk (1 M)

*Lunch*
- 1 small whole-wheat pita bread (3-inch; 1 S) sliced open and filled with 1 hard-boiled egg (1 P) crumbled and mixed with 1 teaspoon mayonnaise (1 Fa) combined with ½ teaspoon mustard
- 1 cup string beans (2 V), cooked and chilled (marinated overnight with balsamic vinegar and whole cloves of garlic—freebie)

*Dinner*
- Tri-Color Pasta and Shrimp—see recipe section; use 1 pound of shrimp for 4 servings (2 P, 2 S, 1 V, 1 Fa)
- 1½ cups steamed broccoli (3 V)

*Snack*
- 1 cup plain low-fat yogurt (1 M) topped with 4 dried apricot halves (1 Fr) and 6 almonds (1 Fa)

# DAY 4

*Breakfast*
- ¾ cup whole-grain cereal (1 S) with 1¼ cup strawberries (1 Fr), sliced; 2 walnuts (1 Fa), crumbled; and 1 cup 1% milk or plain soymilk (1 M)

Note: *Save 1 Protein Group swap for lunch.*

*Lunch*
- Broccoli Frittata—see recipe section (2 P—1 Protein Group swap borrowed from breakfast, 1 V, 1 Fa)
- 1 cup grape tomatoes (1 V)
- 4–6 whole-wheat crackers (1 S)

*Dinner*
- Pork with Mustard-Dill Sauce—see recipe section; use 8 ounces of pork tenderloin for 4 servings (2 P, 1 V)
- 1½ cups steamed broccoli (3 V)
- 1 cup mashed potatoes (mashed with low-fat milk; salt and pepper to taste—no fat; 2 S)
- 6 almonds (1 Fa)

*Snack*
- ½ banana (1 Fr) with 2 teaspoons of natural peanut butter spread (1 Fa)
- 1 cup 1% milk or plain soymilk (1 M)

# DAY 5

*Breakfast*
- 1 small whole-wheat pita bread (3 inches; 1 S) spread with 2 table-spoons Homemade Yogurt Cheese (1/4 M)—see recipe section
- 1 ounce of smoked salmon on pita bread (1 P), topped with 1 teaspoon capers (freebie)
- ½ grapefruit (1 Fr)
- ¾ cup 1% milk or plain soymilk (¾ M)

*Note: 1 Fat Group swap saved for lunch.*

*Lunch*
- 1 small baked or microwaved potato (3-ounce; 1 S) topped with 1 cup broccoli (2 V), steamed or microwaved, and 1 ounce cheddar cheese (1 P, 2 Fa—1 Fat Group swap borrowed from breakfast)

*Dinner*
- Lemon Chicken with Zucchini—see recipe section; use 8 ounces of chicken breast for 4 servings (2 P, 1 V, 1 Fa)
- 1½ cups string beans (3 V)
- ⅔ cup whole-wheat couscous (2 S)

*Note: Try cooking couscous in low-sodium vegetable broth*

*Snack*
- Simple Smoothie: ½ banana (1 Fr) blended with 2 teaspoons natural peanut butter (1 Fa), 1 cup 1% milk or plain soymilk (1 M), and ice (freebie)

# DAY 6

*Breakfast*
- 1 soft-boiled egg (1 P) with 2 slices whole-wheat light bread (1 S) and 1 teaspoon butter (1 Fa)
- ½ cup cantaloupe (1/2 Fr—save ½ Fruit Group swap for dinner)
- 1 cup 1% milk or plain soymilk (1 M)

Lunch
- Simple Pasta Salad: ½ cup whole-wheat pasta (1 S), cooked and chilled, tossed with 1 large diced tomato, ¼ cup tuna fish (light and packed in water, 1 P), drained, and mixed with 1 teaspoon mayonnaise (1 Fa) and ½ teaspoon mustard and minced red onion (freebie)
- ½ cup baby carrots (1 V)

Dinner
- Turkey-Apple Salad—see recipe section; use 8 ounces of turkey breast for 4 servings (2 P, 1 Fa, ½ Fr—saved from breakfast) and serve on a small whole-wheat bun (2 S) with lettuce (freebie)
- 1 cup grape tomatoes (1 V)
- Steamed and Chilled Vegetables: 1 cup asparagus (2 V) and ½ cup baby carrots (1 V)

Snack
Once in a while, you can combine the calories from your snack swaps to have a typical dessert food. In this case, you have 1 Fruit Group swap, 1 Fat Group swap and 1 Milk & Yogurt Group swap (60 calories + 45 calories + 90 calories), or 195 calories, to spend on a dessert. Use food labels to determine the amount of a particular food you can have that provides 195 calories. For example, you can have about ¾ cup of ice cream (depending on the flavor and brand) OR have 2 cookies and 1 cup of 1% milk.

## DAY 7

Breakfast
- ¾ cup whole-grain cereal (1 S) with 1¼ cups strawberries (1 Fr), sliced; 6 almonds (1 Fa), slivered; and 1 cup 1% milk or plain soymilk (1 M)

Note: Save 1 Protein Group swap for lunch.

Lunch
- 1 veggie burger (2 P—1 Protein Group swap borrowed from breakfast, ½ S) on 1 slice of whole-wheat light bread (½ S) and topped with spinach leaves, red onion slices, and ½ tomato (1 V), sliced, and ⅛ avocado (1 Fa), sliced
- 1 sliced red pepper (1 V)

*Dinner*
- 4 ounces of flounder fillet (2 P), baked and brushed lightly with olive oil, 1 teaspoon capers, and 1 tablespoon red onion, chopped (freebies)
- Peach Bulgur Salad—see recipe section (2 S, 1 Fa)
- 1 cup steamed asparagus (2 V) and 1 cup beets (2 V), boiled, peeled, and sliced

*Snack*
- Peanut Butter Smoothie: ½ banana (1 Fr) blended with 1 cup 1% milk or plain soymilk (1 M), 2 teaspoons natural peanut butter (2 Fa), and ice (freebie)

# 1500 Calories per Day

## DAY 1

*Breakfast*
- 2 slices whole-wheat bread (2 S) with 4 teaspoons of natural peanut butter (1 P, 1 Fa) and ½ banana sliced on top (1 Fr)
- 1 cup 1% milk or plain soymilk (1 M)

*Lunch*
- Salad: lettuce (freebie), ¼ cup sliced carrots, ¼ cup diced red pepper, ¼ tomato, sliced, ½ cup broccoli (2 V); ⅔ cup garbanzo beans (2 S); 1-ounce chicken breast (1 P), cooked and cubed; 1 teaspoon olive oil (1 Fa); and balsamic vinegar, salt, and pepper to taste (freebies)
- 2 plums (1 Fr)

*Dinner*
On nights that you do not want to follow a recipe, use the swap lists and this suggested guideline to create a simple dinner menu.
- 3 ounces of baked or grilled white-meat chicken or turkey; OR 3 ounces of salmon or fatty fish; OR 6 ounces of baked or grilled flounder, other white fish, or shellfish; OR 3 ounces lean meat (3 P)
- 2 cups vegetables sautéed (4 V) with 2 teaspoon olive oil (2 Fa) and garlic (freebie)
- 1 medium baked potato (6-ounce); OR 1 cup whole-wheat pasta tossed with sautéed vegetables; OR ⅔ cup brown rice topped with sautéed vegetables (2 S)

*Snack*
- Simple Smoothie: 1½ cup sliced strawberries (1 Fr) blended with 1 cup 1% milk (1 M) and ice (freebie)
- 6 almonds (1 Fa)

# DAY 2

*Breakfast*
- Breakfast Protein Smoothie: ½ banana (1 Fr) blended with 1 scoop soy protein powder (1 P), 1 cup 1% milk or plain soymilk (1 M), 2 teaspoons natural peanut butter (1 Fa), and ice (freebie)
- 1½ cup whole-grain cereal squares OR 8–12 whole-wheat crackers (2 S)

*Lunch*
- 2 slices whole-wheat bread (2 S) with 1 ounce thinly sliced turkey breast (1 P), lettuce (freebie), and ⅛ avocado (1 Fa), sliced
- ½ cup baby carrots (1 V) and 1 cup red pepper slices (1 V)
- 1 orange (1 Fr)

*Dinner*
- Beef Stir-Fry—see recipe section; use 12 ounces of eye round steak for 4 servings (3 P, 4 V, ½ S, 1 Fa) over ½ cup brown rice (1½ S)
- 6 cashews sprinkled on top of stir-fry (1 Fa)

*Snack*
- 1 apple (1 Fr), sliced, and 6 cashews (1 Fa)
- 1 cup 1% milk or plain soymilk (1 M)

# DAY 3

*Breakfast*
- ¼ cup cottage cheese (1 P) topped with ¾ cup blueberries (1 Fr)
- 8–12 whole-wheat crackers (2 S)
- 2 walnuts (1 Fa)
- 1 cup 1% milk or plain soymilk (1 M)

*Lunch*

- 1 large whole-wheat pita bread (6-inch; 2 S) sliced open and filled with 1 hard-boiled egg (1 P) crumbled and mixed with 1 teaspoon mayonnaise (1 Fa) combined with ½ teaspoon mustard
- 1 cup string beans (2 V), cooked and chilled (marinated overnight with balsamic vinegar and whole cloves of garlic—freebie)
- 1¼ cup watermelon (1 Fr), cubed

*Dinner*

- Tri-Color Pasta and Shrimp—see recipe section; use 1½ pounds of shrimp for 4 servings (3 P, 2 S, 1 V, 1 Fa)
- 1½ cups steamed broccoli (3 V)
- 6 almonds (1 Fa)

*Snack*

- 1 cup plain low-fat yogurt (1 M) topped with 4 dried apricot halves (1 Fr) and 6 almonds (1 Fa)

## DAY 4

*Breakfast*

- 1½ cup whole-grain cereal (2 S) with 1½ cups strawberries (1 Fr), sliced; 2 walnuts (1 Fa), crumbled; and 1 cup 1% milk or plain soymilk (1 M)

Note: *Save 1 Protein Group swap for lunch.*

*Lunch*

- Broccoli Frittata—see recipe section (2 P—1 Protein Group swap borrowed from breakfast, 1 V, 1 Fa)
- 1 cup grape tomatoes (1 V)
- 8–12 whole-wheat crackers (2 S)
- 1 pear (1 Fr)

*Dinner*

- Pork with Mustard-Dill Sauce—see recipe section; use 12 ounces of pork tenderloin for 4 servings (3 P, 1 V)
- 1½ cups steamed broccoli (3 V)
- 1 cup mashed potatoes (mashed with low-fat milk; salt and pepper to taste—no fat; 2 S)
- 12 almonds (2 Fa)

*Snack*
- ½ banana (1 Fr) with 2 teaspoons of natural peanut butter spread (1 Fa)
- 1 cup 1% milk or plain soymilk (1 M)

# DAY 5

*Breakfast*
- 1 large whole-wheat pita bread (6-inch; 2 S) spread with 2 tablespoons Homemade Yogurt Cheese (¼ M)—see recipe section
- 1 ounce of smoked salmon on pita bread (1 P), topped with 1 teaspoon capers (freebie)
- ½ grapefruit (1 Fr)
- ¾ cup 1% milk or plain soymilk (¾ M)

*Note: 1 Fat Group swap saved for lunch.*

*Lunch*
- 1 medium baked or microwaved potato (6-ounce; 2 S) topped with 1 cup broccoli (2 V), steamed or microwaved, and 1 ounce cheddar cheese (1 P, 2 Fa—1 Fat Group swap borrowed from breakfast)
- ¾ cup fresh fruit salad (1 Fr)

*Dinner*
- Lemon Chicken with Zucchini—see recipe section; use 12 ounces of chicken breast for 4 servings (3 P, 1 V, 1 Fa)
- 1½ cups string beans (3 V)
- ⅔ cup whole-wheat couscous (2 S) fluffed with a fork to combine 1 teaspoon olive oil (1 Fa)

*Note: Try cooking couscous in low-sodium vegetable broth.*

*Snack*
- Simple Smoothie: ½ banana (1 Fr) blended with 2 teaspoons natural peanut butter (1 Fa), 1 cup 1% milk or plain soymilk (1 M), and ice (freebie)

# DAY 6

*Breakfast*
- 1 soft-boiled egg (1 P) with 2 slices whole-wheat bread (2 S) and 1 teaspoon butter (1 Fa)

- ½ cup cantaloupe (½ Fr—save ½ Fruit Group swap for dinner)
- 1 cup 1% milk or plain soymilk (1 M)

*Lunch*
- Simple Pasta Salad: 1 cup whole-wheat pasta (2 S), cooked and chilled, tossed with 1 large diced tomato (1 V), ¼ cup tuna fish (light and packed in water, 1 P), drained, and mixed with 1 teaspoon mayonnaise (1 Fa) and ½ teaspoon mustard and minced red onion (freebie)
- ½ cup baby carrots (1 V)
- ½ mango (1 Fr), cubed

*Dinner*
- Turkey-Apple Salad—see recipe section; use 12 ounces of turkey breast for 4 servings (3 P, 1 Fa, ½ Fr—saved from breakfast) and serve on a small whole-wheat bun (2 S) with lettuce (freebie)
- 1 cup grape tomatoes (1 V)
- Steamed and Chilled Vegetables: 1 cup asparagus (2 V) and ½ cup baby carrots (1 V)
- 2 walnuts (1 Fa)

*Snack*
Once in a while, you can combine the calories from your snack swaps to have a typical dessert food. In this case, you have 1 Fruit Group swap, 1 Fat Group swap, and 1 Milk & Yogurt Group swap (60 calories + 45 calories + 90 calories), or 195 calories, to spend on a dessert. Use food labels to determine the amount of a particular food you can have that provides 195 calories. For example, you can have about ¾ cup ice cream (depending on the flavor and brand) OR have 2 cookies and 1 cup of 1% milk.

## DAY 7

*Breakfast*
- 1½ cups whole-grain cereal (2 S) with 1¼ cups strawberries (1 Fr), sliced; 6 almonds (1 Fa), slivered; and 1 cup 1% milk or plain soymilk (1 M)
*Note: Save 1 Protein Group swap for lunch.*

*Lunch*
- 1 veggie burger (2 P—1 Protein Group swap borrowed from breakfast, ½ S) on 2 slices of whole-wheat light bread (1 S) and topped with spinach leaves, red onion slices, and ½ tomato (1 V), sliced, and ⅛ avocado (1 Fa), sliced
- 1 sliced red pepper (1 V)
- 1 kiwi (1 Fr)

*Note: ½ Grain & Starch Group swap saved for snack.*

*Dinner*
- 6 ounces of flounder fillet (3 P), baked, drizzled with 1 teaspoon olive oil (1 Fa), and topped with 1 teaspoon capers and 1 tablespoon red onion, chopped (freebies)
- Peach Bulgur Salad—see recipe section (2 S, 1 Fa)
- 1 cup steamed asparagus (2 V) and 1 cup beets, boiled, peeled, and sliced (2 V)

*Snack*
- Peanut Butter Smoothie: ½ banana (1 Fr) blended with 1 cup 1% milk or plain soymilk (1 M), 2 teaspoons natural peanut butter (1 Fa), and ice (freebie)
- 2–3 whole-wheat crackers (½ S)

# 1800 Calories per Day

## DAY 1

*Breakfast*
- 2 slices whole-wheat bread (2 S) with 4 teaspoons natural peanut butter (1 P, 1 Fa) and ½ banana sliced on top (1 Fr)
- 1 cup 1% milk or plain soymilk (1 M)

*Lunch*
- Salad: lettuce (freebie), ¼ cup sliced carrots, ¼ cup diced red pepper, ¼ tomato, sliced, ½ cup broccoli (2 V); ⅔ cup garbanzo beans (2 S); 2-ounce chicken breast (2 P), cooked and cubed; 2 teaspoons olive oil (2 Fa); and balsamic vinegar, salt, and pepper to taste (freebies)
- 2 plums (1 Fr)

*Dinner*

On nights that you do not want to follow a recipe, use the swap lists and this suggested guideline to create a simple dinner menu.

- 4 ounces of baked or grilled white-meat chicken or turkey; OR 4 ounces of salmon or fatty fish; OR 8 ounces of baked or grilled flounder, other white fish, or shellfish; OR 4 ounces of lean meat (4 P)
- 2 cups vegetables sautéed (4 V) with 2 teaspoons olive oil (2 Fa) and garlic (freebie)
- 1 medium baked potato (6-ounce); OR 1 cup whole-wheat pasta tossed with sautéed vegetables; OR ⅔ cup brown rice topped with sautéed vegetables (2 S)

*Snack*

- Simple Smoothie: 1¼ cup sliced strawberries (1 Fr) blended with 1 cup 1% milk (1 M) and ice (freebie)
- 6 almonds (1 Fa) mixed with 1½ cup whole-grain cereal squares (2 S)

## DAY 2

*Breakfast*

- Breakfast Protein Smoothie: ½ banana (1 Fr) blended with 1 scoop soy protein powder (1 P), 1 cup 1% milk or plain soymilk (1 M), 2 teaspoons natural peanut butter (1 Fa), and ice (freebie)
- 1½ cup whole-grain cereal squares OR 8–12 whole-wheat crackers (2 S)

*Lunch*

- 2 slices whole-wheat bread (2 S) with 2 ounces thinly sliced turkey breast (2 P), lettuce (freebie), and ¼ avocado (2 Fa), sliced
- ½ cup baby carrots (1 V) and 1 cup red pepper slices (1 V)
- 1 orange (1 Fr)

*Dinner*

- Beef Stir-Fry—see recipe section; use 1 pound of eye round steak for 4 servings (4 P, 4 V, ½ S, 1 Fa) over ½ cup brown rice (1½ S)
- 6 cashews sprinkled on top of stir-fry (1 Fa)

*Snack*

- Homemade Trail Mix: 1½ cups whole-grain cereal squares (2 S) mixed with 2 tablespoons raisins (1 Fr) and 10 peanuts (1 Fa)
- 1 cup 1% milk or plain soymilk (1 M)

## DAY 3

*Breakfast*
- ¼ cup cottage cheese (1 P) topped with ¾ cup blueberries (1 Fr)
- 8–12 whole-wheat crackers (2 S)
- 2 walnuts (1 Fa)
- 1 cup 1% milk or plain soymilk (1 M)

*Lunch*
- 1 large whole-wheat pita bread (6-inch; 2 S) sliced open and filled with 2 hard-boiled eggs (2 P) crumbled and mixed with 2 teaspoons mayonnaise (2 Fa) combined with ½ teaspoon mustard
- 1 cup string beans (2 V), cooked and chilled (marinated overnight with balsamic vinegar and whole cloves of garlic—freebie)
- 1¼ cup watermelon (1 Fr), cubed

*Dinner*
- Tri-Color Pasta and Shrimp—see recipe section; use 2 pounds of shrimp for 4 servings (4 P, 2 S, 1 V, 1 Fa)
- 1½ cups steamed broccoli (3 V)
- 6 almonds (1 Fa)

*Snack*
- 1 cup plain low-fat yogurt (1 M) topped with Homemade Trail Mix including 4 dried apricot halves (1 Fr), 1½ cups whole-grain cereal squares (2 S), and 6 almonds (1 Fa)

## DAY 4

*Breakfast*
- 1½ cup whole-grain cereal (2 S) with 1½ cup strawberries (1 Fr), sliced; 2 walnuts (1 Fa), crumbled; and 1 cup 1% milk or plain soymilk (1 M)

Note: *Save 1 Protein Group swap for lunch.*

*Lunch*
- Broccoli Frittata—see recipe section (2 P—1 Protein Group swap borrowed from breakfast, 1 V, 1 Fa)
- 1 cup grape tomatoes (1 V)

- 8–12 whole-wheat crackers (2 S) with 1 ounce low-fat cheese (1 P)
- 1 pear (1 Fr)
- 6 almonds (1 Fa)

### Dinner
- Pork with Mustard-Dill Sauce—see recipe section; use 1 pound of pork tenderloin for 4 servings (4 P, 1 V)
- 1½ cups steamed broccoli (3 V)
- 1 cup mashed potatoes (mashed with low-fat milk; salt and pepper to taste—no fat; 2 S)
- 12 almonds (2 Fa)

### Snack
- 2 slices whole-wheat bread (2 S) with 2 teaspoons of natural peanut butter spread (1 Fa) and ½ banana (1 Fr), sliced
- 1 cup 1% milk or plain soymilk (1 M)

# DAY 5

### Breakfast
- 1 large whole-wheat pita bread (6-inch; 2 S) spread with 2 tablespoons Homemade Yogurt Cheese (¼ M)
- 1 ounce of smoked salmon on pita bread (1 P) topped with 10 green olives (1 Fa), diced
- ½ grapefruit (1 Fr)
- ¾ cup 1% milk or plain soymilk (¾ M)

### Lunch
- 1 medium baked or microwaved potato (6-ounce; 2 S) topped with 1 cup broccoli (2 V), steamed or microwaved; 1 ounce ham, diced (1 P); and 1 ounce cheddar cheese (1 P, 2 Fa)
- ¾ cup fresh fruit salad (1 Fr)

### Dinner
- Lemon Chicken with Zucchini—see recipe section; use 1 pound of chicken breast for 4 servings (4 P, 1 V, 1 Fa)

- 1½ cups string beans (3 V)
- ⅔ cup whole-wheat couscous (2 S) fluffed with a fork to combine 1 teaspoon olive oil (1 Fa)

Note: *Try cooking couscous in low-sodium vegetable broth.*

*Snack*
- Simple Smoothie: ½ banana (1 Fr) blended with 2 teaspoons natural peanut butter (1 Fa), 1 cup 1% milk or plain soymilk (1 M), and ice (freebie)
- 8–12 whole-wheat crackers (2 S)

# DAY 6

*Breakfast*
- 1 soft-boiled egg (1 P) with 2 slices whole-wheat bread (2 S) and 1 teaspoon butter (1 Fa)
- ½ cup cantaloupe (½ Fr—save ½ Fruit Group swap for dinner)
- 1 cup 1% milk or plain soymilk

*Lunch*
- Simple Pasta Salad: 1 cup whole-wheat pasta (2 S), cooked and chilled, tossed with 1 teaspoon olive oil (1 Fa), 1 large diced tomato (1 V), ½ cup tuna fish (light and packed in water, 2 P), drained, and mixed with 1 teaspoon mayonnaise (1 Fa) and ½ teaspoon mustard and minced red onion (freebie)
- ½ cup baby carrots (1 V)
- ½ mango (1 Fr), cubed

*Dinner*
- Turkey-Apple Salad—see recipe section; use 1 pound of turkey breast for 4 servings (4 P, 1 Fa, ½ Fr—saved from breakfast) and serve on a small whole-wheat bun (2 S) with lettuce (freebie)
- 1 cup grape tomatoes (1 V)
- Steamed and Chilled Vegetables: 1 cup asparagus (2 V) and ½ cup baby carrots (1 V)
- 2 walnuts (1 Fa)

*Snack*

Once in a while, you can combine some of the calories from your snack swaps to have a typical dessert food. In this case, you have the following swaps for snacks throughout the day: 1 Fa, 1 Fr, 1 M, 2 S. For your first snack you can use 2 Grain & Starch Group swaps and 1 Milk & Yogurt Group swap (160 calories + 90 calories), or 250 calories, on typical dessert foods. Use food labels to determine the amount of a particular food you can have that provides 250 calories. For example, you can have about 1 cup of ice cream (depending on the flavor and brand) OR 3 cookies and 1 cup of 1% milk. Then for a second snack you can use your other snack swaps to have 2 tablespoons raisins (1 Fr) and 6 almonds (1 Fa).

# DAY 7

*Breakfast*
- 1½ cups whole-grain cereal (2 S) with 1¼ cups strawberries (1 Fr), sliced; 6 almonds (1 Fa), slivered; and 1 cup 1% milk or plain soymilk (1 M)

*Note: Save 1 Protein Group swap for lunch.*

*Lunch*
- 1 veggie burger (2 P—1 Protein Group swap borrowed from breakfast, ½ S) with 1 ounce soy cheese (1 P) melted overtop on 2 slices of whole-wheat light bread (1 S) and topped with spinach leaves, red onion slices, and ½ tomato (1 V), sliced, and ¼ avocado (2 Fa), sliced
- 1 sliced red pepper (1 V)
- 1 kiwi (1 Fr)

*Note: ½ Grain & Starch Group swap saved for snack.*

*Dinner*
- 8 ounces of flounder fillet (4 P), baked, drizzled with 1 teaspoon olive oil (1 Fa), and topped with 1 teaspoon capers and 1 tablespoon red onion, chopped (freebies)
- Peach Bulgur Salad—see recipe section (2 S, 1 Fa)
- 1 cup steamed asparagus (2 V) and 1 cup beets (2 V), boiled, peeled, and sliced

*Snack*
- Simple Smoothie: ½ banana (1 Fr) blended with 1 cup 1% milk or plain soymilk (1 M) and ice (freebie); ¾ cup whole-grain cereal squares (1 S)
- 6–9 whole-wheat crackers (1½ S) dipped in 2 teaspoons natural peanut butter (1 Fa)

# 2100 Calories per Day

## DAY 1

*Breakfast*
- 2 slices whole-wheat bread (2 S) with 4 teaspoons of natural peanut butter (1 P, 1 Fa) and ½ banana sliced on top (1 Fr)
- 1 cup 1% milk or plain soymilk (1 M)

*Lunch*
- Salad: lettuce (freebie), ¼ cup sliced carrots, ¼ cup diced red pepper, ¼ tomato, sliced, ½ cup broccoli (2 V); ⅔ cup garbanzo beans (2 S); 2-ounce chicken breast (2 P), cooked and cubed; 2 teaspoons olive oil (2 Fa); and balsamic vinegar, salt, and pepper to taste (freebies)
- 2 plums (1 Fr)

*Dinner*
On nights that you do not want to follow a recipe, use the swap lists and this suggested guideline to create a simple dinner menu.
- 4 ounces of baked or grilled white-meat chicken or turkey; OR 4 ounces of salmon or fatty fish; OR 8 ounces of baked or grilled flounder, other white fish, or shellfish; OR 4 ounces of lean meat (4 P)
- 2 cups vegetables sautéed (4 V) with 2 teaspoons olive oil (2 Fa) and garlic (freebie)
- 2 cups mashed potato; OR 2 cups whole-wheat pasta tossed with sautéed vegetables; OR 1⅓ cups brown rice topped with sautéed vegetables (4 S)

*Snack*
- Protein Smoothie: 1¼ cup sliced strawberries (1 Fr) blended with 1 scoop soy protein powder (1 P), 1 cup 1% milk (1 M), and ice (freebie)
- Homemade Trail Mix: 6 almonds (1 Fa) mixed with 1½ cups whole-grain cereal squares (2 S) and 2 tablespoons raisins (1 Fr)

## DAY 2

*Breakfast*
- Protein Smoothie: ½ banana (1 Fr) blended with 1 scoop soy protein powder (1 P), 1 cup 1% milk or plain soymilk (1 M), 2 teaspoons natural peanut butter (1 Fa), and ice (freebie)
- 1½ cup whole-grain cereal squares OR 8–12 whole-wheat crackers (2 S)

*Lunch*
- 2 slices whole-wheat bread (2 S) with 2 ounces turkey breast (2 P), thinly sliced; lettuce (freebie); and ¼ avocado (2 Fa), sliced (2 Fa)
- ½ cup baby carrots (1 V) and 1 cup red pepper slices (1 V)
- 1 orange (1 Fr)

*Dinner*
- Beef Stir-Fry—see recipe section; use 1 pound eye round steak for 4 servings (4 P, 4 V, ½ S, 1 Fa) over 1 cup brown rice plus 2 tablespoons (3½ S)
- 6 cashews sprinkled on top of stir-fry (1 Fa)

*Snack*
- Homemade Train Mix: 1½ cups whole-grain cereal (2 S) mixed with 10 peanuts (1 Fa) and 2 tablespoons raisins (1 Fr); 1 cup plain low-fat yogurt (1 M)
- ¾ cup fresh fruit salad (1 Fr) with 1 ounce low-fat cheese (1 P)

## DAY 3

*Breakfast*
- ¼ cup cottage cheese (1 P) topped with ¾ cup blueberries (1 Fr)
- 8–12 whole-wheat crackers (2 S)
- 2 walnuts (1 Fa)
- 1 cup 1% milk or plain soymilk (1 M)

*Lunch*
- 1 large whole-wheat pita bread (6-inch; 2 S) sliced open and filled with 2 hard-boiled eggs (2 P) crumbled and mixed with 2 teaspoons mayonnaise (2 Fa) combined with ½ teaspoon mustard (freebie)

- 1 cup string beans (2 V), cooked and chilled (marinated overnight with balsamic vinegar and whole cloves of garlic—freebie)
- 1¼ cup watermelon (1 Fr), cubed

*Dinner*
- Tri-Color Pasta and Shrimp—see recipe section; use 2 pounds of shrimp for 4 servings (4 P, 2 S, 1 V, 1 Fa)
- 1½ cups steamed broccoli (3 V)
- 4, 4-inch bread sticks (2 S)
- 6 almonds (1 Fa)

*Snack*
- 1 cup plain low-fat yogurt (1 M) topped with Homemade Trail Mix including 4 dried apricot halves (1 Fr), ¾ cup whole-grain cereal squares (1 S), and 6 almonds (1 Fa)
- ½ cup soybeans (1 S, 1P) and 12 cherries (1 Fr)

# DAY 4

*Breakfast*
- 1½ cup whole-grain cereal (2 S) with 1½ cup strawberries (1 Fr), sliced; 2 walnuts (1 Fa), crumbled; and 1 cup 1% milk or plain soymilk (1 M)
Note: *Save 1 Protein Group swap for lunch.*

*Lunch*
- Broccoli Frittata—see recipe section (2 P—1 Protein Group swap borrowed from breakfast, 1 V, 1 Fa)
- 1 cup grape tomatoes (1 V)
- 8–12 whole-wheat crackers (2 S) with 1 ounce low-fat cheese (1 P)
- 1 pear (1 Fr)
- 6 almonds (1 Fa)

*Dinner*
- Pork with Mustard-Dill Sauce—see recipe section; use 1 pound of pork tenderloin for 4 servings (4 P, 1 V)
- 1½ cups steamed broccoli (3 V)
- 2 cups mashed potatoes (mashed with low-fat milk; salt and pepper to taste—no fat; 4 S)
- 12 almonds (2 Fa)

*Snack*
- 2 slices whole-wheat light bread (1 S) with 2 teaspoons of natural peanut butter spread (1 Fa) and 1/2 banana (1 Fr), sliced; 1 cup 1% milk or plain soymilk (1 M)
- 4–6 whole-wheat crackers (1 S) with 1 ounce low-fat cheese (1 P) and 10 grapes (1 Fr)

# DAY 5

*Breakfast*
- 1 large whole-wheat pita bread (6-inch; 2 S) spread with 2 tablespoons Homemade Yogurt Cheese (¼ M)—see recipe section
- 1 ounce of smoked salmon on pita bread (1 P) topped with 10 green olives (1 Fa), diced
- ½ grapefruit (1 Fr)
- ¾ cup 1% milk or plain soymilk (¾ M)

*Lunch*
- 1 medium baked or microwaved potato (6-ounce; 2 S) topped with 1 cup broccoli (2 V), steamed or microwaved; 1 ounce ham (1 P), diced; and 1 ounce cheddar cheese (1 P, 2 Fa)
- ¾ cup fresh fruit salad (1 Fr)

*Dinner*
- Lemon Chicken with Zucchini—see recipe section; use 1 pound of chicken breast for 4 servings (4 P, 1 V, 1 Fa)
- 1½ cups string beans (3 V)
- 1⅓ cups whole-wheat couscous (4 S) fluffed with a fork to combine 1 teaspoon olive oil (1 Fa)

Note: *Try cooking couscous in low-sodium vegetable broth.*

*Snack*
- Simple Smoothie: ½ banana (1 Fr) blended with 4 teaspoons natural peanut butter (1 P, 1 Fa), 1 cup 1% milk or plain soymilk (1 M), and ice (freebie)
- 8–12 whole-wheat crackers (2 S) and ½ cup applesauce (1 Fr)

# DAY 6

*Breakfast*
- 1 soft-boiled egg (1 P) with 2 slices whole-wheat bread (2 S) and 1 teaspoon butter (1 Fa)
- ½ cup cantaloupe (½ Fr—save ½ Fruit Group swap for dinner)
- 1 cup 1% milk or plain soymilk (1 M)

*Lunch*
- Simple Pasta Salad: 1 cup whole-wheat pasta (2 S), cooked and chilled, tossed with 1 teaspoon olive oil (1 Fa), 1 large diced tomato (1 V), ½ cup tuna fish (light and packed in water, 2 P), drained, and mixed with 1 teaspoon mayonnaise (1 Fa) and ½ teaspoon mustard and minced red onion (freebie)
- ½ cup baby carrots (1 V)
- ½ mango (1 Fr), cubed

*Dinner*
- Turkey-Apple Salad—see recipe section; use 1 pound of turkey breast for 4 servings (4 P, 1 Fa, ½ Fr—saved from breakfast) and serve on a small whole-wheat bun (2 S) with lettuce (freebie)
- 1 cup grape tomatoes (1 V)
- Steamed and Chilled Vegetables: 1 cup asparagus (2 V) and ½ cup baby carrots (1 V)
- ⅔ cup garbanzo beans (2 S) tossed with 1 teaspoon olive oil (1 Fa) and 1 tablespoon red onion, minced, balsamic vinegar, salt, and pepper to taste (freebies)

*Snack*
Once in a while, you can combine some of the calories from your snack swaps to have a typical dessert food. In this case, you have the following swaps for snacks throughout the day: 1 Fa, 2 Fr, 1 M, 1 P, and 2 S. For your first snack you can use 2 Grain & Starch Group swaps and 1 Protein Group swap (160 calories + 55 calories), or 215 calories, on typical dessert foods. Use food labels to determine the amount of a particular food you can have that provides 215 calories. For example, you can have about ¾ cup of ice cream (depending on the flavor and brand) OR 2–3 cookies and 1 cup of 1% milk. Then for a second snack you can use your other snack swaps to have 1 cup plain low-fat yogurt (1 M) topped with 4 tablespoons raisins (2 Fr) and 6 almonds (1 Fa).

# DAY 7

*Breakfast*
- 1½ cups whole-grain cereal (2 S) with 1¼ cups strawberries (1 Fr), sliced; 6 almonds (1 Fa), slivered; and 1 cup 1% milk or plain soymilk (1 M)

Note: *Save 1 Protein Group swap for lunch.*

*Lunch*
- 1 veggie burger (2 P—1 Protein Group swap borrowed from breakfast, ½ S) with 1 ounce soy cheese (1 P) melted overtop on 2 slices of whole-wheat light bread (1 S) and topped with spinach leaves, red onion slices, and ½ tomato (1 V), sliced, and ¼ avocado (2 Fa), sliced
- 1 sliced red pepper (1 V)
- 1 kiwi (1 Fr)

Note: *½ Grain & Starch Group swap saved for snack.*

*Dinner*
- 8 ounces of flounder fillet (4 P), baked, drizzled with 1 teaspoon olive oil (1 Fa), and topped with 1 teaspoon capers and 1 tablespoon red onion, chopped (freebies)
- Peach Bulgur Salad—see recipe section (2 S, 1 Fa)
- 1 cup steamed asparagus (2 V) and 1 cup beets (2 V), boiled, peeled, and sliced
- 1 cup corn (2 S)

*Snack*
- Simple Smoothie: ½ banana (1 Fr) blended with 1 cup 1% milk or plain soymilk (1 M) and ice (freebie); ¾ cup whole-grain cereal squares (1 S)
- 2–3 whole-wheat crackers (½ S—saved from lunch) dipped in 2 teaspoons natural peanut butter (1 Fa)
- ½ cup soybeans (1 P, 1 S) with 1 apple (1 Fr)

# 2400 Calories per Day

## DAY 1

*Breakfast*
- 3 slices whole-wheat bread (3 S) with 4 teaspoons of natural peanut butter (1 P, 1 Fa) and ½ banana sliced on top (1 Fr)
- 1 cup 1% milk or plain soymilk (1 M)

*Lunch*
- Salad: lettuce (freebie), ¼ cup sliced carrots, ¼ cup diced red pepper, ¼ tomato, sliced, ½ cup broccoli (2 V); ⅔ cup garbanzo beans (2 S); 2-ounce chicken breast (2 P), cooked and cubed; 2 teaspoons olive oil (2 Fa); and balsamic vinegar, salt, and pepper to taste (freebies)
- 4–6 whole-wheat crackers (1 S)
- 2 plums (1 Fr)

*Dinner*
On nights that you do not want to follow a recipe, use the swap lists and this suggested guideline to create a simple dinner menu.
- 5 ounces of baked or grilled white-meat chicken or turkey; OR 5 ounces of salmon or fatty fish; OR 10 ounces of baked or grilled flounder, other white fish, or shellfish; OR 5 ounces of lean meat (5 P)
- 2 cups vegetables sautéed (4 V) with 2 teaspoons olive oil (2 Fa) and garlic (freebie)
- 2 cups mashed potato; OR 2 cups whole-wheat pasta tossed with sautéed vegetables; OR 1⅓ cup brown rice topped with sautéed vegetables (4 S)
- 6 cashews (1 Fa)

*Snack*
- Protein Smoothie: 1¼ cups sliced strawberries (1 Fr) blended with 1 scoop soy protein powder (1 P), 1 cup 1% milk (1 M), and ice (freebie)
- Homemade Trail Mix: 12 almonds (2 Fa) mixed with 1½ cups whole-grain cereal squares (2 S) and 2 tablespoons raisins (1 Fr)

# DAY 2

*Breakfast*
- Breakfast Protein Smoothie: ½ banana (1 Fr) blended with 1 scoop soy protein powder (1 P), 1 cup 1% milk or plain soymilk (1 M), 2 teaspoons natural peanut butter (1 Fa), and ice (freebie)
- 2¼ cup whole-grain cereal squares OR 12–18 whole-wheat crackers (3 S)

*Lunch*
- 2 slices whole-wheat bread (2 S) with 2 ounces thinly sliced turkey breast (2 P), lettuce (freebie), and 1/4 avocado (2 Fa), sliced
- ½ cup baby carrots (1 V) and 1 cup red pepper slices (1 V)
- 1 corn on the cob OR ¾ ounce pretzels (1 S)
- 1 orange (1 Fr)

Note: *Look for whole-wheat pretzels with 2–3 grams of fiber per serving.*

*Dinner*
- Beef Stir-Fry—see recipe section; use 1¼ pounds of eye round steak for 4 servings (5 P, 4 V, ½ S, 1 Fa) over 1 cup brown rice plus 2 tablespoons (3½ S)
- 12 cashews (2 Fa) sprinkled on top of stir-fry

*Snack*
- Homemade Trail Mix: 1½ cups whole-grain cereal squares (2 S) mixed with 2 teaspoons raisins (1 Fr) and 10 peanuts (1 Fa); 1 cup plain low-fat yogurt (1 M)
- ¾ cup fresh fruit salad (1 Fr) with 1 ounce low-fat cheese (1 P) and 2 walnuts (1 Fa), crumbled

# DAY 3

*Breakfast*
- ¼ cup cottage cheese (1 P) topped with ¾ cup blueberries (1 Fr)
- 12–18 whole-wheat crackers (3 S)
- 2 walnuts (1 Fa)
- 1 cup 1% milk or plain soymilk (1 M)

*Lunch*

- 1 large whole-wheat pita bread (6-inch; 2 S) sliced open and filled with 2 hard-boiled eggs (2 P) crumbled and mixed with 2 teaspoons mayonnaise (2 Fa) combined with ½ teaspoon mustard
- 1 cup string beans (2 V), cooked and chilled (marinated overnight with balsamic vinegar and whole cloves of garlic—freebie)
- 2, 4-inch bread sticks (1 S)
- 1¼ cup watermelon (1 Fr), cubed

*Dinner*

- Tri-Color Pasta and Shrimp—see recipe section; use 2½ pounds of shrimp for 4 servings (5 P, 2 S, 1 V, 1 Fa)
- 1½ cups steamed broccoli (3 V)
- 4, 4-inch bread sticks (2 S)
- 12 almonds (2 Fa)

*Snack*

- 1 cup plain low-fat yogurt (1 M) topped with Homemade Trail Mix including 4 dried apricot halves (1 Fr), ¾ cup whole-grain cereal squares (1 S), and 12 almonds (2 Fa)
- ½ cup soybeans (1 S, 1 P) and 12 cherries (1 Fr)

## DAY 4

*Breakfast*

- 2¼ cups whole-grain cereal (3 S) with 1½ cups strawberries (1 Fr), sliced; 2 walnuts (1 Fa), crumbled; and 1 cup 1% milk or plain soymilk (1 M)

Note: *Save* 1 *Protein Group swap for lunch.*

*Lunch*

- Broccoli Frittata—see recipe section (2 P—1 Protein Group swap borrowed from breakfast, 1 V, 1 Fa)
- 1 cup grape tomatoes (1 V)
- 12–18 whole-wheat crackers (3 S) with 1 ounce low-fat cheese (1 P)
- 1 pear (1 Fr)
- 6 almonds (1 Fa)

*Dinner*

- Pork with Mustard-Dill Sauce—see recipe section; use 1¼ pounds of pork tenderloin for 4 servings (5 P, 1 V)
- 1½ cups steamed broccoli (3 V)
- 2 cups mashed potatoes (mashed with low-fat milk; salt and pepper to taste—no fat; 4 S) with 1 teaspoon butter on top (1 Fa)
- 12 almonds (2 Fa)

*Snack*

- 2 slices whole-wheat light bread (1 S) with 2 teaspoons of natural peanut butter spread (1 Fa) and ½ banana (1 Fr), sliced; 1 cup 1% milk or plain soymilk (1 M)
- 4–6 whole-wheat crackers (1 S) with 1 ounce low-fat cheese (1 P), 10 grapes (1 Fr), and 6 almonds (1 Fa)

## DAY 5

*Breakfast*

- 1½ large whole-wheat pita bread (6-inch; 3 S) spread with 4 tablespoons Homemade Yogurt Cheese (½ M)—see recipe section
- 1 ounce smoked salmon on pita bread (1 P), topped with 10 green olives (1 Fa), diced
- ½ grapefruit (1 Fr)
- ½ cup 1% milk or plain soymilk (½ M)

*Lunch*

- 1 large baked or microwaved potato (9-ounce; 3 S) topped with 1 cup broccoli (2 V), steamed or microwaved; 1 ounce ham (1 P), diced; and 1 ounce cheddar cheese (1 P, 2 Fa)
- ¾ cup fresh fruit salad (1 Fr)

*Dinner*

- Lemon Chicken with Zucchini—see recipe section; use 1¼ pounds of chicken breast for 4 servings (5 P, 1 V, 1 Fa)
- 1½ cups string beans (3 V)
- 1⅓ cups whole-wheat couscous (4 S) fluffed with a fork to combine 2 teaspoons olive oil (2 Fa)

*Note: Try cooking couscous in low-sodium vegetable broth.*

*Snack*
- Simple Smoothie: ½ banana (1 Fr) blended with 4 teaspoons natural peanut butter (1 P, 1 Fa), 1 cup 1% milk or plain soymilk (1 M), and ice (freebie)
- 8–12 whole-wheat crackers (2 S), ½ cup applesauce (1 Fr), and 6 cashews (1 Fa)

# DAY 6

*Breakfast*
- 1 soft-boiled egg (1 P) with 3 slices whole-wheat bread (3 S) and 1 teaspoon butter (1 Fa)
- ½ cup cantaloupe (½ Fr—save ½ Fruit Group swap for dinner)
- 1 cup 1% milk or plain soymilk

*Lunch*
- Simple Pasta Salad: 1½ cup whole-wheat pasta (3 S), cooked and chilled, tossed with 1 teaspoon olive oil (1 Fa), 1 large diced tomato (1 V), ½ cup tuna fish (light and packed in water, 2 P), drained, and mixed with 1 teaspoon mayonnaise (1 Fa) and ½ teaspoon mustard and minced red onion (freebie)
- ½ cup baby carrots (1 V)
- ½ mango (1 Fr), cubed

*Dinner*
- Turkey-Apple Salad—see recipe section; use 1¼ pounds of turkey breast for 4 servings (5 P, 1 Fa, ½ Fr—saved from breakfast) and serve on a small whole-wheat bun (2 S) with lettuce (freebie)
- 1 cup grape tomatoes (1 V)
- Steamed and Chilled Vegetables: 1 cup asparagus (2 V) and ½ cup baby carrots (1 V)
- ⅔ cup garbanzo beans (2 S) tossed with 2 teaspoons olive oil (2 Fa) and 1 tablespoon red onion, minced, balsamic vinegar, salt, and pepper to taste (freebies)

*Snack*
Once in a while, you can combine some of the calories from your snack swaps to have a typical dessert food. In this case, you have the following swaps for snacks throughout the day: 2 Fa, 2 Fr, 1 M, 1 P, and 2 S. For your first snack you can use 2 Grain & Starch Group swaps and 1 Protein

Group swap (160 calories + 55 calories), or 215 calories, on typical dessert foods. Use food labels to determine the amount of a particular food you can have that provides 215 calories. For example, you can have about ¾ cup of ice cream (depending on the flavor and brand) OR 2–3 cookies and 1 cup of 1% milk. Then for a second snack you can use your other snack swaps to have 1 cup plain low-fat yogurt (1 M) topped with 4 tablespoons raisins (2 Fr) and 12 almonds (2 Fa).

## DAY 7

*Breakfast*
- 2¼ cups whole-grain cereal (3 S) with 1¼ cups strawberries (1 Fr), sliced; 6 almonds (1 Fa), slivered; and 1 cup 1% milk or plain soymilk (1 M)

*Note: Save 1 Protein Group swap for lunch.*

*Lunch*
- 1 veggie burger (2 P—1 Protein Group swap borrowed from breakfast, ½ S) with 1 ounce soy cheese melted over top (1 P) on 2 slices of whole-wheat light bread (1 S) and topped spinach leaves, red onion slices, and ½ tomato (1 V), sliced, and 1/4 avocado (2 Fa), sliced
- ½ cup green peas (1 S), fresh or frozen, steamed or microwaved
- 1 sliced red pepper (1 V)
- 1 kiwi (1 Fr)

*Note: ½ Grain & Starch Group swap saved for snack.*

*Dinner*
- 10 ounces of flounder filled (5 P), baked, drizzled with 2 teaspoons olive oil (2 Fa) and topped with 1 teaspoon capers and 1 tablespoon red onion, chopped (freebies)
- Peach Bulgur Salad—see recipe section (2 S, 1 Fa)
- 1 cup steamed asparagus (2 V) and 1 cup beets (2 V), boiled, peeled, sliced
- 1 cup corn (2 S)

*Snack*
- Simple Smoothie: ½ banana (1 Fr) blended with 1 cup 1% milk or plain soymilk (1 M) and ice (freebie); ¾ cup whole-grain cereal squares (1 S)
- 2–3 whole-wheat crackers (½ S—saved from lunch) dipped in 2 teaspoons natural peanut butter (1 Fa)
- ½ cup soybeans (1 P, 1 S) with 1 apple (1 Fr) and 2 walnuts (1 Fa)

# RECIPES

### Broccoli Frittata (serves 4)

*Ingredients*

- 1 medium onion, diced
- 2 teaspoons olive oil
- ½ teaspoon dried dill
- 10-ounce package of frozen broccoli
- Dash nutmeg
- ½ cup low-fat cottage cheese
- 4 large eggs
- 8 egg whites
- 2 teaspoons olive oil

*Directions*

In a large nonstick skillet, sauté onion and dill in olive oil until the onion is translucent. Meanwhile, defrost broccoli and squeeze out excess water. Mix in broccoli and nutmeg. When thoroughly mixed and warm, remove the broccoli mixture and set it aside in a bowl. Whisk together eggs, egg whites, and cottage cheese and mix well. Heat additional olive oil in the skillet under low heat and then pour in the egg mixture, shaking the pan to distribute it evenly. As eggs set around the edges, lift up the solid part of the egg and allow the uncooked portions to flow underneath. Continue until all of the egg mixture is set. Add the broccoli mixture, and distribute it evenly overtop. Cover until the egg is dry, taking care not to burn the bottom. Cut into 4 equal pieces.

### Beef Stir-Fry (serves 4)

*Ingredients*

- ¼ cup reduced sodium soy sauce
- ¼ cup water
- ¼ cup vegetarian broth or bouillon
- 2 tablespoons honey
- ½ teaspoon ground ginger
- 4 cloves garlic, crushed
- Eye round steak, trimmed of fat and sliced (amount used depends on calorie level, refer to menu)

- 1 teaspoon canola oil, cold-pressed or mechanically extracted
- 1 onion, chopped
- 2 cups broccoli, chopped and blanched
- 2 cups cauliflower, chopped and blanched
- 1 red pepper, chopped
- 1 cup mushrooms, chopped
- 2 cups water chestnuts, chopped

*Directions*

Make the marinade by whisking together soy sauce, water, honey, ginger, and garlic. Coat beef with half of the marinade, seal the container, and refrigerate for at least 1 hour or overnight. Wipe a nonstick skillet with a paper towel coated with canola oil. Add 1 teaspoon of canola oil and heat the pan under medium-high heat. Add beef, and cook each side 3–5 minutes. Remove and place in warm bowl. Add broccoli and cauliflower, stirring often and adding the other half of the marinade a few teaspoons at a time to keep vegetables from burning. Add onion, red pepper, mushrooms, and water chestnuts. Again, add the marinade a few teaspoons at a time to keep vegetables from burning, and stir the vegetables often. When the vegetables are just tender, add beef and enough marinade to have sauce for the rice. Stir for 1 minute or so until ingredients are mixed and warm.

## **Lemon Chicken with Zucchini** (serves 4)

*Ingredients*
- Chicken breast, no skin, cut in strips (amount used depends on calorie level, refer to menu)
- ½ cup lemon juice
- 4 teaspoons olive oil
- 2 tablespoons water
- 1 tablespoons parsley, dried
- 2 teaspoons chives, dried
- 1 teaspoon dried tarragon
- 1 teaspoon grated lemon peel
- ½ teaspoon dried savory
- Salt and pepper to taste
- 4 cups zucchini

*Directions*

Whisk together all the ingredients into a measuring cup for marinade. Place the chicken strips in a plastic bag. Pour half of the marinade in the bag and shake with the chicken. Marinate for at least 6 hours or overnight. Heat a large nonstick skillet and place chicken strips in the skillet. Discard marinade left over in the bag. Cook on both sides until the chicken is golden brown and cooked through. Remove and place in warm bowl. Add fresh marinade (the half not used with chicken) and heat to simmer. Place the zucchini in marinade and mix to coat. Cook until the zucchini is tender. Add chicken back to the pan and toss it with the zucchini until the chicken is warm.

**Peach Bulgur Salad** (serves 4)

*Ingredients*

- 2 cups boiling water
- 1 cup bulgur wheat
- 1 cup diced peaches
- 3 tablespoons unsweetened orange juice
- 4 teaspoons canola oil
- 1 tablespoon lime juice
- ½ teaspoon grated lime zest
- ½ teaspoon grated fresh ginger
- ¼ teaspoon crushed red pepper
- ⅛ teaspoon ground cinnamon
- ⅛ teaspoon cumin
- 2 cups fresh spinach leaves, cut into thin strips

*Directions*

Pour boiling water over the bulgur. After the water is absorbed, fluff with a fork. Add diced peaches and set aside. Combine orange juice and the next seven ingredients. Mix orange juice dressing with bulgur and peaches. Lastly, add spinach and toss until evenly distributed.

**Pork with Mustard-Dill Sauce** (serves 4)

*Ingredients*

- 2 cups baby carrots, sliced in half
- Pork tenderloin, cut into 1-inch-thick slices (amount used depends on calorie level, refer to menu)

- ½ teaspoon garlic powder or garlic salt
- ⅛ teaspoon pepper
- ½ cup low-fat, plain yogurt
- 4 teaspoons Dijon-style mustard
- ½ teaspoon dill weed, dried
- ½ teaspoon sugar

*Directions*
Microwave or steam the baby carrots. Slice the pork. Sauté the pork in a nonstick frying pan over medium heat for 3–4 minutes per side. Toss the baby carrots and sautéed pork in a warm bowl. Season with garlic powder (or garlic salt) and pepper. Put yogurt, mustard, dill, and sugar in a measuring cup and stir well. Warm in microwave for 30 seconds and stir. Repeat until just warm—do not allow the mixture to cook or curdle. Arrange the pork and carrots on a plate and spoon the mustard-dill sauce on top.

**Tri-Color Pasta and Shrimp** (serves 4)
*Ingredients*
- 6 ounces dry tri-color whole-wheat pasta
- 4 teaspoons olive oil
- 4 cloves of garlic, crushed
- Salt and pepper to taste
- 1 yellow bell pepper, diced
- 1 red bell pepper, diced
- ¾ cup vegetable broth or bouillon
- Shrimp, large, peeled and de-veined (amount used depends on calorie level, refer to menu)

*Directions*
Cook pasta according to the package directions. While the pasta is cooking, heat olive oil in a large nonstick skillet over medium heat. Add garlic and sauté until golden color. Add bell peppers, salt and pepper and cook for 3–5 minutes, stirring. Add vegetable broth and heat to simmer. Add shrimp and simmer until shrimp are done. Drain pasta and add to shrimp mixture. Toss and serve.

**Turkey-Apple Salad** (serves 4)

*Ingredients*

- Turkey breast, cooked, no skin, cubed (amount used depends on calorie level, refer to menu)
- 2 cups apples, cored and diced
- 2 cups celery, diced
- ¼ cup red onion, minced
- ¼ cup raisins
- 4 teaspoons mayonnaise
- 2 tablespoons low-fat plain yogurt
- ¼ teaspoon freshly grated nutmeg
- ¼ teaspoon ground cinnamon
- Salt and pepper to taste

*Directions*

In a large bowl, combine turkey, apples, celery, red onion, and raisins. In a small bowl, whisk together mayonnaise, low-fat yogurt, nutmeg, cinnamon, salt, and pepper. Combine with the turkey and apple mixture.

# HIGH-CARB
# DAILY

## MENUS

### 1200 Calories

#### DAY 1

*Breakfast*
- ¾ cup whole-grain cereal (1 S) with ¾ cup blueberries (1 Fr) and 1 cup 1% milk or plain soymilk (1 M)

*Lunch*
- Salad: lettuce (freebie), ¼ cup sliced carrots, ¼ cup diced red pepper, ¼ tomato, sliced, ½ cup broccoli (2 V); ⅓ cup garbanzo beans (1 S); 1-ounce chicken breast (1 P), cooked and cubed; 1 teaspoon olive oil (1 Fa); and balsamic vinegar, salt, and pepper to taste (freebies)
- 1 orange (1 Fr)

*Dinner*
On nights that you do not want to follow a recipe, use the swap lists and this suggested guideline to create a simple dinner menu.
- 2 ounces of baked or grilled white-meat chicken or turkey; OR 2 ounces of salmon or fatty fish; OR 4 ounces of baked or grilled flounder, other white fish, or shellfish; OR 2 ounces of lean meat (2 P)
- 2 cups vegetables sautéed (4 V) with 1 teaspoon olive oil (1 Fa) and garlic (freebie)

- 1 medium baked potato (6-ounce); OR 1 cup whole-wheat pasta tossed with sautéed vegetables; OR ⅔ cup brown rice topped with sautéed vegetables (2 S)

*Snack*
- Simple Smoothie: 1¼ cups sliced strawberries (1 Fr) blended with 1 cup 1% milk (1 M) and ice (freebie)
- 4–6 whole-wheat low-fat crackers (1 S)

## DAY 2

*Breakfast*
- ½ cup plain oatmeal (1 S), cooked, with 1 peach (1 Fr), sliced on top
- 1 cup 1% milk or plain soymilk (1 M)

*Lunch*
- 2 slices whole-wheat light bread (1 S) with 1 ounce thinly sliced turkey breast (1 P), lettuce (freebie), ⅛ avocado (1 Fa), sliced, and mustard (freebie)
- ½ cup baby carrots (1 V) and 1 cup red pepper slices (1 V)
Note: *Save 1 Fruit Group swap for dinner.*

*Dinner*
- Tofu Stir-Fry—see recipe section; use 1½ pounds of tofu for 4 servings (2 P, 2 V, 1 Fr, 1 Fa) and serve over ⅔ cup brown rice (2 S)
- 1 cup steamed baby carrots (2 V)

*Snack*
- 1, ½-inch slice of Apricot-Orange Bread (1 S)—see recipe section
- 1 cup cantaloupe (1 Fr), cubed, topped with 1 cup plain low-fat yogurt (1 M)
Note: *You can mix 1 tablespoon vanilla yogurt into the plain yogurt until you get accustomed to plain low-fat yogurt.*

## DAY 3

*Breakfast*
- 1 whole-grain waffle (less than 3 grams of fat; 1S) topped with ½ cup apple sauce (1 Fr) and ½ cup plain low-fat yogurt (½ M)
- ½ cup 1% milk or plain soymilk (½ M)

*Lunch*
- 1 cup baby carrots (2 V) and celery sticks (freebie) dipped in ⅓ cup hummus (1 S, 1 Fa)
- 1 ounce low-fat cheese (1 P)
- 10 grapes (1 Fr)

*Dinner*
- Shrimp Vegetable Kabobs—see recipe section; use 1 pound (or 24 jumbo) shrimp (2 P, 2 V, 1 Fa)
- 1 cup grilled asparagus (2 V) lightly brushed with olive oil and seasoned with salt and pepper to taste (freebies)
- ⅔ cup brown rice (2 S)

*Snack*
- 1, ½-inch slice of Banana-Nut Bread (1 S)—see recipe section—with 1 cup 1% milk or plain soymilk (1 M)
- 1¼ cups strawberries (1 Fr), sliced

# DAY 4

*Breakfast*
- Simple Smoothie: ½ banana (1 Fr) blended with 1 cup 1% milk or plain soymilk (1 M) and ice (freebie)
- 4–6 whole-wheat crackers (1 S)

*Lunch*
- ½ cup whole-wheat pasta (1 S), cooked and topped with Ratatouille—see recipe section (4 V—extra vegetables are freebies, 1 Fa)
- 1 ounce low-fat cheese (1 P) and 1 pear (1 Fr)

*Dinner*
- 4 ounces of flounder fillet (2 P), baked, lightly brushed with olive oil, and topped with 1 teaspoon capers and 1 tablespoon red onion chopped (freebies)
- Tabbouleh—see recipe section (1 S, 1 V, 1 Fa)
- ½ cup green peas (1 S)
- 1½ cups asparagus (3 V)

*Snack*
- 1, ½-inch slice of Banana Nut Bread (1 S)—see recipe section
- 1 cup honeydew melon (1 Fr), cubed, topped with 1 cup plain low-fat yogurt (1 M)

# DAY 5

*Breakfast*
- ½ cup oatmeal (1 S), cooked, topped with 2 tablespoons raisins (1 Fr)
- 1 cup 1% milk or plain soymilk (1 M)

*Lunch*
- 1 ounce low-fat soy- or rice-based cheese (1 P) with 4–6 whole-wheat crackers (1 S)
- ½ cup baby carrots (1 V) and 1 sliced red pepper (1 V)
- 1 apple

Note: *Save 1 Fat Group swap for dinner. Soy-based cheeses are more common than cheeses made from rice milk, but both are available.*

*Dinner*
- Warm Pork and Pear Salad—see recipe section; use 8 ounces of pork for 4 servings (2 P, 1 Fr—borrowed from snack, 2 Fa—1 Fat Group swap borrowed from lunch)
- 1 cup string beans (2 V) and 1 cup beets (2 V), boiled and peeled
- ⅔ cup whole-wheat couscous (2 S)

*Snack*
- ¾ cup whole-grain cereal (1 S) with 1 cup 1% milk or plain soymilk (1 M)

Note: *1 Fruit Group swap borrowed for dinner.*

# DAY 6

*Breakfast*
- 1 cup plain low-fat yogurt (1 M) topped with 1 cup fresh fruit salad (1 Fr) and ¾ cup whole-grain cereal (1 S)

*Lunch*
- 1 small whole-wheat pita bread (3-inch; 1 S) sliced open and stuffed with 1 hard-boiled egg (1 P) crumbled and mixed with 1 teaspoon mayonnaise (1 Fa), ½ teaspoon mustard, and 1 teaspoon minced red onion (freebies)
- 1 cup green beans (2 V) blanched and marinated overnight with balsamic vinegar and 2 cloves of garlic cut in small chunks
- 12 cherries (1 Fr)

*Dinner*
- Chicken and Tomato Basil Sauce over Pasta—see recipe section; use 8 ounces of chicken breast, no skin, for 4 servings (2 P, 2 S, 2 V, 1 Fa)
- 1 cup spinach (2 V), cooked

*Snack*
Once in a while, you can combine the calories from your snack swaps to have a typical dessert food. In this case, you have 1 Fruit Group swap, 1 Grain & Starch Group swap, and 1 Milk & Yogurt Group swap (60 calories + 80 calories + 90 calories), or 230 calories, to spend on a dessert. Use food labels to determine the amount of a particular food you can have that provides 230 calories. For example, you can have about ¾ cup of ice cream (depending on the flavor and brand) OR 3 cookies and 1 cup of 1% milk.

## DAY 7

*Breakfast*
- 1, ½-inch slice of Apricot and Orange Bread (1 S)—see recipe section
- 1 cup 1% milk or plain soymilk (1M)
- ½ grapefruit (1 Fr)

*Lunch*
- 1 large tomato (1 V), top sliced off and seeds scooped out, stuffed with ¼ cup tuna fish (light, packed in water, 1 P) and mixed with 1 teaspoon mayonnaise (1 Fa), ½ teaspoon mustard, 1 tablespoon minced celery, 1 teaspoon minced red onion, and salt and pepper to taste (freebies)
- ½ cup baby carrots (1 V) and 1 cup zucchini sticks (1 V—extra vegetables are freebies)

- 4–6 whole-wheat crackers (1 S)
- ½ cup cantaloupe (½ Fr—other ½ Fruit Group swap saved for dinner), cubed

*Dinner*
- Turkey Mango Wrap—see recipe section; use 8 ounces of turkey breast for 4 servings (2 P, 2 S, 1 V, ½ Fr borrowed from breakfast, 1 Fa)
- 1½ cups jicama (3 V), cut into thick sticks

*Snack*
- 1 cup plain low-fat yogurt (1 M) topped with ¾ cup blueberries (1 Fr) and 3 tablespoons Grape-Nuts cereal (1 S)

# 1500 Calories

## DAY 1

*Breakfast*
- 1½ cups whole-grain cereal (2 S) with ¾ cup blueberries (1 Fr) and 1 cup 1% milk or plain soymilk (1 M)

*Lunch*
- Salad: lettuce (freebie), ¼ cup sliced carrots, ¼ cup diced red pepper, ¼ tomato, sliced, ½ cup broccoli (2 V); ⅔ cup garbanzo beans (2 S); 2-ounce chicken breast (2 P), cooked and cubed; 1 teaspoon olive oil (1 Fa); and balsamic vinegar, salt, and pepper to taste (freebies)
- 1 orange (1 Fr)

*Dinner*
On nights that you do not want to follow a recipe, use the swap lists and this suggested guideline to create a simple dinner menu.
- 3 ounces of baked or grilled white-meat chicken or turkey; OR 3 ounces of salmon or fatty fish; OR 6 ounces of baked or grilled flounder, other white fish, or shellfish; OR 3 ounces of lean meat (3 P)
- 2 cups vegetables sautéed (4 V) with 1 teaspoon olive oil (1 Fa) and garlic (freebie)
- 1 medium baked potato (6-ounce); OR 1 cup whole-wheat pasta tossed with sautéed vegetables; OR ⅔ cup brown rice topped with sautéed vegetables (2 S)

*Snack*
- Simple Smoothie: 1¼ cups sliced strawberries (1 Fr) blended with 1 cup 1% milk (1 M) and ice (freebie)
- 4–6 whole-wheat low-fat crackers (1 S) and 12 cherries (1 Fr)

# DAY 2

*Breakfast*
- 1 cup plain oatmeal (2 S), cooked, with 1 peach (1 Fr), sliced on top
- 1 cup 1% milk or plain soy milk (1 M)

*Lunch*
- 2 slices whole-wheat bread (2 S) with 2 ounces thinly sliced turkey breast (2 P), lettuce (freebie), ⅛ avocado (1 Fa), sliced, and mustard (freebie)
- ½ cup baby carrots (1 V) and 1 cup red pepper slices (1 V)

Note: *Save 1 Fruit Group swap for dinner.*

*Dinner*
- Tofu Stir-Fry—see recipe section; use 1½ pounds of tofu for 4 servings (2 P, 2 V, 1 Fr, 1 Fa) and serve over ⅓ cup brown rice (1 S)
- 1 cup steamed baby carrots (2 V)
- ½ cup soybeans (1 S, 1 P)

*Snack*
- 1, ½-inch slice of Apricot-Orange Bread (1 S)—see recipe section—and ½ cup apple sauce (1 Fr)
- 1 cup cantaloupe (1 Fr), cubed, topped with 1 cup plain low-fat yogurt (1 M)

Note: *You can mix 1 tablespoon vanilla yogurt into the plain yogurt until you get accustomed to plain low-fat yogurt.*

# DAY 3

*Breakfast*
- 2 whole-grain waffles (less than 3 grams of fat; 2 S) topped with ½ cup apple sauce (1 Fr) and ½ cup plain low-fat yogurt (½ M)
- ½ cup 1% milk or plain soymilk (½ M)

*Lunch*
- 1 cup baby carrots (2 V) and celery sticks (freebie) dipped in ⅓ cup hummus (1 S, 1 Fa)
- 4–6 whole-wheat crackers (1 S)
- 2 ounces low-fat cheese (2 P)
- 10 grapes (1 Fr)

*Dinner*
- Shrimp Vegetable Kabobs—see recipe section; use 1½ pounds (or 36 jumbo) shrimp (3 P, 2 V, 1 Fa)
- 1 cup grilled asparagus (2 V) lightly brushed with olive oil and seasoned with salt and pepper to taste (freebies)
- ⅔ cup brown rice (2 S)

*Snack*
- 1, ½-inch slice of Banana-Nut Bread (1 S)—see recipe section—with 1 cup 1% milk or plain soymilk (1 M)
- 1¼ cups strawberries (1 Fr), sliced, and ½ banana (1 Fr), sliced

## DAY 4

*Breakfast*
- Simple Smoothie: ½ banana (1 Fr) blended with 1 cup 1% milk or plain soymilk (1 M) and ice (freebie)
- 8–12 whole-wheat crackers (2 S)

*Lunch*
- 1 cup whole-wheat pasta (2 S), cooked and topped with Ratatouille— see recipe section (4 V—extra vegetables are freebies, 1 Fa)
- 2 ounces low-fat cheese (2 P) and 1 pear (1 Fr)

*Dinner*
- 6 ounces of flounder fillet (3 P), baked, lightly brushed with olive oil, and topped with 1 teaspoon capers and 1 tablespoon red onion chopped (freebies)
- Tabbouleh—see recipe section (1 S, 1 V, 1 Fa)
- ½ cup green peas (1 S)
- 1½ cups asparagus (3 V)

*Snack*
- 1, ½-inch slice of Banana Nut Bread (1 S)—see recipe section—with 1¼ cup watermelon (1 Fr), cubed
- 1 cup honeydew melon (1 Fr), cubed, topped with 1 cup plain low-fat yogurt (1 M)

# DAY 5

*Breakfast*
- 1 cup oatmeal (2 S), cooked, topped with 2 tablespoons raisins (1 Fr)
- 1 cup 1% milk or plain soymilk (1 M)

*Lunch*
- 2 ounces low-fat soy- or rice-based cheese (2 P) with 8–12 whole-wheat crackers (2 S)
- ½ cup baby carrots (1 V) and 1 sliced red pepper (1 V)
- 1 apple (1 Fr)

Note: *Save 1 Fat Group swap for dinner. Soy-based cheeses are more common than cheeses made from rice milk, but both are available.*

*Dinner*
- Warm Pork and Pear Salad—see recipe section; use 12 ounces of pork for 4 servings (3 P, 1 Fr—borrowed from snack, 2 Fa—1 Fat Group swap borrowed from lunch)
- 1 cup string beans (2 V) and 1 cup beets (2 V), boiled and peeled
- ⅔ cup whole-wheat couscous (2 S)

*Snack*
- ¾ cup whole-grain cereal (1 S) with 1 cup 1% milk or plain soymilk (1 M) and ¾ cup blueberries (1 Fr)

Note: *1 Fruit Group swap borrowed for dinner.*

# DAY 6

*Breakfast*
- 1 cup plain low-fat yogurt (1 M) topped with 1 cup fresh fruit salad (1 Fr) and 1½ cups whole-grain cereal (2 S)

*Lunch*
- 1 large whole-wheat pita bread (6-inch; 2 S) sliced open and stuffed with 2 hard-boiled eggs (2 P) crumbled and mixed with 1 teaspoon mayonnaise (1 Fa), ½ teaspoon mustard, and 1 teaspoon minced red onion (freebies)
- 1 cup green beans (2 V) blanched and marinated overnight with balsamic vinegar and 2 cloves of garlic cut in small chunks
- 12 cherries (1 Fr)

*Dinner*
- Chicken and Tomato Basil Sauce over Pasta—see recipe section; use 12 ounces of chicken breast, no skin, for 4 servings (3 P, 2 S, 2 V, 1 Fa)
- 1 cup spinach (2 V), cooked

*Snack*
Once in a while, you can combine the calories from your snack swaps to have a typical dessert food. In this case, you have the following swaps for snacks throughout the day: 2 Fr, 1 M, and 2 S. For your first snack you can use 1 Fruit Group swap, 1 Grain & Starch Group swap, and 1 Milk & Yogurt Group swap (60 calories + 80 calories + 90 calories), or 230 calories, on typical dessert foods. Use food labels to determine the amount of a particular food you can have that provides 230 calories. For example, you can have about ¾ cup of ice cream (depending on the flavor and brand) OR 3 cookies and 1 cup of 1% milk. Then for a seconds snack you can use your other snack swap to have 1 pear (1 Fr) and 4–6 whole-wheat crackers (1 S).

# DAY 7

*Breakfast*
- 2, ½-inch slices of Apricot and Orange Bread (2 S)—see recipe section
- 1 cup 1% milk or plain soymilk (1M)
- ½ grapefruit (1 Fr)

*Lunch*
- 1 large tomato (1 V), top sliced off and seeds scooped out, stuffed with ½ cup tuna fish (light, packed in water, 2 P) and mixed with 1 teaspoon mayonnaise (1 Fa), ½ teaspoon mustard, 1 tablespoon minced celery, 1 teaspoon minced red onion, and salt and pepper to taste (freebies)

- ½ cup baby carrots (1 V) and 1 cup zucchini sticks (1 V—extra vegetables are freebies)
- 8–12 whole-wheat crackers (2 S)
- ½ cup cantaloupe (½ Fr—other ½ Fruit Group swap saved for dinner), cubed

*Dinner*
- Turkey Mango Wrap—see recipe section; use 12 ounces of turkey breast for 4 servings (3 P, 2 S, 1 V, ½ Fr borrowed from breakfast, 1 Fa)
- 1½ cups jicama (3 V), cut into thick sticks

*Snack*
- 1 cup plain low-fat yogurt (1 M) topped with ¾ cup blueberries (1 Fr) and 3 tablespoons Grape-Nuts cereal (1 S)
- 1 nectarine (1 Fr)

# 1800 Calories

## DAY 1

*Breakfast*
- 2¼ cups whole-grain cereal (3 S) with ¾ cup blueberries (1 Fr) and 1 cup 1% milk or plain soymilk (1 M)

*Lunch*
- Salad: lettuce (freebie), ¼ cup sliced carrots, ¼ cup diced red pepper, ¼ tomato, sliced, ½ cup broccoli (2 V); ⅔ cup garbanzo beans (2 S); 2-ounce chicken breast (2 P), cooked and cubed; 1 teaspoon olive oil (1 Fa); and balsamic vinegar, salt, and pepper to taste (freebies)
- 1 orange (1 Fr)

*Dinner*
On nights that you do not want to follow a recipe, use the swap lists and this suggested guideline to create a simple dinner menu.
- 3 ounces of baked or grilled white-meat chicken or turkey; OR 3 ounces of salmon or fatty fish; OR 6 ounces of baked or grilled flounder, other white fish, or shellfish; OR 3 ounces of lean meat (3 P)

- 2 cups vegetables sautéed (4 V) with 1 teaspoon olive oil (1 Fa) and garlic (freebie)
- 1 large baked potato (9-ounce); OR 1½ cups whole-wheat pasta tossed with sautéed vegetables; OR 1 cup brown rice topped with sautéed vegetables (3 S)

*Snack*
- Simple Smoothie: 1¼ cups sliced strawberries (1 Fr) blended with 1 cup 1% milk (1 M) and ice (freebie)
- 8–12 whole-wheat low-fat crackers (2 S) with 12 cherries (1 Fr) and 6 almonds (1 Fa)

# DAY 2

*Breakfast*
- 1½ cups plain oatmeal (3 S), cooked, with 1 peach (1 Fr), sliced on top
- 1 cup 1% milk or plain soymilk (1 M)

*Lunch*
- 2 slices whole-wheat bread (2 S) with 2 ounces thinly sliced turkey breast (2 P), lettuce (freebie), ⅛ avocado (1 Fa), sliced, and mustard (freebie)
- ½ cup baby carrots (1 V) and 1 cup red pepper slices (1 V)
*Note: Save 1 Fruit Group swap for dinner.*

*Dinner*
- Tofu Stir-Fry—see recipe section; use 1½ pounds of tofu for 4 servings (2 P, 2 V, 1 Fr, 1 Fa) and serve over ⅔ cup brown rice (2 S)
- 1 cup steamed baby carrots (2 V)
- ½ cup soybeans (1 S, 1 P)

*Snack*
- 2, ½-inch slices of Apricot-Orange Bread (2 S)—see recipe section—and ½ cup apple sauce (1 Fr)
- 1 cup cantaloupe (1 Fr), cubed, topped with 1 cup plain low-fat yogurt (1 M) and 6 almonds (1 Fa)
*Note: You can mix 1 tablespoon vanilla yogurt into the plain yogurt until you get accustomed to plain low-fat yogurt.*

# DAY 3

*Breakfast*
- 3 whole-grain waffles (less than 3 grams of fat; 3 S) topped with ½ cup apple sauce (1 Fr) and ½ cup plain low-fat yogurt (½ M)
- ½ cup 1% milk or plain soymilk (½ M)

*Lunch*
- 1 cup baby carrots (2 V) and celery sticks (freebie) dipped in ⅓ cup hummus (1 S, 1 Fa)
- 4–6 whole-wheat crackers (1 S)
- 2 ounces low-fat cheese (2 P)
- 10 grapes (1 Fr)

*Dinner*
- Shrimp Vegetable Kabobs—see recipe section; use 1½ pounds (or 36 jumbo) shrimp (3 P, 2 V, 1 Fa)
- 1 cup grilled asparagus (2 V) lightly brushed with olive oil and seasoned with salt and pepper to taste (freebies)
- 1 cup brown rice (3 S)

*Snack*
- 2, ½-inch slices of Banana-Nut Bread (2 S)—see recipe section—with 1 cup 1% milk or plain soymilk (1 M)
- 1¼ cups strawberries (1 Fr), sliced, and ½ banana (1 Fr), sliced, and 6 cashews (1 Fa)

# DAY 4

*Breakfast*
- Simple Smoothie: ½ banana (1 Fr) blended with 1 cup 1% milk or plain soymilk (1 M) and ice (freebie)
- 12–18 whole-wheat crackers (3 S)

*Lunch*
- 1 cup whole-wheat pasta (2 S), cooked and topped with Ratatouille—see recipe section (4 V—extra vegetables are freebies, 1 Fa)
- 2 ounces low-fat cheese (2 P) and 1 pear (1 Fr)

*Dinner*
- 6 ounces of flounder fillet (3 P), baked, lightly brushed with olive oil, and topped with 1 teaspoon capers and 1 tablespoon red onion chopped (freebies)
- Tabbouleh—see recipe section (1 S, 1 V, 1 Fa)
- 1 cup green peas (2 S)
- 1½ cups asparagus (3 V)

*Snack*
- 2, ½-inch slices of Banana Nut Bread (2 S)—see recipe section—with 1 ¼ cups watermelon (1 Fr), cubed
- 1 cup honeydew melon (1 Fr), cubed, topped with 1 cup plain low-fat yogurt (1 M) and 10 peanuts (1 Fa)

# DAY 5

*Breakfast*
- 1½ cups oatmeal (3 S), cooked, topped with 2 tablespoons raisins (1 Fr)
- 1 cup 1% milk or plain soymilk (1 M)

*Lunch*
- 2 ounces low-fat soy- or rice-based cheese (2 P) with 8–12 whole-wheat crackers (2 S)
- ½ cup baby carrots (1 V) and 1 sliced red pepper (1 V)
- 1 apple (1 Fr)

Note: *Save 1 Fat Group swap for dinner. Soy-based cheeses are more common than cheeses made from rice milk, but both are available.*

*Dinner*
- Warm Pork and Pear Salad—see recipe section; use 12 ounces of pork for 4 servings (3 P, 1 Fr—borrowed from snack, 2 Fa—1 Fat Group swap borrowed from lunch)
- 1 cup string beans (2 V) and 1 cup beets (2 V), boiled and peeled
- 1 cup whole-wheat couscous (3 S)

*Snack*
- 1½ cups whole-grain cereal (2 S) with 1 cup 1% milk or plain soymilk (1 M)
- 4 dried apricot halves (1 Fr) with 6 almonds (1 Fa)

Note: *1 Fruit Group swap borrowed for dinner.*

## DAY 6

*Breakfast*
- 1 cup plain low-fat yogurt (1 M) topped with 1 cup fresh fruit salad (1 Fr) and 2¼ cups whole-grain cereal (3 S)

*Lunch*
- 1 large whole-wheat pita bread (6-inch; 2 S) sliced open and stuffed with 2 hard-boiled eggs (2 P) crumbled and mixed with 1 teaspoon mayonnaise (1 Fa), ½ teaspoon mustard, and 1 teaspoon minced red onion (freebies)
- 1 cup green beans (2 V) blanched and marinated overnight with balsamic vinegar and 2 cloves of garlic cut in small chunks
- 12 cherries (1 Fr)

*Dinner*
- Chicken and Tomato Basil Sauce over Pasta—see recipe section; use 12 ounces of chicken breast, no skin, for 4 servings (3 P, 2 S, 2 V, 1 Fa)
- 1 cup spinach (2 V), cooked
- 2, 4-inch breadsticks (1 S)

*Snack*
Once in a while, you can combine the calories from your snack swaps to have a typical dessert food. In this case, you have the following swaps for snacks throughout the day: 1 Fa, 2 Fr, 1 M, and 2 S. For your first snack you can use 2 Grain & Starch Group swaps and 1 Milk & Yogurt Group swap (160 calories + 90 calories), or 250 calories, on typical dessert foods. Use food labels to determine the amount of a particular food you can have that provides 250 calories. For example, you can have about ¾ cup of ice cream (depending on the flavor and brand) OR 3 cookies and 1 cup of 1% milk. Then for a second snack have 1 pear (1 Fr) and 6 almonds (1 Fa). For a third snack you can use your other snack swap to have 10 grapes (1 Fr).

## DAY 7

*Breakfast*
- 3, ½-inch slices of Apricot and Orange Bread (2 S)—see recipe section
- 1 cup 1% milk or plain soymilk (1 M)
- ½ grapefruit (1 Fr)

*Lunch*
- 1 large tomato (1 V), top sliced off and seeds scooped out, stuffed with ½ cup tuna fish (light, packed in water, 2 P) and mixed with 1 teaspoon mayonnaise (1 Fa), ½ teaspoon mustard, 1 tablespoon minced celery, 1 teaspoon minced red onion, and salt and pepper to taste (freebies)
- ½ cup baby carrots (1 V) and 1 cup zucchini sticks (1 V—extra vegetables are freebies)
- 12–18 whole-wheat crackers (3 S—1 Grain & Starch Group swap borrowed from dinner)
- ½ cup cantaloupe (½ Fr—other ½ Fruit Group swap saved for dinner), cubed

*Dinner*
- Turkey Mango Wrap—see recipe section; use 12 ounces of turkey breast for 4 servings (3 P, 2 S, 1 V, ½ Fr borrowed from lunch, 1 Fa)
- 1½ cups jicama (3 V), cut into thick sticks

*Note:* 1 *Grain & Starch Group swap borrowed for lunch.*

*Snack*
- 1 cup plain low-fat yogurt (1 M) topped with ¾ cup blueberries (1 Fr) and 6 tablespoons Grape-Nuts cereal (2 S)
- 1 nectarine (1 Fr) and 10 peanuts (1 Fa)

# 2100 Calories

## DAY 1

*Breakfast*
- 2¼ cups whole-grain cereal (3 S) and 1 cup 1% milk or plain soymilk (1 M)
- ¾ cup blueberries (1 Fr) and ¼ cup cottage cheese (1 P)

*Lunch*
- Salad: lettuce (freebie), ¼ cup sliced carrots, ¼ cup diced red pepper, ¼ tomato, sliced, ½ cup broccoli (2 V); ⅔ cup garbanzo beans (2 S); 2-ounce chicken breast (2 P), cooked and cubed; 1 teaspoon olive oil (1 Fa); and balsamic vinegar, salt, and pepper to taste (freebies)
- 2, 4-inch bread sticks (1 S)
- 1 orange (1 Fr)

*Dinner*

On nights that you do not want to follow a recipe, use the swap lists and this suggested guideline to create a dinner simple menu.

- 3 ounces of baked or grilled white-meat chicken or turkey; OR 3 ounces of salmon or fatty fish; OR 6 ounces of baked or grilled flounder, other white fish, or shellfish; OR 3 ounces of lean meat (3 P)
- 2 cups vegetables sautéed (4 V) with 1 teaspoon olive oil (1 Fa) and garlic (freebie)
- 2 cups mashed potatoes; OR 2 cups whole-wheat pasta tossed with sautéed vegetables; OR 1⅓ cups brown rice topped with sautéed vegetables (4 S)
- 1 apple (1 Fr)

*Snack*

- Simple Smoothie: 1¼ cups sliced strawberries (1 Fr) blended with 1 cup 1% milk (1 M) and ice (freebie)
- 8–12 whole-wheat low-fat crackers (2 S) with 12 cherries (1 Fr) and 6 almonds (1 Fa)

# DAY 2

*Breakfast*
- 1 cup plain oatmeal (2 S), cooked, with 1 peach (1 Fr), sliced on top
- 2 slices whole-wheat light bread (1 S) with 1 soft-boiled egg (1 P)
- 1 cup 1% milk or plain soymilk (1 M)

*Lunch*
- 2 slices whole-wheat bread (2 S) with 2 ounces thinly sliced turkey breast (2 P), lettuce (freebie), ⅛ avocado (1 Fa), sliced, and mustard (freebie)
- ½ cup baby carrots (1 V) and 1 cup red pepper slices (1 V)
- 2 tablespoons raisins (1 Fr) tossed with ¾ cup whole-grain cereal squares (1 S) for a crunchy side dish.

*Dinner*
- Tofu Stir-Fry—see recipe section; use 1½ pounds of tofu for 4 servings (2 P, 2 V, 1 Fr, 1 Fa) and serve over 1 cup brown rice (3 S)
- 1 cup steamed baby carrots (2 V)
- ½ cup soybeans (1 S, 1 P)

*Snack*
- 2, ½-inch slices of Apricot-Orange Bread (2 S)—see recipe section—and ½ cup apple sauce (1 Fr)
- 1 cup cantaloupe (1 Fr), cubed, topped with 1 cup plain low-fat yogurt (1 M) and 6 almonds (1 Fa)

*Note: You can mix 1 tablespoon vanilla yogurt into the plain yogurt until you get accustomed to plain low-fat yogurt.*

# DAY 3

*Breakfast*
- French Toast: 3 slices whole-wheat bread (3 S) coated with 1 egg scrambled (1 P), cooked on nonstick skillet and topped with ½ cup apple sauce (1 Fr) and ½ cup plain low-fat yogurt (½ M)
- ½ cup 1% milk or plain soymilk (½ M)

*Lunch*
- 1 cup baby carrots (2 V) and celery sticks (freebie) dipped in ⅓ cup hummus (1 S, 1 Fa)
- 8–12 whole-wheat crackers (2 S)
- 2 ounces low-fat cheese (2 P)
- 10 grapes (1 Fr)

*Dinner*
- Shrimp Vegetable Kabobs—see recipe section; use 1½ pounds (or 36 jumbo) shrimp (3 P, 2 V, 1 Fa)
- 1 cup grilled asparagus (2 V) lightly brushed with olive oil and seasoned with salt and pepper to taste (freebies)
- 1⅓ cups brown rice (4 S)
- 1¼ cups watermelon (1 Fr), cubed

*Snack*
- 2, ½-inch slices of Banana-Nut Bread (2 S)—see recipe section—with 1 cup 1% milk or plain soymilk (1 M)
- 1¼ cups strawberries (1 Fr), sliced, ½ banana (1 Fr), sliced, and 6 cashews (1 Fa)

# DAY 4

*Breakfast*
- Protein Smoothie: ½ banana (1 Fr) blended with 1 scoop soy protein powder (1 P), 1 cup 1% milk or plain soymilk (1 M), and ice (freebie)
- 12–18 whole-wheat crackers (3 S)

*Lunch*
- 1½ cups whole-wheat pasta (3 S), cooked and topped with Ratatouille— see recipe section (4 V—extra vegetables are freebies, 1 Fa)
- 2 ounces low-fat cheese (2 P) and 1 pear (1 Fr)

*Dinner*
- 6 ounces of flounder fillet (3 P), baked, lightly brushed with olive oil, and topped with 1 teaspoon capers and 1 tablespoon red onion chopped (freebies)
- Tabbouleh—see recipe section (1 S, 1 V, 1 Fa)
- 1 cup green peas (2 S)
- 2, 4-inch bread sticks (1 S)
- 1½ cups asparagus (3 V)
- 1 cup papaya (1 Fr), cubed

*Snack*
- 2, ½-inch slices of Banana Nut Bread (2 S)—see recipe section—with 1¼ cups watermelon (1 Fr), cubed
- 1 cup honeydew melon (1 Fr), cubed, topped with 1 cup plain low-fat yogurt (1 M) and 10 peanuts (1 Fa)

# DAY 5

*Breakfast*
- 1½ cups oatmeal (3 S), cooked, topped with 2 tablespoons raisins (1 Fr)
- 1 cup 1% milk or plain soymilk (1 M)
Note: *1 Protein Group swap saved for lunch.*

*Lunch*
- 3 ounces low-fat soy- or rice-based cheese (3 P—1 Protein Group swap borrowed from breakfast) with 12–18 whole-wheat crackers (3 S)
- ½ cup baby carrots (1 V) and 1 sliced red pepper (1 V)
- 1 apple (1 Fr)

*Note: Save 1 Fat Group swap for dinner. Soy-based cheeses are more common than cheeses made from rice milk, but both are available.*

*Dinner*
- Warm Pork and Pear Salad—see recipe section; use 12 ounces of pork for 4 servings (3 P, 1 Fr, 2 Fa—1 Fat Group swap borrowed from lunch)
- 1 cup string beans (2 V) and 1 cup beets (2 V), boiled and peeled
- 1⅓ cups whole-wheat couscous (4 S)

*Snack*
- 1½ cups whole-grain cereal (2 S) with 2 tablespoons raisins (1 Fr) and 1 cup 1% milk or plain soymilk (1 M)
- 4 dried apricot halves (1 Fr) with 6 almonds (1 Fa)

# DAY 6

*Breakfast*
- Omelet: sauté onion, tomatoes, and mushrooms in a nonstick skillet wiped with olive oil from a paper towel (extra vegetables and this small amount of olive oil are freebies) and scramble with 3 egg whites (1 P); place on 3 slices whole-wheat bread (3 S)
- 1 cup fresh fruit salad (1 Fr) topped with 1 cup plain low-fat yogurt (1 M)

*Lunch*
- 1½ large whole-wheat pita breads (6-inch; 3 S) sliced open and stuffed with 2 hard-boiled eggs (2 P) crumbled and mixed with 1 teaspoon mayonnaise (1 Fa), ½ teaspoon mustard and 1 teaspoon minced red onion (freebies)
- 1 cup green beans (2 V) blanched and marinated overnight with balsamic vinegar and 2 cloves of garlic cut in small chunks
- 12 cherries (1 Fr)

*Dinner*
- Chicken and Tomato Basil Sauce over Pasta—see recipe section; use 12 ounces of chicken breast, no skin, for 4 servings (3 P, 2 S, 2 V, 1 Fa)
- 1 cup spinach (2 V), cooked
- 4, 4-inch breadsticks (2 S)
- 1 peach (1 Fr)

*Snack*
Once in a while, you can combine the calories from your snack swaps to have a typical dessert food. In this case, you have the following swaps for snacks throughout the day: 1 Fa, 2 Fr, 1 M, and 2 S. For your first snack you can use 2 Grain & Starch Group swaps and 1 Milk & Yogurt Group swap (160 calories + 90 calories), or 250 calories, on typical dessert foods. Use food labels to determine the amount of a particular food you can have that provides 250 calories. For example, you can have about ¾ cup ice cream (depending on the flavor and brand) OR 3 cookies and 1 cup of 1% milk. Then for a second snack you can have 1 pear (1 Fr) and 6 almonds (1 Fa). For a third snack you can use your other snack swap to have 10 grapes (1 Fr).

# DAY 7

*Breakfast*
- 3, ½-inch slices of Apricot and Orange Bread (3 S)—see recipe section
- 1 cup 1% milk or plain soymilk (1 M)
- ¼ cup cottage cheese (1 P) topped with 1 cup honeydew melon (1 Fr), cubed

*Lunch*
- 1 large tomato (1 V), top sliced off and seeds scooped out, stuffed with ½ cup tuna fish (light, packed in water, 2 P) and mixed with 1 teaspoon mayonnaise (1 Fa), ½ teaspoon mustard, 1 tablespoon minced celery, 1 teaspoon minced red onion, and salt and pepper to taste (freebies)
- ½ cup baby carrots (1 V) and 1 cup zucchini sticks (1 V—extra vegetables are freebies)
- 12–18 whole-wheat crackers (3 S)
- 1 apple ( 1 Fr)

*Dinner*
- Turkey Mango Wrap—see recipe section; use 12 ounces turkey breast for 4 servings (3 P, 2 S, 1 V, ½ Fr, 1 Fa)
- 1 cup sweet potato (2 S)
- 1½ cups jicama (3 V), cut into thick sticks
- ½ cup cantaloupe (½ Fr), cubed

*Snack*
- 1 cup plain low-fat yogurt (1 M) topped with ¾ cup blueberries (1 Fr) and 6 tablespoons Grape-Nuts cereal (2 S)
- 1 nectarine (1 Fr) and 10 peanuts (1 Fa)

# 2400 Calories

## DAY 1

*Breakfast*
- 2¼ cups whole-grain cereal (3 S) and 1 cup 1% milk or plain soymilk (1 M)
- ¾ cup blueberries (1 Fr) and ¼ cup cottage cheese (1 P)

*Lunch*
- Salad: lettuce (freebie), ¼ cup sliced carrots, ¼ cup diced red pepper, ¼ tomato, sliced, ½ cup broccoli (2 V); ⅔ cup garbanzo beans (2 S); 2-ounce chicken breast (2 P), cooked and cubed; 1 teaspoon olive oil (1 Fa); and balsamic vinegar, salt, and pepper to taste (freebies)
- 2, 4-inch bread sticks (1 S)
- 1 orange (1 Fr)
- 1 cup 1% milk or plain soymilk (1 M)

*Dinner*
On nights that you do not want to follow a recipe, use the swap lists and this suggested guideline to create a simple dinner menu.
- 4 ounces of baked or grilled white-meat chicken or turkey; OR 4 ounces of salmon or fatty fish; OR 8 ounces of baked or grilled flounder, other white fish, or shellfish; OR 4 ounces of lean meat (4 P)
- 2 cups vegetables sautéed (4 V) with 1 teaspoon olive oil (1 Fa) and garlic (freebie)

- 2½ cups mashed potatoes; OR 2½ cups whole-wheat pasta tossed with sautéed vegetables; OR 1⅔ cups brown rice topped with sautéed vegetables (5 S)
- 1 apple (1 Fr)

*Snack*
- Simple Smoothie: 1¼ cups sliced strawberries (1 Fr) blended with 1 cup 1% milk (1 M) and ice (freebie)
- 12–18 whole-wheat low-fat crackers (3 S) with 12 cherries (1 Fr) and 6 almonds (1 Fa)

# DAY 2

*Breakfast*
- 1 cup plain oatmeal (2 S), cooked, with 1 peach (1 Fr), sliced on top
- 2 slices whole-wheat light bread (1 S) with 1 soft-boiled egg (1 P)
- 1 cup 1% milk or plain soymilk (1 M)

*Lunch*
- 2 slices whole-wheat bread (2 S) with 2 ounces thinly sliced turkey breast (2 P), lettuce (freebie), ⅛ avocado (1 Fa), sliced, and mustard (freebie)
- ½ cup baby carrots (1 V) and 1 cup red pepper slices (1 V)
- 1 cup plain low-fat yogurt (1 M) topped with 2 tablespoons raisins (1 Fr) and ¾ cup whole-grain cereal squares (1 S)

*Dinner*
- Tofu Stir-Fry—see recipe section; use 1½ pounds of tofu for 4 servings (2 P, 2 V, 1 Fr, 1 Fa) and serve over 1 cup brown rice (3 S)
- 1 cup steamed baby carrots (2 V)
- 1 cup soybeans (2 S, 2 P)

*Snack*
- 3, ½-inch slices of Apricot-Orange Bread (3 S)—see recipe section—and ½ cup apple sauce (1 Fr)
- 1 cup cantaloupe (1 Fr), cubed, topped with 1 cup plain low-fat yogurt (1 M) and 6 almonds (1 Fa)

*Note: You can mix 1 tablespoon vanilla yogurt into the plain yogurt until you get accustomed to plain low-fat yogurt.*

# DAY 3

*Breakfast*
- French Toast: 3 slices whole-wheat bread (3 S) coated with 1 egg scrambled (1 P), cooked on nonstick skillet and topped with ½ cup apple sauce (1 Fr) and ½ cup plain low-fat yogurt (½ M)
- ½ cup 1% milk or plain soymilk (½ M)

*Lunch*
- 1 cup baby carrots (2 V) and celery sticks (freebie) dipped in ⅓ cup hummus (1 S, 1 Fa)
- 8–12 whole-wheat crackers (2 S)
- 2 ounces low-fat cheese (2 P)
- 10 grapes (1 Fr)
- 1 cup 1% milk or plain soymilk (1 M)

*Dinner*
- Shrimp Vegetable Kabobs—see recipe section; use 2 pounds (or 48 jumbo) shrimp (4 P, 2 V, 1 Fa)
- 1 cup grilled asparagus (2 V) lightly brushed with olive oil and seasoned with salt and pepper to taste (freebies)
- 1⅔ cups brown rice (5 S)
- 1¼ cups watermelon (1 Fr), cubed

*Snack*
- 3, ½-inch slices of Banana-Nut Bread (3 S)—see recipe section—with 1 cup 1% milk or plain soymilk (1 M)
- 1¼ cups strawberries (1 Fr), sliced, and ½ banana (1 Fr), sliced, and 6 cashews (1 Fa)

# DAY 4

*Breakfast*
- Protein Smoothie: ½ banana (1 Fr) blended with 1 scoop soy protein powder (1 P), 1 cup 1% milk or plain soymilk (1 M), and ice (freebie)
- 12–18 whole-wheat crackers (3 S)

*Lunch*
- 1½ cups whole-wheat pasta (3 S), cooked and topped with Ratatouille—see recipe section (4 V—extra vegetables are freebies, 1 Fa)
- 2 ounces low-fat cheese (2 P) and 1 pear (1 Fr)
- 1 cup 1% milk or plain soymilk (1 M)

*Dinner*
- 8 ounces of flounder fillet (4 P), baked, lightly brushed with olive oil, and topped with 1 teaspoon capers and 1 tablespoon red onion chopped (freebies)
- Tabbouleh—see recipe section (1 S, 1 V, 1 Fa)
- 1 cup green peas (2 S)
- 4, 4-inch bread sticks (2 S)
- 1½ cups asparagus (3 V)
- 1 cup papaya (1 Fr), cubed

*Snack*
- 2, ½-inch slices of Banana Nut Bread (2 S)—see recipe section—with 1 ¼ cups watermelon (1 Fr), cubed
- 1 cup honeydew melon (1 Fr), cubed, topped with 1 cup plain low-fat yogurt (1 M), 3 tablespoons wheat germ (1 S), and 10 peanuts (1 Fa)

# DAY 5

*Breakfast*
- 1½ cups oatmeal (3 S), cooked, topped with 2 tablespoons raisins (1 Fr)
- 1 cup 1% milk or plain soymilk (1 M)

*Note: 1 Protein Group swap saved for lunch.*

*Lunch*
- 3 ounces low-fat soy- or rice-based cheese (3 P—1 Protein Group swap borrowed from breakfast) with 12–18 whole-wheat crackers (3 S)
- ½ cup baby carrots (1 V) and 1 sliced red pepper (1 V)
- 1 cup plain low-fat yogurt (1 M) topped with ¾ cup fresh fruit salad (1 Fr)

*Note: Save 1 Fat Group swap for dinner. Soy-based cheeses are more common than cheeses made from rice milk, but both are available.*

*Dinner*
- Warm Pork and Pear Salad—see recipe section; use 1 pound of pork for 4 servings (4 P, 1 Fr, 2 Fa—1 Fat Group swap borrowed from lunch)
- 1 cup string beans (2 V) and 1 cup beets (2 V), boiled and peeled
- 1⅔ cups whole-wheat couscous (5 S)

*Snack*
- 2¼ cups whole-grain cereal (3 S) with 2 tablespoons raisins (1 Fr) and 1 cup 1% milk or plain soymilk (1 M)
- 4 dried apricot halves (1 Fr) with 6 almonds (1 Fa)

# DAY 6

*Breakfast*
- Omelet: sauté onion, tomatoes, and mushrooms in a nonstick skillet wiped with olive oil from a paper towel (extra vegetables and this small amount of olive oil are freebies) and scramble with 3 egg whites (1 P); place on 3 slices whole-wheat bread (3 S)
- 1 cup fresh fruit salad (1 Fr) topped with 1 cup plain low-fat yogurt (1 M)

*Lunch*
- 1½ large whole-wheat pita breads (6-inch; 3 S) sliced open and stuffed with 2 hard-boiled eggs (2 P) crumbled and mixed with 1 teaspoon mayonnaise (1 Fa), ½ teaspoon mustard, and 1 teaspoon minced red onion (freebies)
- 1 cup green beans (2 V) blanched and marinated overnight with balsamic vinegar and 2 cloves of garlic cut in small chunks
- 12 cherries (1 Fr)
- 1 cup 1% milk or plain soymilk (1 M)

*Dinner*
- Chicken and Tomato Basil Sauce over Pasta—see recipe section; use 1 pound of chicken breast, no skin, for 4 servings (4 P, 2 S, 2 V, 1 Fa)
- 1 cup spinach (2 V), cooked
- 6, 4-inch breadsticks (3 S)
- 1 peach (1 Fr)

*Note*: If you prefer to have more pasta and less breadsticks, use 12 ounces of dry pasta in the recipe. The Chicken and Tomato Basil Sauce over Pasta recipe would then count as 4 P, 4 S, 2 V, 1 Fa). You would then have 2 breadsticks (1 S) instead of 6 breadsticks.

*Snack*
Once in a while, you can combine the calories from your snack swaps to have a typical dessert food. In this case, you have the following swaps for snacks throughout the day: 1 Fa, 2 Fr, 1 M, and 3 S. For your first snack you can use 2 Grain & Starch Group swaps and 1 Milk & Yogurt Group swap (160 calories + 90 calories), or 250 calories, on typical dessert foods. Use food labels to determine the amount of a particular food you can have that provides 250 calories. For example, you can have about ¾ cup of ice cream (depending on the flavor and brand) OR 3 cookies and 1 cup of 1% milk. Then for a second snack you can have 1 pear (1 Fr) and 6 almonds (1 Fa). For a third snack you can use your other snack swaps to have 10 grapes (1 Fr) and 4–6 whole-wheat crackers (1 S).

# DAY 7

*Breakfast*
- 3, ½-inch slices of Apricot and Orange Bread (3 S)—see recipe section
- 1 cup 1% milk or plain soymilk (1M)
- ¼ cottage cheese (1 P) topped with 1 cup honeydew melon (1 Fr), cubed

*Lunch*
- 1 large tomato (1 V), top sliced off and seeds scooped out, stuffed with ½ cup tuna fish (light, packed in water, 2 P) and mixed with 1 teaspoon mayonnaise (1 Fa), ½ teaspoon mustard, 1 tablespoon minced celery, 1 teaspoon minced red onion, and salt and pepper to taste (freebies)
- ½ cup baby carrots (1 V) and 1 cup zucchini sticks (1 V—extra vegetables are freebies)
- 12–18 whole-wheat crackers (3 S)
- 1 apple ( 1 Fr)
- 1 cup 1% milk or plain soymilk (1 M)

*Dinner*

- Turkey Mango Wrap—see recipe section; use 1 pound of turkey breast for 4 servings (4 P, 2 S, 1 V, ½ Fr, 1 Fa)
- 1½ cup sweet potato (3 S)
- 1½ cups jicama, cut into thick sticks (3 V)
- ½ cup cantaloupe (½ Fr), cubed

*Snack*

- 1 cup plain low-fat yogurt (1 M) topped with ¾ cup blueberries (1 Fr) and 6 tablespoons Grape-Nuts cereal (2 S)
- Homemade Trail Mix: 2 tablespoons raisins (1 Fr), 1½ cups whole-grain cereal squares (2 S), and 10 peanuts (1 Fa)

# RECIPES

## Apricot-Nut Bread

*Ingredients*
- 6 ounces dried apricots, cut into small pieces
- 2 cups water
- 2 tablespoons butter
- 1 cup sugar
- 1 egg, slightly beaten
- 1 tablespoon orange peel, freshly grated
- 2 cups all-purpose flour
- 1½ cups whole-wheat flour
- ½ cup fat-free dry milk powder
- 2 teaspoons baking powder
- 1 teaspoon baking soda
- 1 teaspoon salt
- ½ cup orange juice
- ½ cup pecans, chopped (or another type of nut)

*Directions*
Preheat oven to 350°F. Grease two, 9 x 5–inch loaf pans. Cook the apricots in water in a covered pot over medium heat for 10–15 minutes or until the apricots are just tender. Drain and reserve ¾ cup of cooking liquid, mixing with orange juice in a large measuring cup. Set apricots aside to cool. Cream together butter and sugar; beat in egg and orange peel using a whisk. Whisk together dry ingredients, including all-purpose flour, whole-wheat flour, dry milk powder, baking powder, baking soda, and salt. Add ⅓ of the flour mixture to butter mixture and incorporate. Add ⅓ of the orange juice mixture and mix in thoroughly. Continue alternating the addition of flour mixture and juice mixture, mixing each time. Fold in apricot and pecan pieces. Put half of batter in each of the two greased loaf pans. Bake for 40 to 45 minutes or until bread springs back when lightly touched in center. Let stand and cool for 5 minutes. Remove from pans and cool completely on a wire rack.

## Banana-Nut Bread

*Ingredients*

- 1 cup ripe banana, mashed
- ⅓ cup low-fat buttermilk
- ½ cup brown sugar, packed
- ¼ cup butter
- 1 egg, slightly beaten
- 1 cup all-purpose flour
- 1 cup whole-wheat flour
- 1 teaspoon baking powder
- ½ teaspoon baking soda
- ½ teaspoon salt
- ½ cup walnuts, chopped (or another type of nut)

*Directions*

Preheat oven to 350°F. Lightly grease two, 9 x 5–inch loaf pans. Stir together the mashed banana and buttermilk, and set aside. Cream brown sugar and butter together. Beat in egg and banana mixture thoroughly and mix with sugar and butter. Whisk together all-purpose flour, whole-wheat flour, baking powder, baking soda, and salt. Add the dry ingredients to the banana mixture. Stir well until blended. Fold in walnuts. Bake for 50–55 minutes or until the bread springs back lightly when pressed in the center. (An inserted toothpick may not come out clean, because the warm banana may be mushy until the bread is cooled.) Cool for 5 minutes in pans. Remove from pans and place on wire rack to cool completely.

## Chicken and Tomato Basil Sauce over Pasta (serves 4)

*Ingredients*

- 6 ounces dry whole-wheat pasta
- 1 teaspoon olive oil
- ¼ teaspoon salt and pepper to taste
- Chicken breast, no skin, cut into strips (amount used depends on calorie level, refer to menu)
- ⅓ cup thinly sliced fresh basil or 2 teaspoons dried basil
- ¼ cup grated Parmesan cheese

*Sauce*
- 3 teaspoons olive oil
- 1 cup onion chopped
- 4 cloves garlic, crushed
- 6 cups plum tomatoes (fresh or canned—if canned purchase with paste included)
- 1 teaspoon sugar
- 1 tablespoon parsley
- Salt and pepper to taste

*Directions*

Make the sauce first. Heat olive oil in a large pot over medium heat. Add onions and garlic and sauté until tender, stirring often. Add tomatoes, sugar, parsley, salt, and pepper. Simmer for 30 minutes. If the sauce is thin, uncover while simmering. In the meantime, boil water for pasta and cook pasta according to package directions. In a nonstick skillet heat 1 teaspoon olive oil over medium heat. Add the chicken strips and sauté, stirring often. Season with salt and pepper to taste. Set aside in a warm bowl. When the pasta is cooked, drain and pour it into the sauce when the sauce is cooked. Toss. Divide equally into 4 bowls. Equally divide chicken onto pasta and top with equal portions of basil. Sprinkle 1 tablespoon Parmesan cheese on top of each bowl.

**Ratatouille** (serves 4)

*Ingredients*
- 4 teaspoons olive oil
- 2 cloves garlic, crushed
- 1 onion, thinly sliced
- 2 teaspoons dried basil
- ½ teaspoon dried oregano
- ½ teaspoon dried thyme
- 1 teaspoon dried parsley
- 1 eggplant, peeled and cubed
- 2 green peppers, coarsely chopped
- 4 large tomatoes, coarsely chopped
- 3 zucchini, peeled and sliced

*Directions*

Heat olive oil in a large pot under medium heat. Add garlic, onions, and herbs. Cook until tender, stirring often. Add eggplant, stirring to coat with oil. Mix in peppers. Cook for approximately 10 minutes, stirring often to prevent the vegetables from sticking. Add tomatoes and zucchini, mixing to evening distribute them. Cover and cook over lower heat about 15 to 20 minutes, or until vegetables are tender but not mushy.

## Shrimp Vegetable Kabobs (Serves 4)

*Ingredients*

- 2 tablespoons light soy sauce
- 2 tablespoons lemon juice
- 1 clove garlic, crushed
- ⅛ teaspoon pepper
- 2 tablespoons dry white wine, vegetable broth or water
- 2 teaspoons grated fresh ginger
- 4 teaspoons canola oil, cold-pressed or mechanically extracted
- Jumbo shrimp, peeled with tails left on, deveined, washed (amount used depends on calorie level, refer to menu)
- 1½ red pepper, cut into large chunks
- 2 zucchini, peeled and cut into thick slices
- Approximately 24 mushrooms, cleaned
- 2 large onions, cut into chunks

*Directions*

Make the marinade by combining the first seven ingredients and whisking them together vigorously. Place the shrimp in a container; pour half the marinade over the shrimp. Close the container and refrigerate for at least 1 hour or overnight. Reserve the rest of the marinade for barbequing. Soak 12 wooden skewers to allow them to expand, making it easier to remove the shrimp after it is cooked. Place the grate 4 to 5 inches from heat and preheat barbeque. Plan for 12 skewers, 3 per person. Alternate shrimp (2 per skewer) and vegetables on skewers. Brush vegetables on skewers with remaining marinade. Place skewers on moderately hot barbeque. Cook approximately 2 minutes on each side, or until shrimp are done.

### **Tabbouleh** (serves 4)

*Ingredients*

- ½ cup dry bulgur
- 4 cups water
- 4 tomatoes, chopped
- 1 red bell pepper, seeded and chopped
- ½ cup parsley
- 4 teaspoons olive oil
- 3 tablespoons lemon juice
- Salt and pepper to taste

*Directions*

Soak bulgur in boiling water for 60 minutes. In the meantime, prepare the vegetables. Mix together the tomatoes, red pepper, parsley, olive oil, lemon juice, salt, and pepper. Line a strainer with a paper towel or cheese cloth, and pour the bulgur in it to drain. Pick up the corners of the towel or cheese cloth and squeeze out the excess water. Combine bulgur with vegetables and mix thoroughly.

### **Tofu Stir-Fry** (serves 4)

*Ingredients*

- 4 teaspoons canola oil
- 2 cloves garlic
- 2 tablespoons fresh ginger, grated
- Tofu (see menus for amount)
- 1 cup broccoli florets, chopped
- 1 cup cauliflower florets, chopped
- 2 scallions, sliced
- 1½ cups water chestnuts, sliced
- 1 cup mushrooms, sliced
- 10 ounces pineapple chunks, canned in own juices
- ¼ cup low sodium soy sauce
- 1 tablespoon cornstarch

*Directions*

Heat canola oil in skillet under medium-high heat. Add garlic, ginger, and tofu and cook until tofu is lightly browned on both sides. Remove tofu and set aside in warm bowl. Add broccoli, cauliflower, scallions, mushrooms, and water chestnuts, stirring often. Cook until vegetables are just tender. In the meantime, whisk together pineapple juice, soy sauce, and cornstarch thoroughly. When smooth, pour into skillet, stirring to coat vegetables. Add pineapple and tofu to skillet to warm.

**Turkey Mango Wrap** (serves 4)
*Ingredients*
- 3 teaspoons canola oil, cold-pressed or mechanically extracted
- 1 yellow bell pepper, seeded and chopped
- ½ cup red onion, chopped
- 1 chili pepper, minced (optional)
- ½ teaspoon ground cinnamon
- ½ teaspoon ground coriander
- ½ teaspoon cumin
- ½ teaspoon ground oregano
- Turkey breast, no skin, cubed (amount used depends on calorie level, refer to menu)
- ¾ cup fresh salsa
- ¼ cup raisins
- 1 cup chopped mango
- 1⅓ cup chickpeas
- 4, 6-inch tortillas (no fat added)

*Directions*
Heat oil in a large skillet. Sauté pepper, onions, and chili with cinnamon, coriander, cumin, and oregano. Add turkey and continue to sauté. Stir often until pepper and onion are tender and turkey is cooked. (You could also use cooked, leftover turkey cubes and simply reheat.) Reduce heat and mix in salsa, raisins, mango, and chickpeas. Cook for about another 3–5 minutes until warm. Warm tortillas in toaster oven—don't overcook. Scoop equal amounts of turkey mixture in the center of each of four tortillas. Fold bottom of tortilla up and roll.

**Warm Pork and Pear Salad** (serves 4)

*Ingredients*
- Pork tenderloin (amount used depends on calorie level, refer to menu)
- 2 ripe pears, cored, peeled, each sliced into 8 pieces
- 2 teaspoons butter
- 2 teaspoons canola oil, cold-pressed or mechanically extracted
- ¼ cup cider vinegar
- 4 teaspoons sugar
- ½ teaspoon salt
- ¼ cup raisins
- ¼ cup walnuts, chopped
- 6 cups salad greens

*Directions*
Cut pork into strips and set aside. In a large nonstick skillet, heat butter. Sauté pear slices until they are just tender. Remove them from the pan and place them in a warm bowl. Add oil to the pan and heat under medium heat. Add pork and stir-fry until lightly browned on both sides, about 3–5 minutes. Remove pork and set aside with pears. Add vinegar, sugar, and salt to pan, stir until sugar dissolves. Add raisins. Then return pork and pears to pan and gently coat and warm pork and pears. Equally divide greens onto four plates, and top with equal amounts of pork and pear mixture. Top with walnuts.

# Appendix 1
## Body Mass Index Table

| | Normal | | | | | | Overweight | | | | | Obese | | | | | |
|---|---|---|---|---|---|---|---|---|---|---|---|---|---|---|---|---|---|
| **BMI** | 19 | 20 | 21 | 22 | 23 | 24 | 25 | 26 | 27 | | 29 | | 31 | | 33 | | 35 |
| **Height (inches)** | | | | | | | | | **Body Weight (pounds)** | | | | | | | | |
| 58 | 91 | 96 | 100 | 105 | 110 | 115 | 119 | 124 | 129 | 134 | 138 | 143 | 148 | 153 | 158 | 162 | 167 |
| 59 | 94 | 99 | 104 | 109 | 114 | 119 | 124 | 128 | 133 | 138 | 143 | 148 | 153 | 158 | 163 | 168 | 173 |
| 60 | 97 | 102 | 107 | 112 | 118 | 123 | 128 | 133 | 138 | 143 | 148 | 153 | 158 | 163 | 168 | 174 | 179 |
| 61 | 100 | 106 | 111 | 116 | 122 | 127 | 132 | 137 | 143 | 148 | 153 | 158 | 164 | 169 | 174 | 180 | 185 |
| 62 | 104 | 109 | 115 | 120 | 126 | 131 | 136 | 142 | 147 | 153 | 158 | 164 | 169 | 175 | 180 | 186 | 191 |
| 63 | 107 | 113 | 118 | 124 | 130 | 135 | 141 | 146 | 152 | 158 | 163 | 169 | 175 | 180 | 186 | 191 | 197 |
| 64 | 110 | 116 | 122 | 128 | 134 | 140 | 145 | 151 | 157 | 163 | 169 | 174 | 180 | 186 | 192 | 197 | 204 |
| 65 | 114 | 120 | 126 | 132 | 138 | 144 | 150 | 156 | 162 | 168 | 174 | 180 | 186 | 192 | 198 | 204 | 210 |
| 67 | 121 | 127 | 134 | 140 | 146 | 153 | 159 | 166 | 172 | 178 | 185 | 191 | 198 | 204 | 211 | 217 | 223 |
| 68 | 125 | 131 | 138 | 144 | 151 | 158 | 164 | 171 | 177 | 184 | 190 | 197 | 203 | 210 | 216 | 223 | 230 |
| 69 | 128 | 135 | 142 | 149 | 155 | 162 | 169 | 176 | 182 | 189 | 196 | 203 | 209 | 216 | 223 | 230 | 236 |
| 70 | 132 | 139 | 146 | 153 | 160 | 167 | 174 | 181 | 188 | 195 | 202 | 209 | 216 | 222 | 229 | 236 | 243 |
| 71 | 136 | 143 | 150 | 157 | 165 | 172 | 179 | 186 | 193 | 200 | 208 | 215 | 222 | 229 | 236 | 243 | 250 |
| 72 | 140 | 147 | 154 | 162 | 169 | 177 | 184 | 191 | 199 | 206 | 213 | 221 | 228 | 235 | 242 | 250 | 258 |
| 73 | 144 | 151 | 159 | 166 | 174 | 182 | 189 | 197 | 204 | 212 | 219 | 227 | 235 | 242 | 250 | 257 | 265 |
| 74 | 148 | 155 | 163 | 171 | 179 | 186 | 194 | 202 | 210 | 218 | 225 | 233 | 241 | 249 | 256 | 264 | 272 |
| 75 | 152 | 160 | 168 | 176 | 184 | 192 | 200 | 208 | 216 | 224 | 232 | 240 | 248 | 256 | 264 | 272 | 279 |
| 76 | 156 | 164 | 172 | 180 | 189 | 197 | 205 | 213 | 221 | 230 | 238 | 246 | 254 | 263 | 271 | 279 | 287 |

## Appendix 1
### Body Mass Index Table

| | | | | Extreme Obesity | | | | | | | | | | | | | | |
|---|---|---|---|---|---|---|---|---|---|---|---|---|---|---|---|---|---|---|
| 36 | 37 | 38 | 39 | 40 | 41 | 42 | 43 | 44 | 45 | 46 | 47 | 48 | 49 | 50 | 51 | 52 | 53 | 54 |

**Body Weight (pounds)**

| 36 | 37 | 38 | 39 | 40 | 41 | 42 | 43 | 44 | 45 | 46 | 47 | 48 | 49 | 50 | 51 | 52 | 53 | 54 |
|---|---|---|---|---|---|---|---|---|---|---|---|---|---|---|---|---|---|---|
| 172 | 177 | 181 | 186 | 191 | 196 | 201 | 205 | 210 | 215 | 220 | 224 | 229 | 234 | 239 | 244 | 248 | 253 | 258 |
| 178 | 183 | 188 | 193 | 198 | 203 | 208 | 212 | 217 | 222 | 227 | 232 | 237 | 242 | 247 | 252 | 257 | 262 | 267 |
| 184 | 189 | 194 | 199 | 204 | 209 | 215 | 220 | 225 | 230 | 235 | 240 | 245 | 250 | 255 | 261 | 266 | 271 | 276 |
| 190 | 195 | 201 | 206 | 211 | 217 | 222 | 227 | 232 | 238 | 243 | 248 | 254 | 259 | 264 | 269 | 275 | 280 | 285 |
| 196 | 202 | 207 | 213 | 218 | 224 | 229 | 235 | 240 | 246 | 251 | 256 | 262 | 267 | 273 | 278 | 284 | 289 | 295 |
| 203 | 208 | 214 | 220 | 225 | 231 | 237 | 242 | 248 | 254 | 259 | 265 | 270 | 278 | 282 | 287 | 293 | 299 | 304 |
| 209 | 215 | 221 | 227 | 232 | 238 | 244 | 250 | 256 | 262 | 267 | 273 | 279 | 285 | 291 | 296 | 302 | 308 | 314 |
| 216 | 222 | 228 | 234 | 240 | 246 | 252 | 258 | 264 | 270 | 276 | 282 | 288 | 294 | 300 | 306 | 312 | 318 | 324 |
| | | | | | | | | | | | | | | | | | | |
| 230 | 236 | 242 | 249 | 255 | 261 | 268 | 274 | 280 | 287 | 293 | 299 | 306 | 312 | 319 | 325 | 331 | 338 | 344 |
| 236 | 243 | 249 | 256 | 262 | 269 | 276 | 282 | 289 | 295 | 302 | 308 | 315 | 322 | 328 | 335 | 341 | 348 | 354 |
| 243 | 250 | 257 | 263 | 270 | 277 | 284 | 291 | 297 | 304 | 311 | 318 | 324 | 331 | 338 | 345 | 351 | 358 | 365 |
| 250 | 257 | 264 | 271 | 278 | 285 | 292 | 299 | 306 | 313 | 320 | 327 | 334 | 341 | 348 | 355 | 362 | 369 | 376 |
| 257 | 265 | 272 | 279 | 286 | 293 | 301 | 308 | 315 | 322 | 329 | 338 | 343 | 351 | 358 | 365 | 372 | 379 | 386 |
| 265 | 272 | 279 | 287 | 294 | 302 | 309 | 316 | 324 | 331 | 338 | 346 | 353 | 361 | 368 | 375 | 383 | 390 | 397 |
| 272 | 280 | 288 | 295 | 302 | 310 | 318 | 325 | 333 | 340 | 348 | 355 | 363 | 371 | 378 | 386 | 393 | 401 | 408 |
| 280 | 287 | 295 | 303 | 311 | 319 | 326 | 334 | 342 | 350 | 358 | 365 | 373 | 381 | 389 | 396 | 404 | 412 | 420 |
| 287 | 295 | 303 | 311 | 319 | 327 | 335 | 343 | 351 | 359 | 367 | 375 | 383 | 391 | 399 | 407 | 415 | 423 | 431 |
| 295 | 304 | 312 | 320 | 328 | 336 | 344 | 353 | 361 | 369 | 377 | 385 | 394 | 402 | 410 | 418 | 426 | 435 | 443 |

# BIBLIOGRAPHY

### Chapter 1

1. Nestle, M. 2002. *Food Politics*. Berkeley: University of California Press, 457.
2. Schlosser, E. 2001. *Fast Food Nation*. New York City: Houghton Mifflin, 367.

### Chapter 3

1. Backstrand, J. R.. 2003. Quantitative approaches to nutrient density for public health nutrition. *Public Health Nutrition*, 6:829–837.
2. USDA. 2002. Caloric sweeteners, http://ers.usda.gov/Data/FoodConsumption/ (accessed July 8, 2004).
3. Putnam, J.P., J. Allshouse, L. Scott Kantor. 2002. U.S. per capita food supply trends: more calories, refined carbohydrates, and fats. *Food Review*, 25(3):2–15.
4. Jacobson, M.F. Liquid candy: how soft drinks are harming Americans' health. http://www.cspinet.org/sodapop/liquid_candy.htm (accessed 2004).
5. Whole Grains Council. Reaping the benefits of whole grains: A consumers' guide. http://www.wholegrainscouncil.org/Consumer%20Guide.html (accessed 2003).
6. Foster-Powell, K., S. H. A. Holt, and J. C. Brand-Miller. 2002. International table of glycemic index and glycemic load values: 2002. *American Journal of Clinical Nutrition*, 76:5–56.
7. Ascherio, A., M. J. Stampfer, and W. C. Willett. 2000. Trans fatty acids and coronary heart disease. Havard School of Public Health, http://www.hsph.edu/reviews/transfats.html (accessed July 8, 2004).

8. Lada, A. T., and L. L. Rudel. 2003. Dietary monunsaturated versus polyunsaturated fatty acids: Which is better for protection from conorary heart disease? *Current Opinion in Lipidology*, 14:41–46.

9. Institute of Medicine. 2002. Dietary reference intakes for energy, carbohydrate, fiber, fat, fatty acids, cholesterol, protein, and amino acids. Washington D.C.: National Academies Press, 936.

10. Simopolous, A. P. 1999. Essential fatty acids in health and chronic disease. *American Journal of Clinical Nutrition*, 70:560S–569S.

11. Vessby, B. 2003. Dietary fat, fatty acid composition in plasma and the metabolic syndrome. *Current Opinion in Lipidology*, 14:15–19.

12. Clifton, P., M. Noakes, and B. Parker. 2002. The effect of a high protein weight loss diet in overweight subjects with type 2 diabetes. *American Journal of Clinical Nutrition*, 75:343S(1).

13. Layman, D. K. 2003 The role of leucine in weight loss diets and glucose homeostasis. *Journal of Nutrition*, 133:261S–267S.

14. National Academy of Sciences. 2004. Dietary reference intakes for water, potassium, sodium, chloride, and sulfate.

15. Craig, J. W. 2002. Phytochemicals: Guardians of our health. *Vegetarian Nutrition*, A Dietetic Practice Group of ADA http://www.andrews.edu/NUFS/phyto.html (accessed March 12, 2004).

**Chapter 4**

1. Hu, F. 2003. Plant-based foods and prevention of cardiovascular disease: An overview. *American Journal of Clinical Nutrition*, 78(3S):544S–551S.

2. Lampe, J. 2003. Spicing up a vegetarian diet: Chemopreventive effects of phytochemicals. *American Journal of Clinical Nutrition*, 78:579S–583S.

3. Park, E., and Pezzuto, J. 2002. Botanicals in cancer chemoprevention. *Cancer and Metastasis Reviews*, 21(3–4):231–255.

4. Seaman, D. 2002. The diet-induced proinflammatory state: A cause of chronic pain and other degenerative diseases? *Journal of Manipulative and Physiological Therapeutics*, 25(3):168–179.

5. Surh, Y. 2003. Cancer chemoprevention with dietary phytochemicals. *Nature Reviews Cancer*, 3(10):768–780.

**Chapter 5**

1. American Diabetes Association and American College of Cardiology. 2002. So many nutrition recommendations—contradictory or compatible. *Diabetes and Cardiovascular Disease Review*, 4:1–4.

2. Bonora, E., S. Kiechl, *et al*. 1998. Prevalence of insulin resistance in metabolic disorders: the Bruneck study. *Diabetes*, 47(10):1643–1650.
3. Bonow, R. O., and R. H. Eckel. 2003. Diet, obesity and cardiovascular risk. *New England Journal of Medicine*, 348(21):2057–2058.
4. American Diabetes Association and American College of Cardiology. 2002. Redefining diabetes control. *Diabetes and Cardiovascular Disease Review*, 1:1–3.
5. American Diabetes Association. 2004. Diagnosis and classification of diabetes mellitus. *Diabetes Care*, 27(S1):S5–S10.

**Chapter 6**

1. Bonora, E., et al. 1998. Prevalence of insulin resistance in metabolic disorders: The Bruneck study. *Diabetes*, 47(10):1643–1650.
2. Bonow, R. O., and R. H. Eckel. 2003. Diet, obesity and cardiovascular risk. *New England Journal of Medicine*, 348(21):2057–2058.
3. Poirier, P., and J.-P. Despres. 2003. Waist circumference, visceral obesity and cardiovascular risk. *Journal of Cardiopulmonary Rehabilitation*, 23:161–169.
4. Cordain, L., et al. 2002. The paradoxical nature of hunter-gatherer diets: Meat-based, yet non-atherogenic. *European Jounral of Clinical Nutrition*, 56:S42–S52.
5. Samaha, F. F., et al. 2003. A low-carbohydrate as compared with a low fat diet in severe obesity. *New England Journal of Medicine*, 248(21):2074–2081.
6. Foster, G. D., et al. 2003. A randomization trial of a low-carbohydrate diet for obesity. *New England Journal of Medicine*, 348(21):2082–2090.
7. Westman, E., et al. 2002. Effect of a 6-month adherence to a very low carbohydrate diet program. *American Journal of Medicine*, 113:30–36.
8. Brehm, B. J., et al. 2003. A randomized trial comparing a very low carbohydrate diet and a calorie-restricted low fat diet on body weight and cardiovascular risk factors in healthy women. *Journal of Clinical Endocrinology and Metabolism*, 88(4):1617–1623.
9. Hu, F. 2003. Plant-based foods and prevention of cardiovascular disease: An overview. *American Journal of Clinical Nutrition*, 78(3S):544S–551S.
10. Lampe, J. 2003. Spicing up a vegetarian diet: chemopreventive effects of phytochemicals. *American Journal of Clinical Nutrition*, 78:579S–583S.
11. Park, E., and J. Pezzuto. 2002. Botanicals in cancer chemoprevention. *Cancer and Metastasis Reviews*, 21(3–4):231–255.
12. Slavin, J. 2003. Why whole grains are protective: biological mechanisms. *Proceedings of the Nutrition Society*, 62(1):129–134.
13. Surh, Y. 2003. Cancer chemoprevention with dietary phytochemicals. *Nature Reviews Cancer*, 3(10):768–780.

14. American Institute for Cancer Research. 1997. Food, nutrition and the prevention of cancer: A global perspective. American Institute for Cancer Research: Washington DC.

15. Bravata, D. M., et al. 2003. Efficacy and safety of low-carbohydrate diets: A systmatic review. *Journal of the American Medical Association*, 2003. 289(14):1837–1850.

16. Fleming, R. 2000. The effect of high-protein diets on coronary blood flow. *Angiology*, 51(10):817–826.

17. Fleming, R. 2002. The effect of high-, moderate-, and low-fat diets on weight loss and cardiovascular disease risk factors. *Preventive Cardiology*, 5(3):110–118.

18. Go, V., R. Butrum, and D. Wong. 2003. Diet, nutrition, and cancer prevention: The postgemomic era. *Journal of Nutrition*, 133(11S1):3830S–3836S.

19. O'Keefe, J., and J. Cordain. 2004. Cardiovascular disease resulting from a diet and lifestyle at odds with our Paleolithic genome: How to become a 21st-century hunter-gatherer. *Mayo Clinic Proceedings*, 79(1):101–108.

20. Heaney, R. P. 1993. Protein intake and the calcium economy. *Journal of the American Dietetic Association*, 93(11):1259–1260.

21. Catena, C., et al. 2003. Insulin receptors and renal sodium handling in hypertensive fructose-fed rats. *Kidney International*, 64:2163–2171.

22. Shinozaki, K., et al. 2004. Molecular mechanisms of impaired endothelial function associated with insulin resistance. *Current Drug Targets—Cardiovascular and Haematological Disorders*, 4:1–11.

23. Mutch, N., H. M. Wilson, and N. A. Booth 2001. Plasminogen activator inhibitor-1 and haemostasis in obesity. *Proceedings of the Nutrition Society*, 60:341–347.

24. Garg, R., D. Tripathy, and A. Dandona. 2003. Insulin resistance as a proinflammatory state: Mechanisms, mediators and therapeutic interventions. *Current Drug Targets*, 4:487–492.

25. Festa, A., et al. 2003. Inflammation in the prediabetic state is related to increased insulin resistance rather than decreased insulin secretion. *Diabetes*, 52(6):A58.

26. Enstrom, G., et al. 2003. Inflammation-sensitive plasma proteins are associated with future weight gain. *Diabetes*, 52(8):2097–2101.

27. Haffner, S. 2003. Pre-diabetes, insulin resistance, inflammation and CVD risk. *Diabetes Research and Clinical Practice*, 61(1001):9–19.

28. Aronson, D., et al. 2004. Association between fasting glucose and c-reactive protein in middle-aged subjects. *Diabetic Medicine*, 21(1):39–45.

29. Lada, A. T., and L. L. Rudel. 2003. Dietary monounsaturated versus polyunsaturated fatty acids: which is better for protection from conorary heart disease? *Current Opinion in Lipidology*, 14:41–46.

30. Institute of Medicine. 2002. Dietary reference intakes for energy, carbohydrate, fiber, fat, fatty acids, cholesterol, protein, and amino acids. Washington, D.C.: National Academies Press, 936.

31. Vessby, B. 2003. Dietary fat, fatty acid composition in plasma and the metabolic syndrome. *Current Opinion in Lipidology*, 14:15–19.
32. Knight, E., et al. 2003. The impact of protein intake on renal funcion decline in women with normal renal function or mild renal insufficiency. *Annals of Internal Medicine*, 138(6):460–467.
33. Balen, A. 2003. Why polycycstic ovarian syndrome matters. *Pulse*, 2003:50.

## Chapter 7

1. American Institute for Cancer Research. 1997. Food, nutrition and the prevention of cancer: a global perspective, American Institute for Cancer Research: Washington D.C.
2. Go, V., R. Butrum, and D. Wong. 2003. Diet, nutrition, and cancer prevention: The postgemomic era. *Journal of Nutrition*, 133(11S1):3830S–3836S.
3. Hu, F. 2003. Plant-based foods and prevention of cardiovascular disease: An overview. *American Journal of Clinical Nutrition*, 78(3S):544S–551S.
4. Lampe, J. 2003. Spicing up a vegetarian diet: Chemopreventive effects of phytochemicals. *American Journal of Clinical Nutrition*, 78:579S–583S.
5. O'Keefe, J., and J. Cordain. 2004. Cardiovascular disease resulting from a diet and lifestyle at odds with our Paleolithic genome: How to become a 21st-century hunter-gatherer. *Mayo Clinic Proceedings*, 79(1):101–108.
6. Slavin, J. 2003. Why whole grains are protective: Biological mechanisms. *Proceedings of the Nutrition Society*, 62(1):129–134.
7. Surh, Y. 2003. Cancer chemoprevention with dietary phytochemicals. *Nature Reviews Cancer*, 3(10):768–780.
8. Layman, D., et al. 2003. A reduced ratio of dietary carbohydrate to protein improves body composition and blood lipid profiles during weight loss in adult women. *Journal of Nutrition*, 133(2):411–417.
9. Layman, D. K., et al. 2003a. Increased dietary protein modifies glucose and insulin homeostasis in adult women during weight loss. *Journal of Nutrition*, 133:405–410.
10. Clifton, P., M. Noakes, and B. Parker. 2002. The effect of a high protein weight loss diet in overweight subjects with type 2 diabetes. *American Journal of Clinical Nutrition*, 75(2):343S(1).
11. Clifton, P., J. Bowen, and M. Noakes. 2003. High protein weight loss diets and glucose metabolism. *Diabetes*, 52(6):A392.
12. Farnsworth, E., et al. 2003. Effect of a high-protein, energy-restricted diet on body composition, glycemic control, and lipid concentrations in overweight and obese hyperinsulinemic men and women. *American Journal of Clinical Nutrition*, 78(1):31–39.

13. Layman, D. K. 2003b. The role of leucine in weight loss diets and glucose homeostasis. *Journal of Nutrition*, 133:261S–267S.

14. Pelkman, C. L., et al. 2004. Effects of moderate-fat (from monounsaturated fat) and low-fat weight-loss diets on the serum lipid profile in overweight and obese men and women. *American Journal of Clinical Nutrition*, 79:204–212.

15. Esposito, K., et al. 2003. Effect of weight loss and lifestyle changes on vasular inflammatory markers in obese women. *Journal of the American Medical Association*, 289:1799–1804.

16. Park, E., and J. Pezzuto. 2002. Botanicals in cancer chemoprevention. *Cancer and Metastasis Reviews*, 21(3–4):231–255.

17. Caddick, S., et al. 2003. The DASH Diet and blood pressure. *Current Atherosclerosis Reports*, 5(6):484–491.

18. Appel, L., et al. 2003. Effects of comprehensive lifestyle modification on blood pressure control: Main results of the PREMIER clinical trial. *Journal of the American Medical Association*, 289(16):2083–2093.

19. Floch, M. H., and J. Hong-Curtiss. 2001. Probiotics and functional foods in gastrointestinal disorders. *Current Gastroenterology Reports*, 3(4):343–350.

20. Brady, L., D. Gallaher, and F. Busta. 2000. The role of probiotic cultures in the prevention of colon cancer. *Journal of Nutrition*, 130(2S):410S–414S.

21. Roberfroid, M., and J. Slavin. 2000. Nondigestible oligosaccharides. *Critical Reviews in Food Science and Nutrition*, 40(6):461–480.

22. Floch, M., and K. Moussa. 1998. Probiotics and dietary fiber: The clinical coming of age of intestinal microecology. *Journal of Clinical Gastroenterology*, 27(2): 99–100.

23. Liu, S., et al. 2000. A prospective study of dietary glycemic load, carbohydrate intake, and risk of coronary heart disease in US women. *American Journal of Clinical Nutrition*, 71:1455–1461.

24. Ascherio, A., M. J. Stampfer, and W. C. Willett. 2000. Trans fatty acids and coronary heart disease. Harvard School of Public Health.

25. Cordain, L., et al. 2002. The paradoxical nature of hunter-gatherer diets: Meat-based, yet non-atherogenic. *European Jounral of Clinical Nutrition*, 56:S42–S52.

## Chapter 8

1. Bonora, E., et al. 1998. Prevalence of insulin resistance in metabolic disorders: The Bruneck study. *Diabetes*, 47(10):1643–1650.

2. Bonow, R. O., and R. H. Eckel. 2003. Diet, obesity and cardiovascular risk. *New England Journal of Medicine*, 348(21):2057–2058.

3. Ornish, D. 2004. Was Dr. Atkins Right? *Journal of the American Dietetic Association*, 104(4):537–542.

4. Jequier, E., and G. Bray. 2002. Low-fat diets are preferred. *American Journal of Medicine*, 113(Suppl 9B):41S–46S.

5. Pelkman, C. 2001. Effects of the glycemic index of foods on serum concentrations of high-density lipoprotein cholesterol and triglycerides. *Current Atherosclerosis Reports*, 3(6):456–461.

6. United States Department of Health and Human Services. 2004. Trends in intake of energy and macronutrients—United States 1971–2000. *Morbidity and Mortality Weekly Reports*, 53(4):80–82.

7. Kennedy, E., S. Bowman, and R. Powell. 1999. Dietary-fat intake in the US population. *Journal of the American College of Nutrition*, 18(3):207–212.

8. Chanmugam, P., J. F. Guthrie, et al. 2003. Did fat intake in the United States really decline between 1989–1991 and 1994–1996. *Journal of the American Dietetic Association*, 103(7):867–872.

9. Diabetes Prevention Program Research Group. 2002. Reduction in the incidence of type 2 diabetes with lifestyle intervention or metformin. *New England Journal of Medicine*, 346(6):393–403.

10. Tuomilehto, J., et al. 2001. Prevention of type 2 diabetes mellitus by changes in lifestyle among subjects with impaired glucose tolerance. *New England Journal of Medicine*, 344(18):1343–1350.

11. Craddick, S., et al. 2003. The DASH Diet and blood pressure. *Current Atherosclerosis Reports*, 5(6):484–491.

12. Appel, L., et al. 2003. Effects of comprehensive lifestyle modification on blood pressure control: main results of the PREMIER clinical trial. *Journal of the American Medical Association*, 289(16):2083–2093.

13. Liu, S., et al. 2000. A prospective study of dietary glycemic load, carbohydrate intake, and risk of coronary heart disease in US women. *American Journal of Clinical Nutrition*, 71:1455–1461.

14. Liu, S., et al. 1999. Whole-grain consumption and risk of coronary heart disease: results from the Nurses' Health Study. *American Journal of Clinical Nutrition*, 1999. 1999:412–419.

15. Fung, T. T., et al. 2002. Whole-grain intake and the risk of type 2 diabetes: A prospective study in men. *American Journal of Clinical Nutrition*, 76:535–540.

16. Pereira, M. A., et al. 2002. Effect of whole grains on insulin sensitivity in overweight hyperinsulinemic adults. *American Journal of Clinical Nutrition*, 75:848–855.

17. Koertge, J., et al. 2003. Improvement in medical risk factors and quality of life in women and men with coronary artery disease in the Multicenter Lifestyle Demonstration Project. *American Journal of Cardiology*, 91(11):1316–1322.

18. Ornish, D. 1998. Avoiding revascularization with lifestyle changes: the Multicenter Lifestyle Demonstration Project. *American Journal of Cardiology*, 82(10B):72T–76T.

19. Ornish, D., et al. 1998. Intensive lifestyle changes for reversal of coronary heart disease: Five year follow-up of the Lifestyle Heart Trial. *Journal of the American Medical Association*, 280(23):2001–2007.

20. Fleming, R. 2002. The effect of high-, moderate-, and low-fat diets on weight loss and cardiovascular disease risk factors. *Preventive Cardiology*, 5(3):110–118.

21. Shick, S., et al. 1998. Persons successful at long term weight loss and maintenance continue to consume a low-energy low-fat diet. *Journal of the American Dietetic Association*, 98(4):408–413.

22. American Institute for Cancer Research. 1997. Food, nutrition and the prevention of cancer: A global perspective, American Institute for Cancer Research: Washington, D.C.

23. Craig, J. W. 2002. Phytochemicals: Guardians of our health. Vegetarian Nutrition: A Dietitic Practice Group of ADA.

24. Go, V., R. Butrum, and D. Wong. 2003. Diet, nutrition, and cancer prevention: the postgemomic era. *Journal of Nutrition*, 133(11S1):3830S–3836S.

25. Hu, F. 2003. Plant-based foods and prevention of cardiovascular disease: an overview. *American Journal of Clinical Nutrition*, 78(3S):544S–551S.

26. Lampe, J. 2003. Spicing up a vegetarian diet: chemopreventive effects of phytochemicals. *American Journal of Clinical Nutrition*, 78:579S–583S.

27. Park, E., and J. Pezzuto 2002. Botanicals in cancer chemoprevention. *Cancer and Metastasis Reviews*, 21(3–4):231–255.

28. Slavin, J. 2003. Why whole grains are protective: biological mechanisms. *Proceedings of the Nutrition Society*, 62(1):129–134.

29. Surh, Y. 2003. Cancer chemoprevention with dietary phytochemicals. *Nature Reviews Cancer*, 3(10):768–780.

30. Fleming, R. 2000. Reversing heart disease in the new millennium—the Fleming unified theory. *Angiology*, 51(8):617–629.

31. Ornish, D. 1999. Very-low-fat diets. *Circulation*, 100(9):1013–1014.

32. Floch, M. H., and J. Hong-Curtiss. 2001. Probiotics and functional foods in gastrointestinal disorders. *Current Gastroenterology Reports*, 3(4):343–350.

33. Brady, L., D. Gallaher, and F. Busta. 2000. The role of probiotic cultures in the prevention of colon cancer. *Journal of Nutrition*, 130(2S):410S–414S.

34. Roberfroid, M., and J. Slavin. 2000. Nondigestible oligosaccharides. *Critical Reviews in Food Science and Nutrition*, 40(6):461–480.

35. Floch, M., and K. Moussa. 1998. Probiotics and dietary fiber: the clinical coming of age of intestinal microecology. *Journal of Clinical Gastroenterology*, 27(2): 99–100.

36. United States Department of Agriculture Economic Research Service. 2004. Sugar and sweeteners. http://ers.usda.gov/publications/so/view.asp?f=specialty/sss-bb/&arc=_ (accessed March 4, 2004).

37. Fried, S., and S. Rao. 2003. Sugars, hypertriglyceridemia, and cardiovascular disease. *American Journal of Clinical Nutrition*, 78(4):873S–880S.

## Chapter 10

1. Utah State University Cooperative Extension Service. Palatability—More than a matter of taste. Behavioral Principles & Practices Feedback, No.1.3.1. http://www.extension.usu.edu/files/factsheets/Palatblty (accessed May 10, 2004).
2. Wang, G., N. Volkow, and J. Fowler. 2002. The role of dopamine in motivation for food in humans: Implications for obesity. *Expert Opinion on Therapeutic Targets*, 6(5):601–609.
3. Wang, G., et al. 2004. Exposure to appetitive food stimuli markedly activates the human brain. *Neuroimage*, 21(4):1790–1797.
4. Alcalay, R. and R. Bell. 2000. Promoting nutrition and physical activity through social marketing: Current practices and recommendations. Center for Advanced Studies in Nutrition and Social Marketing, University of California at Davis: Davis.
5. National Institutes of Health National Cancer Institute. 1997. Theory at a Glance: A guide for health promotion practice.
6. Barrows, K., and B. Jacobs. 2002. Mind-body medicine. An introduction and review of the literature. *Medical Clinics of North America*, 86(1):11–31.
7. Astin, J., et al. 2003. Mind-body medicine: State of the science, implications for practice. *Journal of the American Board of Family Practice*, 16(2):131–147.
8. Labarthe, D., and C. Ayala. 2002. Nondrug interventions in hypertension prevention and control. *Cardiology Clinics*, 20(2):249–263.
9. King, M., T. Carr, and C. d'Cruz. 2002. Transcendental meditation, hypertension and heart disease. *Australian Family Physician*, 31(2):164–168.
10. Smyth, J., et al. 1999. Effects of writing about stressful experiences on symptom reduction in patients with asthma or rheumatoid arthritis. *Journal of the American Medical Association*, 281:1304–1309.
11. Berry, D., and J. Pennebaker. 1993. Nonverbal and verbal emotional expression and health. *Psychother Psychosom*, 59:11–19.
12. Gruzelier, J. 2002. A review of the impact of hypnosis, relaxation, guided imagery and individual differences on aspects of immunity and health. *Stress*, 5(2):147–163.
13. Bakke, A., M. Purtzer, and P. Newton. 2002. The effect of hypnotic-guided imagery on psychological well-being and immune function in patients with prior breast cancer. *Journal of Psychosomatic Research*, 53(6):1131–1137.

14. Hawks, S., et al. 1995. Review of spiritual health: definition, role, and intervention strategies in health promotion. *American Journal of Health Promotion*, 9(5):371–378.
15. Prochaska, J. Summary overview of the transtheoretical model. Cancer Prevention Research Center at the University of Rhode Island. http://www.uri.edu/research/cprc/transtheoretical.htm (accessed May 12, 2004).

## Chapter 11

1. Leibel, R. L., M. Rosenbaum, and J. Hirsch. 1995. Changes in energy expenditure resulting from altered body weight. *New England Journal of Medicine*, 332(10):621–628.
2. Rosenbaum, M., et al. 2000. Effects of changes in body weight on carbohydrate metabolism, catecholamine excretion and thyroid function. *American Journal of Clinical Nutrition*, 71:1421–1432.
3. Weinsier, R. L., et al. 2000. Do adaptive changes in metabolic rate favor weight regain in weight-reduced individuals? An examination of the set-point theory. *American Journal of Clinical Nutrition*, 72:1088–1094.
4. Weinsier, R., G. Hunter, and Y. Schutz. 2001. Metabolic response to weight loss. *American Journal of Clinical Nutrition*, 73(3):655–657.
5. Wyatt, H. R., et al. 1999. Resting metabolic rate in reduced-obese subjects in the National Weight Control Registry. *American Journal of Clinical Nutrition*, 69:1189–1193.
6. Hunter, G. 2002. Women and resistance training. ACSM *Fit Society*, Fall: 4, 13.
7. Poehlman, E., et al. 2002. Effects of endurance and resistance training on total daily energy expenditure in young women: A controlled randomized trial. *Journal of Clinical Endocrinology and Metabolism*, 87:1004–1009.
8. Kraemer, W., et al. 1999. Influence of exercise training on physiological and performance changes with weight loss in men. *Medicine and Science in Sports and Exercise*, 31(9):1320–1329.
9. Lemmer, J. T., et al. 2001. Effect of strength training on resting metabolic rate and physical activity: age and gender comparisons. *Medicine and Science in Sports and Exercise*, 33(4):532–541.
10. Dionne, I., et al. 2004. Age-related differences in metabolic adaptations following resistance training in women. *Experimental Gerontology*, 39(1):133–138.

## Chapter 12

1. Foster, G. D., et al. 2001. Obese patients' perceptions of treatment outcomes and the factors that influence them. *Archives of Internal Medicine*, 161(17):2133–2139.

2. Westenhoefer, J. 2001. The therapeutic challenge: behavioral changes for long-term weight maintenance. *International Journal of Obesity and Related Metabolic Disorders*, 25(Suppl 1):S85–S88.

3. Kern, L., et al. 2002. Changing eating behavior: a preliminary study to consider broader measures of weight control treatment success. *Eating Behaviors*, 3(2):113–121.

4. Westenhoefer, J. 1991. Dietary restraint and disinhibition: is restraint a homogeneous construct? *Appetite*, 16:45–55.

5. Westenhoefer, J., A. Stunkard, and V. Pudel. 1999. Validation of the flexible and rigid control dimensions of dietary restraint. *International Journal of Eating Disorders*, 26:53–64.

6. Westenhoefer, J., et al. 2004. Behavioural correlates of successful weight reduction over 3 y. Results from the Lean Habits Study. *Journal of Consulting and Clinical Psychology*, 72(2):341–348.

7. Kearney, M. and J. O'Sullivan. 2003. Identify shifts as turning points in health behavior change. *Western Journal of Nursing Research*, 25(2):134–152.

8. Wing, R. and J. O. Hill. 2001. Successful weight loss maintenance. *Annual Review of Nutrition*, 21:323–341.

# INDEX

INDEX